Modern Radiotherapy

CARCINOMA OF THE BRONCHUS

Modern Radiotherapy

CARCINOMA OF THE BRONCHUS

Edited by

THOMAS J. DEELEY

M.B., Ch.B., F.F.R., D.M.R.T.

Director, South Wales and Monmouthshire Radiotherapy Service, Velindre Hospital, University Hospital of Wales, Cardiff; Lecturer, Welsh National School of Medicine, Cardiff

NEW YORK
APPLETON-CENTURY-CROFTS
Division of Meredith Corporation

LONDON
BUTTERWORTHS

Suggested U.D.C. Number 615·849: 616·233–006·6

Suggested Additional Number 616·24–006·6

ISBN 0 407 27540 1

Printed and bound in Great Britain by R. J. Acford Ltd., Industrial Estate, Chichester, Sussex.

Contents

Contributors

GERALD ANDERSON, M.B., M.R.C.P.
Consultant Physician, Newport and East Monmouthshire Group of Hospitals

P. J. BANGMA, M.D.
Physician in Lung Diseases, Kliniek voor Longziekten, Utrecht, Holland

SAMUEL CICCIO, M.D.
Instructor, Division of Radiotherapy and Radioisotopes, University of Rochester School of Medicine and Dentistry, Strong Memorial Hospital, Rochester, New York

W. P. CLELAND, F.R.C.S., F.R.C.P., F.A.C.S.
Director, Department of Surgery, Institute of Diseases of the Chest; Consultant Cardiothoracic Surgeon, The Brompton Hospital and Hammersmith Hospital, London

THOMAS J. DEELEY, M.B., CH.B., F.F.R., D.M.R.T.
Director, South Wales and Monmouthshire Radiotherapy Service, Velindre Hospital, University Hospital of Wales, Cardiff; Lecturer, Welsh National School of Medicine, Cardiff

P. C. ELMES, F.R.C.P.
Whitla Professor of Pharmacology and Therapeutics, The Queen's University of Belfast

WALLACE FOX, M.D., F.R.C.P.
Director, Medical Research Council Tuberculosis and Chest Diseases Unit, The Brompton Hospital; Honorary Consultant Physician, The Brompton Hospital, London

D. GREENE, PH.D., F.INST.P.
Physicist, Christie Hospital and Holt Radium Institute, Manchester

RUTH GUTTMANN, M.D.
Professor of Radiology, College of Physicians and Surgeons, Columbia University, New York; Director, Department of Radiotherapy, Francis Delafield Hospital, New York

HURST B. HATCH, JNR., M.D.
Thoracic Medicine Section, Department of Medicine, Ochsner Clinic and Ochsner Foundation Hospital, New Orleans, Louisiana

SHOJI HATTORI, M.D., PH.D.
Director, Department of Lung Cancer, Center for Adult Diseases, Osaka, Japan

J. R. HERON, M.B., CH.B., M.R.C.P.(ED.)
Consultant Neurologist, North Staffordshire Royal Infirmary, Stoke-on-Trent; Visiting Neurologist, Burton-on-Trent General Hospital and Robert Jones and Agnes Hunt Orthopaedic Hospital, Oswestry

LARS R. HOLSTI, M.D.
Professor of Radiotherapy, University of Helsinki; Director of Radiotherapy Clinic, University Central Hospital, Helsinki, Finland

NORMAN HOWARD, M.A., D.M.(OXON.), F.F.R., D.M.R.T.
Consultant Radiotherapist, Charing Cross Group of Hospitals, London; Honorary Consultant Radiotherapist; Royal Marsden Hospital and Wembley Hospital, London

A. M. JELLIFFE, M.D., F.R.C.P., F.F.R., D.C.H.
Deputy Director, Myerstein Institute of Radiotherapy, The Middlesex Hospital, London; Consultant Radiotherapist, Mount Vernon Hospital, Northwood and Hendon Group of Hospitals

KARL P. KLASSEN, M.D.
Professor and Director, Division of Thoracic Surgery, Ohio State University Hospitals, Columbus, Ohio

IVAN LICHTER, F.R.C.S., F.R.A.C.S.
Senior Lecturer in Surgery, University of Otago Medical School; Thoracic Surgeon, Otago Hospital Board, Dunedin, New Zealand

DAPHNE LINE, M.B., B.S.(SYDNEY), D.C.H., M.R.C.P.(LOND.), M.R.C.P.(ED.)
Medical Registrar, Hammersmith Hospital and Royal Postgraduate Medical School, London

J. B. MCEWEN, M.D., D.M.R.T.
Consultant Radiotherapist, St. Mary's General Hospital, Portsmouth

MINORU MATSUDA, M.D., PH.D.
Chief, Laboratory of Diagnostic Cytology, Center for Adult Diseases, Osaka, Japan

CONTRIBUTORS

WILLIAM S. MAXFIELD, M.D.
Professor and Chairman, Louisiana State University School of Medicine, New Orleans; Senior Visiting Radiologist, Charity Hospital, New Orleans, Louisiana

A. B. MILLER, M.B., M.R.C.P.
Member of the Scientific Staff, Medical Reaserch Council Tuberculosis and Chest Diseases Unit, The Brompton Hospital, London

JAMES R. NELSON, M.D.
Resident in Radiology, Ochsner Foundation Hospital, New Orleans, Louisiana

A. H. W. NIAS, M.A., D.M., D.M.R.T.
Senior Radiobiologist, Paterson Laboratories, Christie Hospital and Holt Radium Institute, Manchester

H. C. NOHL-OSER, M.A., D.M.(OXON.), F.R.C.S.
Consultant Thoracic Surgeon, Cardiothoracic Unit, Harefield Hospital, Hillingdon Hospital and West Middlesex Hospital

W. M. ROSS, T.D., M.D., F.R.C.S., F.F.R.
Consultant Radiotherapist, Newcastle Regional Hospital Board and United Newcastle upon Tyne Hospitals

PHILIP RUBIN, M.D.
Chief and Professor, Division of Radiotherapy and Radioisotopes, University of Rochester School Medicine and Dentistry, Strong Memorial Hospital, Rochester, New York

D. K. SAMBROOK, F.R.C.S., D.M.R.T.
Consultant Radiotherapist, Swansea and West Wales Hospitals

ROGER M. E. SEAL, M.R.C.P., F.R.C.PATH.
Consultant Pathologist, Sully Hospital, Penarth; Honorary Lecturer, Department of Tuberculosis and Chest Diseases, Welsh National School of Medicine, Cardiff

G. SIMON, M.D., F.R.C.P., F.F.R.
Radiologist and Demonstrator in Radiological Anatomy, St. Bartholomew's Hospital, London; formerly Director, X-ray Department, The Brompton Hospital, London

S. J. STEEL, M.D., M.R.C.P.
Consultant Physician, The London Chest Hospital and the Romford Group of Hospitals

J. G. STEWART, M.A., M.B., CH.B., F.F.R.
Consultant Radiotherapist, Christie Hospital and Holt Radium Institute, Manchester

CONTRIBUTORS

PETER STRADLING, M.D., F.R.C.P.
Director of the Chest Clinic and Senior Lecturer in Respiratory Diseases, Royal Postgraduate Medical School, Hammersmith Hospital, London

WILLIAM UMIKER, M.D.
Pathologist, St. Joseph Hospital, Lancaster, Pennsylvania; formerly Associate Professor, University of Michigan Medical School

J. C. WAGNER, M.D., M.R.C.PATH.
Senior Scientific Officer, Medical Research Council Pneumoconiosis Research Unit, Llandough Hospital, Penarth; Honorary Consultant Pathologist, Sully Hospital (Thoracic Centre), Penarth

Preface

The *Modern Radiotherapy* volumes are designed to give the established clinician up-to-date knowledge of the advances that are being made in this specialty and to suggest possible ways in which future progress may be achieved. The radiotherapist must have a wide knowledge of all aspects of malignant disease; he is, in fact, a clinical oncologist. With this in mind, contributions have been invited from workers in other specialties. It is hoped that this book will be of interest to all who are concerned with the treatment of patients suffering from carcinoma of the bronchus and will help to bring about a greater co-operation between these workers.

This volume, devoted to carcinoma of the bronchus, includes chapters by pathologists, cytologists, physicians, surgeons, diagnostic radiologists, radiobiologists and physicians as well as radiotherapists. I would like to thank all the contributors for their willing help and co-operation.

I am extremely grateful to Miss J. N. Williams for the secretarial assistance she has given me in the preparation of this volume, and it is a pleasure to acknowledge the considerable help given by the editorial staff of Messrs. Butterworths.

THOMAS J. DEELEY

1—Methods of Controlling the Disease

Thomas J. Deeley

The incidence of lung cancer has shown an increase in almost every country. In the United States of America, the number of deaths from this disease increased from 18,313 in 1950 to 48,583 in 1965 (United States Public Health Service, 1967). Similar reports have been made in other countries, for example Iceland (Dungal, 1950; Thorarinsson and colleagues, 1967), Canada (Phillips, 1966), Finland (Varpela, 1966), Switzerland (Gsell, 1965), Germany (Grimmer, 1968), and France (Flamant, Lasserre and Maujol, 1968). This increase has been shown for both sexes, but there is now some evidence that the rate of increase is beginning to level off for men; women have shown a lower rate than men, possibly due to their lower exposure to tobacco. However, the rate is still rising.

In England and Wales, carcinoma of the bronchus in 1966 accounted for 22,610 deaths in men and 4,415 deaths in women, equivalent to 38·6 and 8·9 per cent of the total cancer deaths for each sex.

Possible ways of combating this increased incidence are by prevention, by earlier diagnosis and by improved methods of treatment.

PREVENTION

The great tragedy is that from the evidence at present available, it would appear that carcinoma of the bronchus is largely preventable. The elimination of cigarette smoking in this country would greatly reduce the incidence of this cancer. It must be admitted that cigarette smoking is not the only causative factor, but it is the major one. Other factors which have been incriminated are air pollution and airborne carcinogens.

The dangers of smoking have been pointed out by many writers almost since its inception in this country. Willson (1956) described the introduction of tobacco to England in the sixteenth century. 'Tobacco was known and used in England probably as early as the 1560s but smoking first became a general practice about 1586, when Drake captured a "great store of tobacco" in the Indies and when Raleigh's unhappy settlers, returning from Roanoke Island, brought the habit with them. The English took to smoking with avidity, and a group of young gallants in London carried the habit to bizarre excess supplying themselves with equipment of gold and silver, seeking instruction from "professors of the art of whiffing", and smoking in public with foppish ostentation. It was perhaps the dissipations of these reeking gallants that first aroused the ire of King James and he doubtless liked smoking the less because it had been made fashionable at court by Raleigh. Whatever the cause, James conceived a violent aversion to tobacco and began a campaign against it which lasted the rest of his life.'

In 1604 King James himself published one of the most noted of anti-tobacco pamphlets, *Counterblaste to Tobacco*. This work, which he described as 'a mere toy', contained some rather unusual medical notions, but with remarkable perspicacity he strongly denounced smoking: 'it often makes a kitchen of a man's inside, dirtying and injecting it with a sticky and oily kind of soot of the kind that has been found in the lungs of heavy smokers who were dissected after death. It is a custom loathsome to the eye, harmful to the brain and dangerous to the lungs.'

There have appeared many further condemnations of the practice. Thus Robert Burton (1577–1640): 'As smoking is commonly abused by most men, which take it as tinkers do ale, 'tis a plague, a mischief, a violent purger of goods, lands, health, hellish, devilish and damned tobacco, the ruin and over-throw of body and soul.' Ben Jonson (1573–1627): 'Neither do thou lust after that tawny weed tobacco.' These censures culminated in the more objective investigations summarized by the Royal College of Physicians (1962) and the United States Department of Health, Education and Welfare (1964, 1967, 1968).

It is now accepted that cigarette smoking is the main cause of lung cancer. The 1964 Report of the United States Public Health Service concluded that:

(1) Cigarette smoking is causally related to lung cancer in men, in whom the magnitude of smoking far outweighs other factors. The data for women, although less extensive, point in the same direction.

(2) The risk of developing the disease increases with the duration

of smoking and the number of cigarettes smoked per day, and is diminished when smoking is discontinued.

(3) The risk for a combined group of pipe, cigar and pipe/cigar smokers is greater than for non-smokers but less than for cigarette smokers. The data are insufficient to warrant a conclusion in each group individually.

Supplementary information contained in the 1967 Report states that:

(1) Additional epidemiological, pathological and experimental data not only confirm the conclusions of the Surgeon General's 1964 Report regarding lung cancer in men but strengthen the causal relationship between smoking and lung cancer in women.

(2) Cessation of cigarette smoking sharply reduces the risk of death from lung cancer relative to the risk if smoking continues.

(3) Although additional experimental studies substantiate the previous experimental data, additional research is needed to specify the tumour-initiating and tumour-promoting agents in tobacco smoke and to elucidate the basic mechanisms of the pathogenesis of lung cancer.

The 1968 Supplement confirms and strengthens the conclusions of the two previous studies that 'Smoking is a serious health hazard in this country, one which is bringing about much unnecessary disease and death within our population'.

Although it has become accepted that smoking is one of the major causes of lung cancer, there is as yet little evidence of any reduction in the amount of tobacco smoked. Programmes aimed at reducing its consumption have been disappointing. One of the difficulties is the lapse of time between cause and effect, which may amount to many years. It is desirable that any educational programme should aim at the child who has not yet started smoking; but the thought of illness or death in 20, 30, 40 or even more years' time is unlikely seriously to affect the habits of the child or teenager. In the adult, long-standing habits are difficult to break, but even in the established smoker the breaking of the habit results in a decreased incidence of lung cancer. Deeley and Cohen (1966) suggested that not only the quantity of tobacco smoked but also the duration of smoking were important factors in the development of the disease.

'We can give advice but we can never prompt behaviour,' to quote the Duc de la Rochefoucauld (1613–80). The advice which we give must be calculated to dissuade the younger generation from starting to smoke and to persuade the established smoker to stop. Smoking and the diseases it causes are no longer mainly medical problems but have become a social and national responsibility. Considerable money is spent on advertising the pleasures of cigarette smoking, but comparatively little is spent on advertising its attendant dangers.

The U.S. Federal Trade Commission (*Report to Congress*, 30 June, 1967) recommended that cigarette packages, cigarette vending machines and all advertisements should carry this statement: 'Warning—Cigarette smoking is dangerous to health and may cause death from cancer and other diseases.'

It has been estimated that the elimination of smoking would greatly reduce the incidence of the disease to the relatively small number of cases due to causes other than tobacco. It would, at the same time, greatly reduce the incidence of other diseases due to smoking: carcinoma of the larynx, the lips and probably the oesophagus, pharynx, mouth, cheek and bladder; certain respiratory diseases such as bronchitis and emphysema; coronary artery disease; peptic ulcer, and sinusitis. While some of these diseases may not cause death, the morbidity materially adds to the number of man-working-days lost to the country.

How can this challenge to the nation's health be met? Four possible lines of approach are suggested:

(1) Reducing tobacco consumption in addicted smokers. There is evidence to suggest that a reduction of his present smoking consumption could delay or avert the development of lung cancer in a patient.

(2) It is difficult, however, to change existing habits, and work must be aimed at discouraging the child or teenager from ever starting. Unfortunately this approach has so far not been encouraging. Much of what a child does is a copy of what his parents do. Future work must therefore be directed not only at the child but at those who influence him—his parents, teachers and friends, health workers and doctors, and in addition other sources of influence such as television, radio, books and films. Factual persuasion is probably of more value than the instilling of fear in the teenager's mind.

(3) Development of a less hazardous cigarette and conversion of the smoking public to it. There is already evidence that some cigarettes have a lower tar content and nicotine level (Smoking and Health Newsletter, 1968).

(4) Finding ways of distinguishing individuals who are more susceptible than the average to the harmful effects of smoking.

If smoking were in some way completely banned it would, of course, be some years before the fall in the death rate was noticeable. In the meantime we, as radiotherapists, would continue to be presented with patients suffering from inoperable disease. Too often the patients referred to us have come 'too late' and all that we offer is palliation of distressing symptoms. The discipline of a radiotherapist demands an attempt at cure. What can be done to increase the survival rate of presenting cases? Can earlier diagnosis produce a patient with a more curable disease? Can improvement in treatment techniques increase the number of cures even where the disease is widespread?

DIAGNOSIS

Symptomatology

There are, of course, no specific symptoms of cancer of the lung. When symptoms do occur, they are those which can be associated with many other chest diseases—cough, sputum, dyspnoea and haemoptysis. About 5 per cent of the patients treated for inoperable carcinoma have no symptoms and the disease is suspected only on a routine chest radiograph (Deeley, 1970). Le Roux (1968) found that only 68 per cent of his patients presented with chest disease; 5 per cent were asymptomatic; 13 per cent complained of symptoms referable to metastases, 12 per cent of non-specific symptoms such as loss of weight or anorexia without respiratory symptoms, and 2 per cent of unusual symptoms such as neurological or endocrine changes secondary to the carcinoma.

The presenting symptom will depend on the site of the primary tumour. On the whole, a peripheral tumour is likely to remain hidden for longer than one in a main bronchus. Erosion of a blood vessel or obstruction of a main airway may produce symptoms at an early stage, and it is to be expected that an undifferentiated tumour will give rise to symptoms before a more slowly growing mass. The presence of superior mediastinal obstruction becomes a medical emergency and treatment is usually instituted immediately.

The association of malignant disease of the chest with an established chronic non-malignant disease may cause delay in diagnosis. Most physicians are aware of the development of lung cancer in the chronic bronchitic. Deeley (1970) reported a history of chronic bronchitis in 270 patients (40 per cent) out of a total of 680 with a histological diagnosis of carcinoma. The case of the unresolved pneumonia is so well known that it does not warrant further elaboration. In recent years there have appeared a number of reports of coexistent pulmonary tuberculosis and bronchogenic carcinoma (Bobrowitz and colleagues, 1961; Larmi, 1967; Sherman, Conant and Peereboon, 1967; Deeley, 1967).

The possibility of coexistent carcinoma of the bronchus must always be borne in mind in patients with known chest disease, particularly in those aged 40 years or over who have a chronic cough and are heavy smokers. The failure of a chest disease to resolve satisfactorily with the appropriate treatment, or the extension of disease in spite of the appropriate therapy, should make the physician suspicious and lead him to investigate further.

The majority of patients attending for treatment have advanced disease. Thompson (1967), in a series of 1,070 patients who were admitted to hospital with bronchogenic carcinoma, found that 50 per cent were unsuitable for surgery on clinical grounds, 20 per cent were inoperable at bronchoscopy, and a further 10 per cent were inoperable at thoracotomy. As Bignall (1966) pointed out, 'more patients would be diagnosed early if they sought advice earlier, but in many cases symptoms are so insidious and unobtrusive that the disease will inevitably be at an advanced stage before this occurs'. With our existing diagnostic procedures, early diagnosis is still largely a matter of chance, depending on the position of the primary growth and on the rate of growth, which in turn is related to the differentiation of the tumour. A greater awareness of the probable seriousness of chest symptoms might result in earlier diagnosis in some cases, but it would be more useful if some method of detection could be applied to the non-symptomatic patient. There are two methods available: cytological examination of sputum and routine chest radiography.

Cytology

Not all cancers of the lung will produce malignant cells in the sputum; the proportion of positive reports will depend on the experience of the cytologist and the number of specimens taken. Several methods have been devised to obtain satisfactory material for examination, and these are described in Chapter 4, including the use of a nylon brush to obtain specimens from a suspicious area seen on x-ray.

There have been several attempts to improve the results of examination of the specimen obtained. The majority of these have aimed at concentrating the number of cells by removing the mucus with various agents such as urea, hydrogen peroxide, detergents, a variety of enzymes, hyaluronidase, lysozyme, papain, trypsin and chymotrypsin

(Pharr and Farber, 1962). Other workers have concentrated the cells by millipore filtration and solution of the filter membrane (Fields and colleagues, 1966; Lin, 1966; Russell and Chang, 1967).

The ease with which sputum specimens can be obtained suggests that this could be a useful screening method for use on asymptomatic patients if some method of automation could be devised for examining the specimens. Until this is achieved, it is suggested that this technique be reserved for high risk patients—that is, males over 40 years of age and heavy smokers.

Radiography

Routine radiography of patient's chests proved to be of immense value in the early diagnosis of pulmonary tuberculosis, but the results of similar surveys applied to cancer of the lung have not been so encouraging. Gilbertsen (1966) reported a detection rate of one lung cancer in 5,378 examinations. Virtama (1962) found a detection rate of 0·41 per thousand, but for people over 60 years of age the rate was 0·89 per thousand. Brett (1968) carried out a prospective study in 29,723 men aged 40 years and over who were radiographed every six months for three years and compared the results with those from 25,311 men who were radiographed at the beginning and end of the three-year period only. He found that the early detection by six-monthly chest radiographs did not significantly reduce the mortality from cancer of the lung, and concluded that a policy of such a large-scale survey was not justified. However, more resectable cases were discovered, and Brett suggested that patients in 'high-risk' groups should be encouraged to have regular radiographic examinations. Nash, Morgan and Tomkins (1968) also suggested that examinations should be limited to this category. They estimated the cost of finding a potential four-year survivor in a group of non-smokers to be £990 and the cost in a group of heavy smokers aged 55 years or over to be £180.

We must conclude that the value of repeated routine chest radiographs has not been demonstrated, and it is not yet possible to carry out large-scale sputum examinations. These diagnostic tests are probably best reserved for patients known to have a high risk of developing lung cancer. Until they have a wider application, we must rely upon a greater appreciation of the importance and implications of chest symptoms.

TREATMENT

The methods of treatment available for carcinoma of the bronchus are surgery, radiotherapy and chemotherapy and various combinations of these. These treatments are described in full in succeeding chapters. It is important that the best possible treatment be given, and this demands consultation and co-operation between all those concerned with diagnosis and therapy.

Where the disease has been diagnosed by histological examination of the tissue obtained at bronchoscopy, it would appear that surgery is preferable to radiotherapy for squamous lesions, there being little difference between the two methods for anaplastic and oat cell tumours (Morrison, Deeley and Cleland, 1963; Medical Research Council Working Party, 1966). Miller, Fox and Tall (1969) reported that radical radiotherapy gave, in terms of survival, better results than surgery in the treatment of small-celled or oat-celled carcinomas of the bronchus diagnosed pre-operatively on bronchial biopsy and judged to be operable.

In small peripheral lesions of the lung, where biopsy is not practicable, a controlled clinical trial of this kind is impossible because histology is only known after thoracotomy. In these cases the method of treatment would appear to be surgical.

Inoperable patients referred for radiotherapy may receive radical treatment aimed at a cure if there is no evidence of spread outside the chest. Where spread has occurred, there may still be a chance of a cure if the metastases are solitary; the remaining patients with widespread metastases may receive palliative therapy for troublesome symptoms.

The introduction of supervoltage therapy made it possible to give an adequate tumour dose to large volumes in the chest, and the results of this method of treatment have produced a small improvement in survival (Deeley and Singh, 1967). It is possible that these results may be further improved by determining the best conditions for irradiating tumours. We need to know the optimum tumour dose, the optimum number of fractions, the best fractionation techniques, the preferred overall time of treatment, the place of hyperbaric oxygen, the application of certain radiosensitizers, and the value of radiation combined with surgery or with chemotherapy. The answers will be obtained only by carefully controlled clinical trials, each designed to answer one specific question. Much work is in progress, and some of the results obtained are given in the chapters of this book.

The high incidence of metastases means that many of the patients presenting with carcinoma of the bronchus are already beyond the reach of radical treatment. Dramatic improvements in survival rates can only be made in two ways: (1) by diagnosing and treating before metastatic spread occurs, and (2) by devising some suitable method of treating widespread disease. At the present stage of our knowledge the only way of dealing with metastases is by some systemic chemotherapeutic agents, but those drugs at present available have proved of very little value and it is hoped that further work may produce more satisfactory compounds.

In carcinoma of the bronchus, new diagnostic methods must be investigated to diagnose the disease at an earlier stage and to determine which individuals are susceptible to the available carcinogens. Serious attempts must be made to improve the existing methods of treatment, but it is incumbent on us as physicians to make every effort to assist any work that will ultimately reduce the incidence. There can be few clinicians who do not believe that the incidence of this disease could be drastically reduced. 'If we believe a thing to be bad, and if we have a right to prevent it, it is our duty to try to prevent it,' said Alfred, Lord Milner (1854–1925).

REFERENCES

Bignall, J. R. (1966). *Br. med. J.* **1,** 341.

Bobrowitz, I. D., Elkin, M., Evans, J. C. and Lin, A. (1961). *Dis. Chest* **40,** 397.

Brett, C. Z. (1968). *Thorax* **23,** 414.

Davies, D. F. (1966). *J. chron. Dis.* **19,** 819.

Deeley, T. J. (1967). *Br. J. Radiol.* **40,** 801.

— (1970). *J. Indian med. Prof.* In the press.

— and Cohen, S. L. (1967). *Bladder Cancer: A Symposium.* Ed. by W. B. Deichman. Alabama: Aesculapius Publishing Co.

— and Singh, S. P. (1967). *Thorax* **22,** 562.

Dungal, N. (1950). *Lancet* **2,** 245.

Fields, M. J., Martin, W. F., Young, B. L. and Tweedale, D. N. (1966). *Acta cytol.* **10,** 220.

Flamant, R., Lasserre, O. and Maujol, L. (1968). *Bull. Inst. natn. Santé Rech. méd.* **23,** 117.

Gilbertsen, V. A. (1966). *J. Am. med. Ass.* **195,** 655.

Grimmer, G. (1968). *Deutsche ApothZtg.* **108,** 529.

Gsell, O. (1965). *Oncologia, Basel* **19,** 194.

Larmi, T. K. I. (1967). *Scand. J. thorac. cardiovasc. Surg.* **1,** 118.

Lawther, P. J. (1963). *Practitioner* **190,** 720.

— (1966). *Postgrad. med. J.* **42,** 703.

Le Roux, B. T. (1968). *Bronchial Carcinoma.* Edinburgh: Livingstone.

Lin, W. (1966). *Acta cytol.* **10,** 368.

Medical Research Council Working Party (1966). *Lancet* **2,** 979.

Miller, A. B., Fox, W. and Tall, R. (1969). *Lancet* **2,** 501.

Morrison, R., Deeley, T. J. and Cleland, W. P. (1963). *Lancet* **1,** 683.
Nash, F. A., Morgan J. M. and Tomkins, J. G. (1968). *Br. med. J.* **2,** 715.
Pharr, S. L. and Farber, S. M. (1962). *Acta cytol.* **6,** 447.
Phillips, A. J. (1966). *Can. med. Ass. J.* **95,** 1172.
Royal College of Physicians (1962). *Smoking and Health, 1962: Summary of a Report on Smoking in Relation to Cancer of the Lung and Other Diseases.* London.
Russell, W. O. and Chang, S. C. (1967). *Cancer, N.Y.* **20,** 681.
Sawicki, E. (1967). *Archs envir. Hlth* **14,** 46.
Sherman, P. H., Conant, J. S. and Peereboon, G. (1967). *Am. Rev. resp. Dis.* **96,** 45.
Smoking and Health Newsletter (1968), Vol. 4, No. 1. Arlington, Va.: National Interagency Council on Smoking and Health.
Thompson, D. T. (1967). *J. thorac. cardiovasc. Surg.* **53,** 159.
Thorarinsson, H., Hallbrimsson, J., Bjarnason, I. O. and Peterson, G. (1967). *Dis. Chest* **52,** 754.
United States Department of Health, Education and Welfare (1964). *Smoking and Health, 1964: Reports of the Advisory Committee to the Surgeon General of the Public Health Service.* Washington, D.C.
— (1967). *Public Health Service Review.* Washington, D.C.
— (1968). *Supplement to the 1967 Public Health Service Review.* Washington, D.C.
United States Public Health Service (1967). *Vital Statistics of the United States, 1965: Mortality 2*, Part A. Washington, D.C.: National Center for Health Statistics.
Varpela, E. (1966). *Annls Chir. Gynaec. Fenn.* **55,** 15.
Virtama, P. (1962). *Annls Med. intern. Fenn.* **51,** Suppl. 37.
Willson, D. H. (1956). *King James VI and I.* London: Jonathan Cape.

2—*Pathology of Lung Cancer*

Roger M. E. Seal

GENERAL CONSIDERATIONS

It is helpful not to consider carcinoma of the lung as a single neoplasm but to regard the general heading as including several neoplasms, each differing in natural history, in aetiology, in rate of development of local and general metastases and in hormonal effects, as well as in histological appearance and radiosensitivity. For example, squamous carcinoma is associated with inhalation of external irritants and probably is the end result of a change in the respiratory epithelial lining of the bronchi, progressing through squamous metaplasia to *in situ* carcinoma before finally becoming locally invasive. The rate of spread of this histological type is slower, accounting for its better surgical prognosis. Oat cell carcinoma, although also associated with inhalation of carcinogens, soon ceases to be merely a locally invasive neoplasm; metastasizing early and widely, it is often surgically inoperable at the time of diagnosis. Adenocarcinomas do not have an association with cigarette smoking or a predominantly male incidence, are often peripheral and are sometimes related to pre-existing lung scars.

Carcinoma of the lung may be diagnosed in a presymptomatic stage by means of routine miniature radiography (Brett, 1969) or by cytological screening of 'high risk' groups (Nasiell, 1969). Patients so found, it is claimed, have a better surgical prognosis. 'Early' diagnosis of symptomatic patients does not imply that the growth is at an early stage in its natural history, as it may already have spread extensively locally or metastasized widely.

In recent years it has been realized that haematogenous spread is not an inevitable consequence of the invasion of vessels but occurs for some time before metastases develop. Many of the circulating malignant cells are dealt with by the host defence mechanism. Mathe (1969) suggests that this immunological mechanism is important and

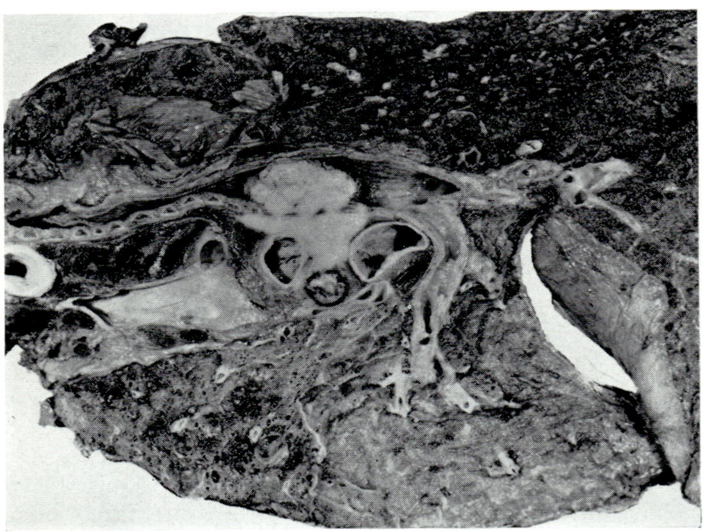

(a)

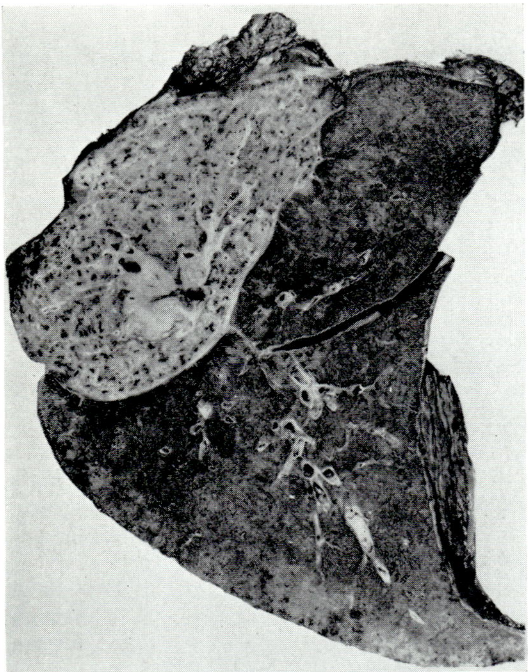

(b)

Figure 1. (*a*) *The growth partly occludes the bronchial lumen and has infiltrated peribronchially. A hilar node is involved.* (*b*) *Right upper lobe consolidation distal to a carcinoma in the upper lobe bronchus growing down the segmental bronchi*

Figure 1. (*c*) *Right upper lobe with central carcinoma causing bronchiectasis distal to the obstruction.* (*d*) *A central lower lobe carcinoma with suppurative pneumonia of a basal segment*

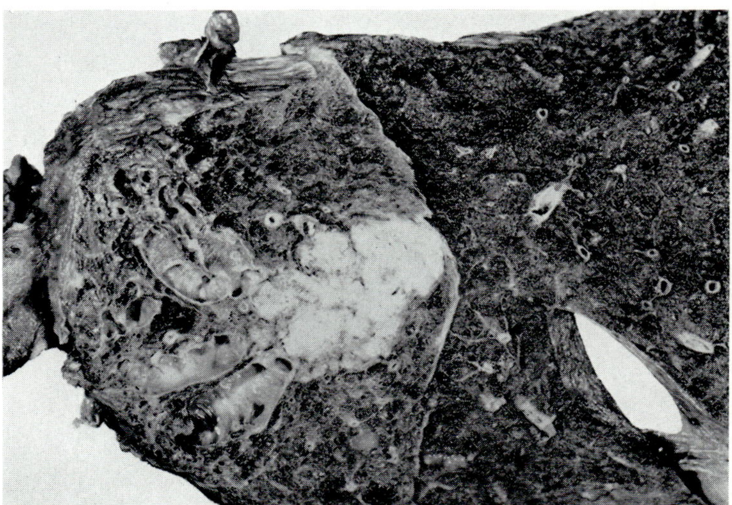

(*c*)

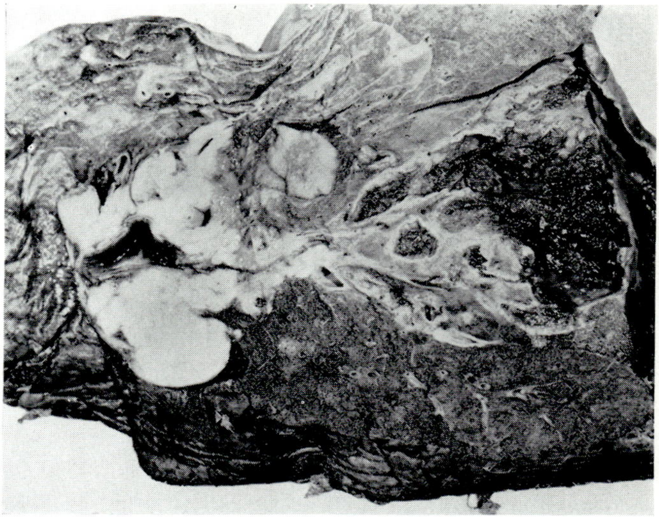

(*d*)

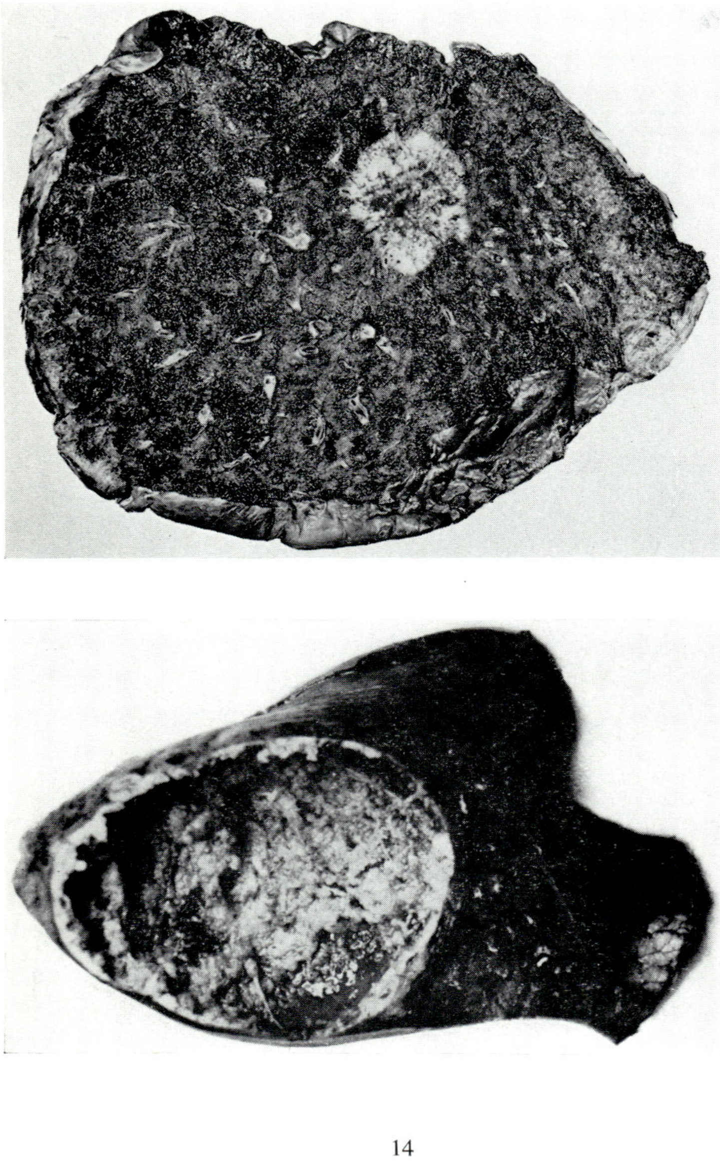

(e) (f)

Figure 1. (e) An excavating necrotic carcinoma. (f) Lobectomy specimen with a peripheral carcinoma growing around a pigmented scar

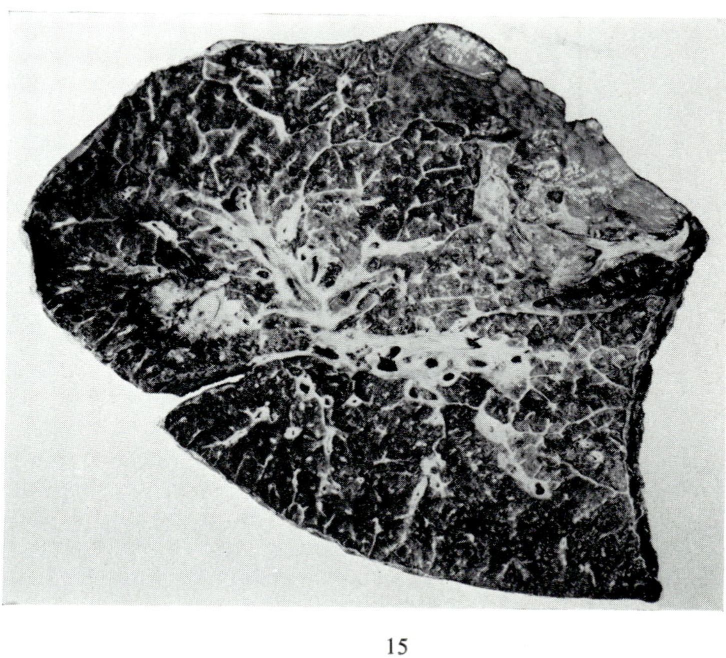

(g)

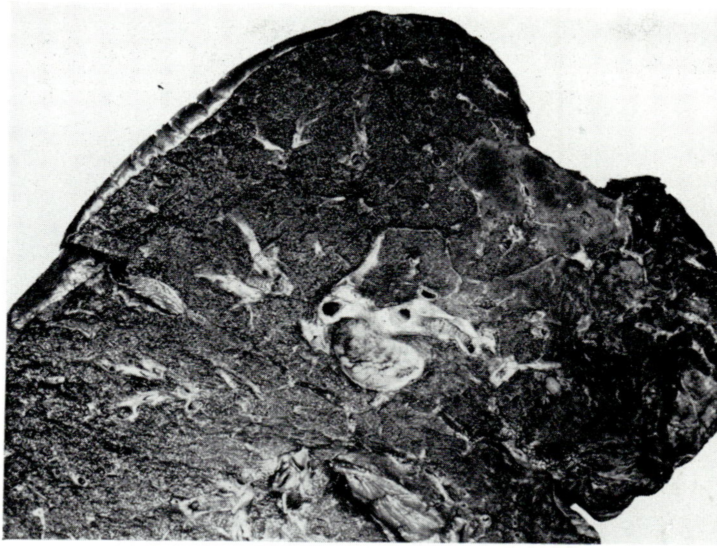

(h)

Figure 1. (*g*) *Permeation of lymphatics clearly delineates the interlobular septa.* (*h*) *A central growth with vascular involvement causing a depressed pulmonary infarct*

feels that immunotherapy may have an important part to play in dealing with malignancy.

PULMONARY SITES AND LOCAL EFFECTS

Pulmonary neoplasms are usually classified as central and peripheral. The macroscopic types and their effects are demonstrated in *Figure 2* and related illustrative photographs (*Figures 1a–f*).

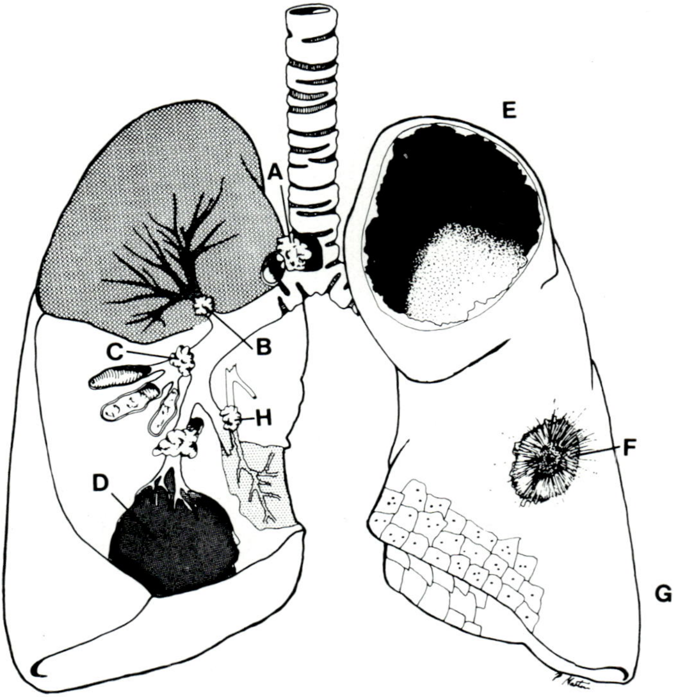

Figure 2

Central growths are best regarded as those which grow in a main, lobar or segmental bronchus or a major division of a segmental bronchus. Rarely, they are no more than a roughening of the epithelial surface and present with haemoptysis; they are then diagnosed by finding squamous carcinoma cells in the sputum while in the *in situ* stage (Canti, 1966). Usually when such 'early' lesions are resected, histological examination clearly demonstrates invasion of submucosa. Sometimes larger growths produce no obstructive effects (*Figures 1a* and *2A*). However, central growths usually soon produce obstructive effects—rarely lobar obstructive emphysema, but commonly collapse consolidation or "obstructive pneumonitis' (*Figures 1b* and *2B*). Bronchiectasis (*Figures 1c* and *2C*), bronchial mucocele and pulmonary suppuration (*Figures 1d* and *2D*) distal to

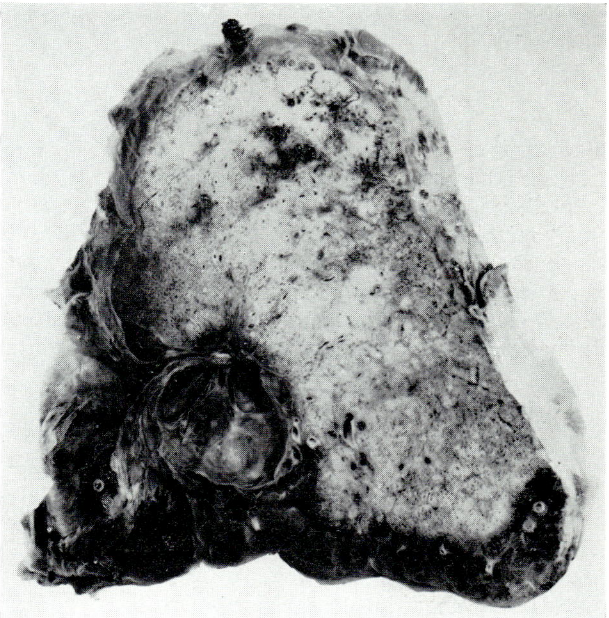

Figure 3. An alveolar cell carcinoma related to an old lung abscess cavity in the right lower lobe

the neoplasm are common consequences. Central growths at the time of diagnosis have usually spread to involve the surrounding parenchyma and closely related intrapulmonary nodes, so that the radiological opacity results from all these components of the growth together with the non-neoplastic lobar or segmental consequences described above. Much of the dramatic improvement seen radiologically after radiotherapy or the use of cytotoxic drugs is due to the resolution of these inflammatory lesions following partial relief of the bronchial obstruction.

Peripheral growths vary from small lesions less than a centimetre in diameter to large spherical growths with an irregular edge occupying much of a lobe. They frequently excavate, thus simulating lung abscess (*Figures 1e* and *2E*), but the irregular wall, varying in thickness, is an important distinguishing feature. Peripheral growths frequently arise in relation to pre-existing lung scars (Raeburn and Spencer, 1953) (*Figures 1f* and *2F*). Such lesions are often subpleural and grow around a puckered scar. This relationship to pre-existing scars is not confined to peripheral growths since occasionally an early invasive carcinoma in a major bronchus may be found in relation to an old bronchial scar (Schwartz, 1952).

The distinction radiologically is sometimes difficult, as a peripheral growth involving only parenchyma may appear radiologically to be in the hilum and central.

Alveolar cell (bronchiolo-alveolar) carcinoma may give rise to multiple small nodular growths resembling secondary deposits and occasionally may involve much of the lobe, radiologically resembling a lobar pneumonia (*Figure 3*). This histological type also may be related to a pre-existing diffuse pulmonary fibrosis, as indeed may other histologically more circumscribed types; post-irradiation fibrosis may be erroneously diagnosed in such cases at autopsy.

HISTOLOGICAL TYPES

The great majority of lung carcinomas have a uniform histological appearance throughout the main tumour and its metastases, although some variation in the degree of differentiation may be encountered. It is not surprising that occasionally a single tumour may combine two distinct histological appearances. Both squamous and oat cell carcinomas are related to smoking, so it is to be expected that malignant change should sometimes simultaneously occur in the epithelial cells of origin of both neoplasms. Similarly, adenocarcinomas of many organs often have squamous areas (adeno-acanthoma) often regarded as a metaplastic change in the glandular epithelium. The rarer occurrence of malignancy in both epithelium and connective tissue (carcinosarcoma) is more difficult to understand.

Since the appearance is fairly uniform in any single patient, it is possible to classify lung tumours into many types using simple cytological, architectural and histochemical criteria. Pathologists have always recognized squamous or epidermoid carcinoma, although different criteria obtain as to inclusion in this group. Well differentiated adenocarcinomas, whether producing mucin or not, are easily recognizable. Other tumours have all given rise to some difficulty. Oat cell carcinomas were considered for many years to be small round cell sarcomas until Barnard (1926) demonstrated their bronchial origin. There are other tumours composed of small malignant cells with no cytological evidence to indicate a squamous nature or any architectural tendency towards an adenocarcinomatous origin. Similarly, large-celled undifferentiated neoplasms have to be classified, in some of which tumour giant cells are a prominent feature.

Evans (1966) classifies carcinoma of the lung simply into (1) adenocarcinoma, (2) carcinoma with squamous characteristics, (3) undifferentiated carcinoma, and (4) oat cell carcinoma.

In view of the important differences already mentioned between the various histological types, it is vital that any comparison between various therapeutic regimens should take histological typing into account. With this object partly in mind, the World Health Organization (Kreyburg, 1967) has classified lung cancer, defining criteria for inclusion in each type or sub-type and providing illustrative transparencies with its publication. This classification is more detailed and has important advantages: it is easier to group together types and sub-types, if deemed justified, when correlations between therapeutic regimens are made, but when the original classification has been simplified, success of therapy in a small sub-group could be so diluted as to be missed. Another obvious advantage of W.H.O. typing is that such an internationally agreed classification is the only one likely to allow comparisons between centres in different countries.

The W.H.O. classification is for all lung tumours, and those involving carcinoma alone are given below.

I. Epidermoid carcinomas.

II. Small cell anaplastic carcinomas:
   1. Fusiform cell type.
   2. Polygonal cell type.
   3. Lymphocyte-like ('oat cell') type.
   4. Others.

III. Adenocarcinomas:
   1. Bronchogenic:
      a. Acinar } with or without mucin formation.
      b. Papillary } with or without mucin formation.
   2. Bronchiolo-alveolar.

IV. Large cell carcinomas:
   1. Solid tumours with mucin-like content.
   2. Solid tumours without mucin-like content.

3. Giant cell carcinomas.
4. 'Clear' cell carcinomas.

V. Combined epidermoid and adenocarcinomas.

Epidermoid Carcinomas

To justify this classification, either definite evidence of keratinization or the presence of intercellular bridges (*Figure 4*) is required. It must be realized that behaviour and therefore prognosis varies with the degree of differentiation, and Goldman (1965) considered

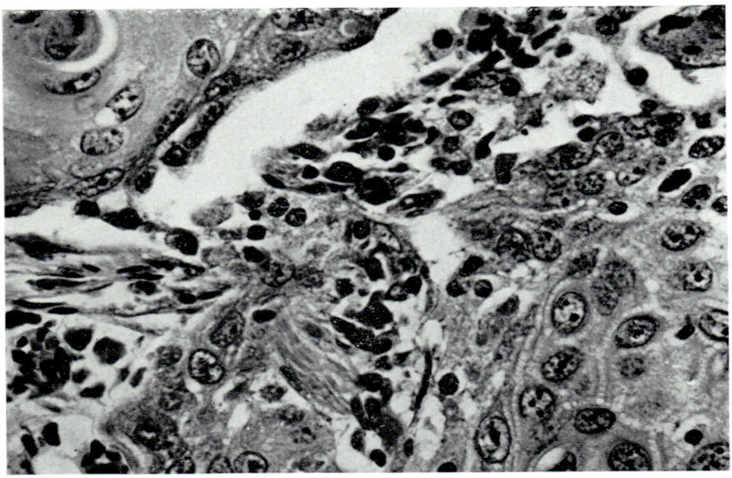

Figure 4. Intercellular bridges in one corner and keratinization in the opposite corner. H and E × 90. W.H.O. I

that from a prognostic viewpoint slightly differentiated squamous carcinomas might be better classified as 'undifferentiated' together with slightly differentiated adenocarcinomas.

Papillary tumours of the surface epithelium, which are mainly squamous, may be regarded as carcinomas by the bronchoscopist, but although some are invasive they carry a good prognosis. The W.H.O. classification includes this epidermoid neoplasm in type VIII.

The results of resection are reasonably good, with 35–45 per cent survival (Bignall and Moon, 1955; Goldman, 1965). A controlled trial of radiotherapy versus surgery showed that surgery was preferable to radiotherapy in operable cases (Morrison, Deeley and Cleland, 1963).

Small Cell Anaplastic Carcinomas

The features necessary for inclusion in this W.H.O. category are well defined by the authors, but much criticism has been levelled at the classification in that it fails to separate the distinctive 'oat cell' neoplasm (*Figure 5*) and to regard it as a type in its own right. Many British pathologists would include the W.H.O. fusiform cell type II (1) in the oat cell category, Spencer (1968) illustrating such a spindle-celled appearance in an oat cell neoplasm. The significance of the tendency to rosette formation and production of mucin described by Azzopardi (1959), sometimes regarded as evidence of differentiation and possibly carrying a better prognosis, has yet to be evaluated.

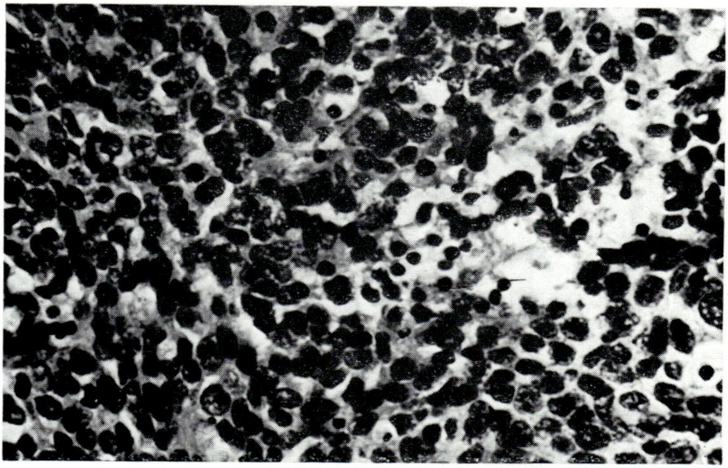

Figure 5. Characteristic small lymphocyte-like cells. H and E × 90

The difficulties and criticisms of the way in which this small-celled group has been arranged does not justify the abandonment or modification of the W.H.O. classification, with its obvious advantage of enabling workers in different countries to evaluate therapy using identical criteria for histological typing.

The treatment of lung cancer of this histological type is disappointing, but the results of a controlled trial of surgery versus radiotherapy give reason to believe radiotherapy to be the treatment of choice (Miller, Fox and Tall, 1969).

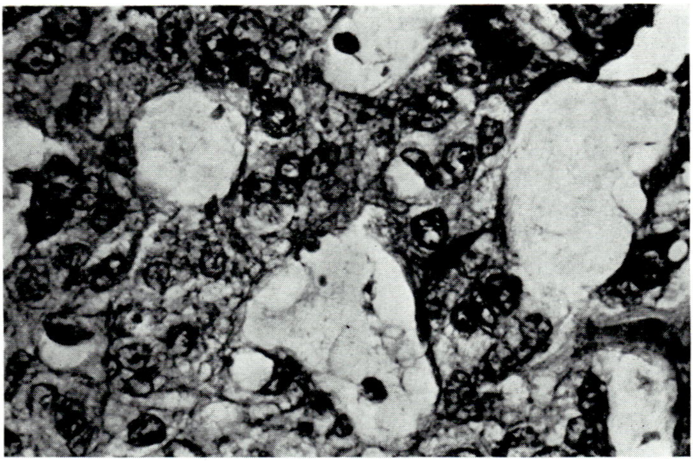

Figure 6. Acinar formation. H and E × 90. W.H.O. III (1a)

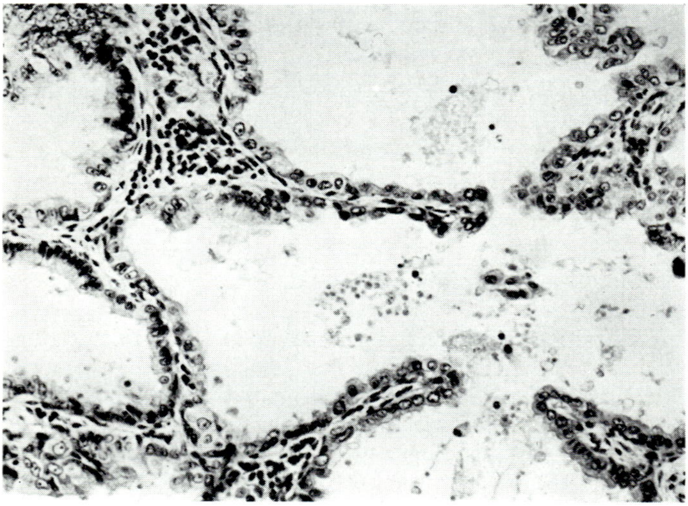

Figure 7. Carcinoma cells growing on the basement membrane of the alveoli. H and E × 70. W.H.O. III (2)

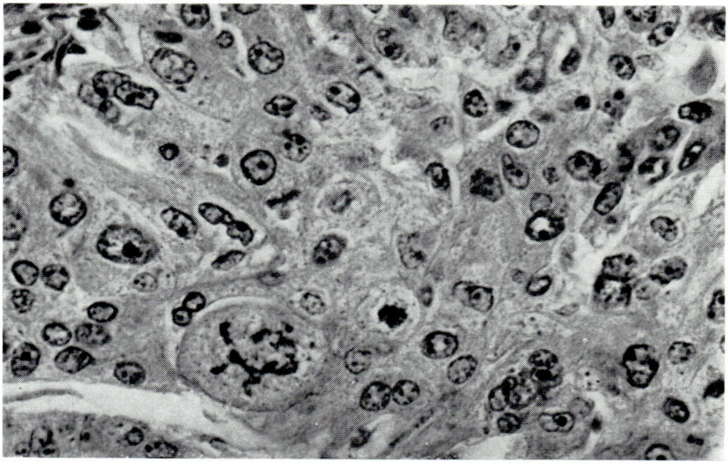

Figure 8. Large cells varying in size and shape without keratinization or acinus formation. H and E × 90. W.H.O. IV (2)

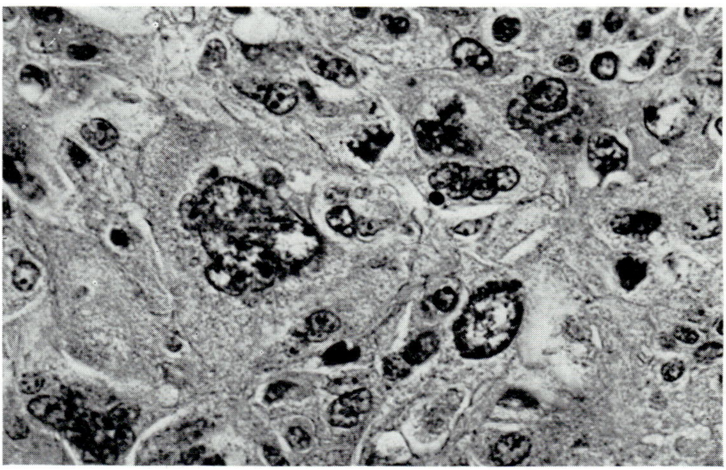

Figure 9. Several bizarre giant cells. H and E × 90. W.H.O. IV (3)

Adenocarcinomas

There is little difficulty in the classification of these tumours, as the presence of tubules and gland-like structures is easily recognizable (*Figure 6*). The production of mucin is not used as a basis for sub-typing. Areas of mucin production within an otherwise characteristic oat cell neoplasm would not warrant classification in this type. Adenocarcinomas are often peripheral and invisible bronchoscopically, but the appearances of exfoliated cells are frequently sufficiently distinctive to enable recognition of this type by this means.

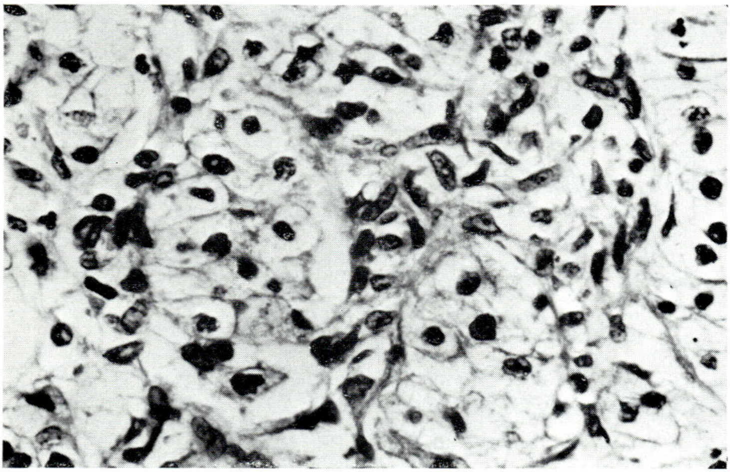

Figure 10. A foam cell or clear cell appearance. H and E × 90

Bronchiolo-alveolar carcinomas, commonly termed alveolar cell carcinomas, are also distinctive (*Figure 7*) and frequently present a distinct clinical picture, with production of much mucoid sputum associated with increasing dyspnoea and cyanosis.

Primary adenocarcinomas of the lung cannot be distinguished on histopathological features from pulmonary deposits, particularly those from an origin in the ovary, stomach or pancreas, although it is surprising how infrequently a search for such a primary growth reveals a non-pulmonary origin.

Large Cell Carcinomas

The criterion for typing in this category is that the neoplasm should consist of large cells without any evidence of epidermidization or formation of gland-like structures (*Figure 8*). The presence of mucin in the cells without glandular structures does not warrant the tumour being typed as an adenocarcinoma. The sub-type 3 (*Figure 9*) may be mimicked by spread from a suprarenal tumour, and sub-type 4 (*Figure 10*) by a deposit from a primary in the kidney. In practice, here again, extensive investigation of this possibility is usually unrewarding and serves merely to delay therapy.

Most of these tumours would be classified as 'undifferentiated' in the many papers reporting on the results of surgery in lung cancer, and in terms of prognosis they fall between the reasonable results for the epidermoid and the poor results for the 'oat cell' group.

SPREAD OF LUNG CANCER

Carcinoma traditionally is considered to spread by direct extension along lymphatic channels and through the blood stream, usually in that sequence. Lesions which appear to be the result of direct spread, such as apical tumours that involve the chest wall, bronchial plexus and sympathetic chain, require formation of lymphatic channels for the extension of the growth across natural anatomical barriers. Similarly, lesions in adrenals, bone and brain may have arisen by a devious spread along lymphatic pathways rather than by haematogenous dissemination. Involvement of lymph nodes is often the result of direct invasion from a neighbouring growth.

In spite of these considerations, it is useful to consider spread under these main headings, realizing the artificiality of such division.

Direct Spread

The earliest direct spread is invasion of the subepithelial structures of the bronchus, followed by invasion of the surrounding parenchyma. Central growths and peripheral growths, particularly of the lingula, may directly involve the pericardium and the phrenic nerve. Peripheral growths may involve the pleura, and subsequent lymphatic extension may produce diffuse neoplastic involvement of visceral and parietal pleura, mimicking a mesothelioma of the pleura.

Direct involvement of pulmonary veins may grow to produce a large mass in the left atrium, and detachment of large fragments has been known to cause sudden death.

Lymphatic Spread

The lymphatic pathways within the lung include bronchial submucosal lymphatics, perivascular lymphatics and a subpleural plexus.

Submucosal lymphatic vessels are often permeated for some distance proximal to the visible intraluminal mass, and their involvement accounts for some of the recurrences after surgical resection. A knowledge of the lymphatic pathways draining the lung and the location of the lymph nodes and their anatomical relationships is essential to an understanding of lung cancer and its clinical manifestations for rational and local treatment, either surgically or with radiotherapy.

The various histological types tend to involve the lymphatics at different times in their natural history and at different rates. Nohl (1962) noted only 32·7 per cent of mediastinal nodes to be involved by epidermoid growths in a surgical series, while adenocarcinomas, undifferentiated growths and oat cell tumours involved these nodes in 54, 57 and 77 per cent of patients respectively. In many cases lymphatic involvement extends beyond the thorax, and the cervical, axillary and supraclavicular nodes must be examined carefully. Lymph nodes around the coeliac axis and along the superior border of the pancreas are frequently the only extrathoracic sites of spread.

Detailed accounts of the lymphatic drainage of the lung include those of Rouvière (1939), Probert in Miller, Seal and Taylor (1963) and, with particular reference to carcinoma of the lung, Borrie (1952) and Nohl (1962). There is general agreement that the spread from the right upper lobe is to hilar nodes on that side, often including nodes between the upper lobe bronchus and the middle and apical lower bronchi. Further extension into the mediastinal nodes involves the right paratracheal and anterior tracheal nodes. Nohl (1962) considered that upper lobe growths seldom involve nodes below a line drawn through the axis of the middle and apical lower lobe bronchi. Right lower lobe growths involve the hilar nodes around the lower part of the right main bronchus and between the lower and middle lobe bronchi. The mediastinal nodes first involved are the subcarinal nodes, the more inferior para-oesophageal nodes and those in the pulmonary ligament. Growths in the left lung metastasize along the lymphatics following the same general principle, except that there is a marked tendency for spread to occur along lymphatic pathways leading to the right paratracheal chain. *Figure 11* illustrates extensive involvement of the right paratracheal group, causing compression of the superior vena cava without invasion or thrombus formation contributing to the obstruction from a left lower lobe primary.

Occasionally the node involvement does not follow the known lymphatic drainage and unusual patterns of node involvement occur, usually regarded as retrograde spread from obstruction of the natural pathways. Extensive involvement of subpleural, perivascular and endobronchial lymphatics produces a characteristic appearance in which the lung is firm and the lymphatics are clearly delineated on

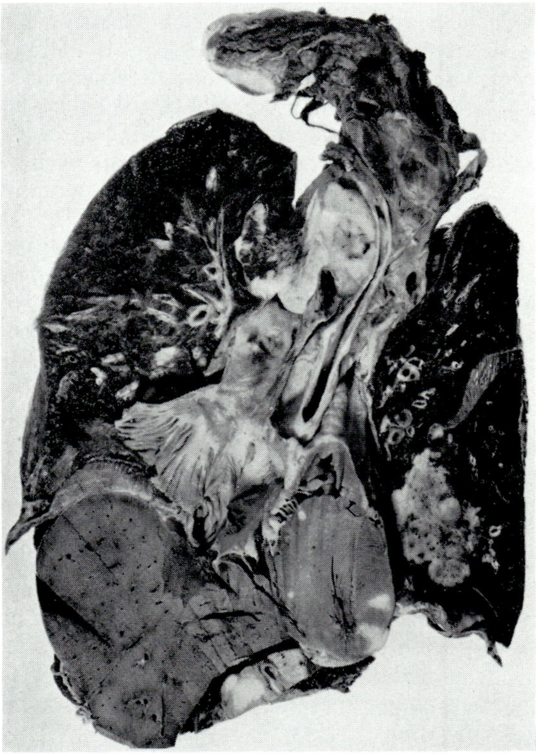

Figure 11. Left lower lobe carcinoma with lymphatic spread to right paratracheal nodes causing superior vena caval obstruction. There are haematogenous myocardial deposits, and lymphatic spread has involved nodes around the coeliac axis

the pleural and cut surface, the lobular structure of the lung being distinct (*see Figures 1g* and *2G*). Pulmonary vessels are thickened, and clinically the lungs are 'stiff' and there is evidence of pulmonary hypertension. This condition, often referred to as lymphangitis carcinomatosa, may result from secondary pulmonary involvement from a primary carcinoma in the stomach or breast.

Haematogenous Dissemination

The first vessels to be affected are the small peripheral pulmonary veins, which are found to be involved in the majority of cases when a careful search is carried out. Hinson and Nohl (1960), after studying resection material, concluded that only involvement of large veins was associated with a poor prognosis from subsequent metastases. Many authors have demonstrated an increase in circulating malignant cells following the inevitable handling and compression involved in surgical removal, and this may contribute to the development of distant metastases in the months following operation. Another mode of access of tumour emboli into the systemic veins is through the lymph venous shunts that are found when lymph nodes are involved by tumour (Edwards and Kinmonth, 1969). Occasionally a central tumour involves related pulmonary vessels, with consequent infarction of the lung distally (*see Figures 1h* and *2H*). Such lesions radiologically resemble segmental obstructive lesions.

The organ most frequently involved is the liver, followed by the adrenals, brain, bones, kidneys and spleen. The factors influencing the likelihood of the development of metastases are ill understood and certainly are not related to the blood flow through an organ; that metastases are to be regarded as a failure of the defence mechanism for dealing with tumour emboli is suggested by the rarity of macroscopic deposits in the spleen although microscopic emboli can frequently be seen.

Occasionally a large solitary metastasis in a distant organ is the only evidence of haematogenous dissemination, and in such instances success has rarely followed surgical removal (Richards and McKissock, 1963). Radiotherapists also have claimed success from this bold approach (Deeley and Rice Edwards, 1968).

Where there is multiple organ involvement, it is sometimes difficult to be sure of the primary site even when histology is available, as some pulmonary tumours mimic those from other sites—for example, clear cell carcinoma of lung and kidney, adenocarcinoma of lung and pancreas, large cell carcinoma of lung and carcinoma of adrenal, and the fact that occasional secondary involvement of the parenchyma of lung and also of the bronchus centrally may resemble a pulmonary primary.

STAGING OF CARCINOMA OF THE LUNG

The assessment of any therapeutic regimen should take into account the stage of the neoplasm at the time of institution of therapy as well as the histological type. All attempts at classification depend on

TABLE 1

Clinical Stage Classification, Union Internationale contre le Cancer, October 1966
Malignant Tumours of the Lung

Regions

1. Hilar.
2. Peripheral.

Hilar tumours	*Peripheral tumours*
T. *Primary tumour*	T. *Primary tumour*
T0. No evidence of primary tumour.	T0. No evidence of primary tumour.
T1. Tumour confined to segmental bronchus.	T1. Tumour confined to a segment of a lobe.
T2. Tumour confined to lobar bronchus.	T2. Tumour confined to one lobe.
T3. Tumour involving the main bronchus.	T3. Tumour involving more than one lobe or extending beyond the lung.
N. *Regional lymph nodes*	N. *Regional lymph nodes*
The regional nodes are the intrathoracic lymph nodes and do not include the cervical lymph nodes.	The regional nodes are the intrathoracic lymph nodes and do not include the cervical lymph nodes.
N0. No clinical, radiological or endoscopic evidence of intrathoracic lymph node enlargement.	N0. No clinical, radiological or endoscopic evidence of intrathoracic lymph node enlargement.
N1. Clinical, radiological or endoscopic evidence of intrathoracic lymph node enlargement.	N1. Clinical, radiological or endoscopic evidence of intrathoracic lymph node enlargement.
Note: Where it is not possible to assess the intrathoracic lymph nodes the symbol NX will be used, permitting eventual addition of histological information, thus: NX– or NX+.	*Note:* Where it is not possible to assess the intrathoracic lymph nodes the symbol NX will be used, permitting eventual addition of histological information, thus: NX– or NX+.
M. *Distant metastases*	M. *Distant metastases*
M0. No distant metastases.	M0. No distant metastases.
M1. Distant metastases including cervical lymph nodes and/or pleural effusion with malignant cells present.	M1. Distant metastases including cervical lymph nodes and/or pleural effusion with malignant cells present.

the degree to which a tumour has spread. Several authors have classified tumours on the basis of tumour extent and degree of spread, but here again an internationally agreed classification exists. This classification depends on a division into peripheral and hilar tumours and acknowledges the difficulty in assessing the extent of lymphatic spread even after full investigation. The classification is given in Table 1.

CONDITIONS THAT MAY MIMIC LUNG CARCINOMA

Many bronchial neoplasms may obstruct the bronchus and produce clinical and radiological features which, in a patient in the cancer age group, can be diagnosed in the absence of biopsy material as carcinoma. The remainder of the W.H.O. classification, given below, includes many of these neoplasms.

VI. Carcinoid tumours.

VII. Bronchial gland tumours:
1. Cylindromas.
2. Muco-epidermoid tumours.
3. Others.

VIII. Papillary tumours of the surface epithelium:
1. Epidermoid.
2. Epidermoid with goblet cells.
3. Others.

IX. 'Mixed' tumours and carcinosarcomas:
1. 'Mixed' tumours.
2. Carcinosarcomas of embryonal type ('blastomas').
3. Other carcinosarcomas.

X. Sarcomas.

XI. Unclassified.

XII. Mesotheliomas:
1. Localized.
2. Diffuse.

XIII. Melanomas.

* * * *

Benign lesions of the lung mimicking malignant tumours:
1. Sclerosing haemangiomas.
2. Plasma cell granulomas.
3. Pseudolymphomas.

Most British clinicians and pathologists have regarded VI and VII (1) as coming under the general term 'bronchial adenoma'. The epidermoid papillary tumours have already been discussed. The 'mixed' tumours include fairly benign growths resembling mixed salivary tumours as well as malignant carcinosarcomas.

Benign connective tissue tumours such as chondromas, lipomas and fibromas may also be misdiagnosed as carcinomas on clinical and radiological grounds.

The fairly common benign chondromatous hamartoma is a peripheral lesion that is often resected, and its benign nature can seldom be proven pre-operatively. Rarely such tumours are multiple.

Malignant lymphomas also occasionally may resemble carcinoma of lung both clinically and radiologically.

Non-neoplastic Conditions

The combination of a 'segmental lesion' with a non-neoplastic bronchial obstruction is fairly common, and in this context the writer has encountered old calcified caseous nodes, various foreign bodies, hydatid hyaline membrane (ectocyst), so-called 'mucoid impaction' and sarcoidosis.

By far the most frequent non-neoplastic condition which may be erroneously regarded as malignant is an organizing pneumonia. Such inflammatory lesions are frequently associated with thickening of the bronchial wall, causing confusing narrowing on bronchography.

The benign neoplastic and non-neoplastic conditions together constitute a large enough proportion to invalidate any conclusions drawn from therapy of any series of lung carcinomas in which a proportion of histologically unproven cases is included.

ACKNOWLEDGEMENTS

Thanks are due to Miss P. Martin, Medical Artist of the Dental School at Cardiff; to Mr. R. Boothby for the photography; and to Miss E. Jackson for the typing.

REFERENCES

Azzopardi, J. G. (1959). 'oat cell carcinoma of bronchus.' *J. Path. Bact.* **78,** 513.

Barnard, W. G. (1926). 'The nature of the "oat cell sarcoma" of the mediastinum.' *J. Path. Bact.* **29,** 241.

Bignall, J. R. and Moon, A. J. (1955). 'Survival after lung resection for bronchial carcinoma.' *Thorax* **19,** 183.

Brett, G. Z. (1969). 'Earlier diagnosis and survival in lung cancer.' *Br. med. J.* **4,** 260.

Borrie, J. (1952). 'Primary carcinoma of the bronchus: prognosis following surgical resection (a clinico-pathological study of 200 patients).' Hunterian Lecture delivered at the Royal College of Surgeons of England on 4 October, 1951, by J. Borrie. *Ann. R. Coll. Surg.* **10,** 165.

Canti, G. (1966). *Carcinoma-in-situ of the Bronchus*, p. 41. Midhurst: King Edward VII Hospital.

Deeley, T. J. and Rice Edwards, J. M. (1968). 'Radiotherapy in the management of cerebral secondaries from bronchial carcinoma.' *Lancet* **1,** 1209.

Edwards, J. M. and Kinmonth, J. B. (1969). 'Lympho-venous shunts in man.' *Br. med. J.* **4,** 579.

Evans, W. (1966). *Histological Appearances of Tumours.* Edinburgh and London: Livingstone.

Goldman, K. P. (1965). 'Histology of lung cancer in relation to prognosis.' *Thorax* **20,** 298.

Hinson, K. F. W. and Nohl, H. C. (1960). 'Involvement of the pulmonary veins by bronchogenic carcinoma.' *Br. J. Dis. Chest.* **54,** 54.

Kreyburg, L. (1967). *International Histological Classification of Tumours, No. 1: Histological Typing of Lung Tumours.* Geneva: World Health Organization.

Mathe, G. (1969). 'Approaches to the immunological treatment of cancer in man.' *Br. med. J.* **4,** 7.

Miller, A. B., Fox, W. and Tall, R. (1969). 'Five-year follow-up of the M.R.C. comparative trial of surgery and radiotherapy for the primary treatment of small-celled or oat-celled carcinoma of the bronchus.' *Lancet* **2,** 501.

Miller, F. J., Seal, R. M. E. and Taylor, M. (1963). *Tuberculosis in Childhood.* London: Churchill.

Morrison, R., Deeley, T. J. and Cleland, W. P. (1963). 'The treatment of carcinoma of the bronchus: a clinical trial to compare surgery and supervoltage radiotherapy.' *Lancet* **1,** 683.

Nasiell, M. (1969). 'Predisposing and prognostic factors in cancer of the respiratory tract.' In *Second Tenovus Cancer Symposium*, Cardiff.

Nohl, H. C. (1962). *The Spread of Carcinoma of the Bronchus.* London: Lloyd-Luke.

Raeburn, C. and Spencer, H. (1953). 'A study of the origin and development of lung cancer.' *Thorax* **8,** 1.

Richards, P. and McKissock, W. (1963). 'Intracranial metastases.' *Br. med. J.* **1,** 15.

Rouvière, H. (1939). *Anatomie des lymphatiques de l'homme.* Paris: Masson.

Schwartz, Ph. (1952). *Advances in Tuberculosis Research*, Vol. V. Basel: Karger.

Spencer, H. (1968). *Pathology of the Lung.* Oxford: Pergamon.

3—Asbestos and Cancer

J. C. Wagner

INTRODUCTION

Due to the tremendous increase in the use of asbestos, there is an urgent need to clarify the link between this group of minerals and malignant neoplasms. The inhalation of asbestos dust may be associated with two types of tumour—bronchial carcinoma and diffuse mesothelioma. It is the only substance which has been associated with mesothelioma of the pleura and peritoneum. Moreover, such tumours have occurred following occupational and environmental exposure, and of the varieties of asbestos used it is possible that only a single type may be implicated in the development of these neoplasms.

Asbestos is the generic name applied to a diverse group of fibrous silicates. A number of these have commercial value, but four types are mainly used in industry: chrysotile, crocidolite, amosite and anthophyllite. Chrysotile is by far the commonest, with a total world annual production of over 3,000,000 tons, the main sources being Canada, the Soviet Union, South Africa and Cyprus. Crocidolite (blue asbestos) is mined in South Africa and was until recently mined in Western Australia, the annual production being around 150,000 tons; the amount imported into Britain has been reduced in recent years and is now about 500 tons. Amosite is found only in South Africa, where 100,000 tons are produced annually; the use of this fibre is increasing in Britain, and about 20,000 tons were brought in during 1968. Anthophyllite is mainly produced from a small mine in Finland with an annual production of 15,000 tons, only a small amount of which is used in Britain. The total production of asbestos has increased about ten times during the last thirty years.

There is evidence that these minerals were first used to strengthen clay pots at least 4,000 years ago. The Egyptians made funeral shrouds from the woven fibres, and the Romans wicks for their lamps. In the Middle Ages, the incombustible nature of these materials was regarded as a curiosity.

The industrial value of asbestos was only appreciated after 1860, when the Canadian deposits were discovered. Initially used for fireproofing and insulation, today asbestos has literally hundreds of important uses in manufactured products in almost every country in the world. In many of these it constitutes an indispensable ingredient without which the product would cease to exist. The major uses of fibre are primarily in the asbestos cement industry and secondly in the manufacture of asphalt and vinyl asbestos floor tiles. Additional important products are asbestos paper, mill boards, roof felting, brake linings, roof coatings, caulking compounds, filters and textiles (Hendry, 1965).

SEQUELAE OF ASBESTOS DUST INHALATION

The inhalation of asbestos dust may lead to the production of asbestos bodies, pleural plaques, asbestosis and later malignant neoplasms.

Asbestos Bodies

Asbestos bodies were first mentioned by Fahr (1914), were clearly described by McDonald (1927), and were studied in detail by Gloyne (1932). They consist of asbestos fibres covered by a golden-brown envelope of iron and protein. These bodies usually have bulbous ends, giving them a drumstick appearance. They vary in length from 10 to 250 μ. They are mostly straight (*Figure 1*), but occasional curved and circular forms have been observed.

When found in the sputum they can be taken as evidence of exposure to asbestos dust, but not of asbestosis without further clinical and radiological evidence. Asbestos bodies in the air spaces of the lung were also thought to be an indication of exposure to asbestos dust, and asbestosis was diagnosed only when asbestos bodies and fibres were incorporated into the interstitial tissues. However, the investigations started by Thomson, Kaschula and MacDonald (1963) in Cape Town, in which they demonstrated asbestos bodies in 25 per cent of adults in a consecutive necropsy series, upset this concept. These findings have been confirmed in most industrial countries, the highest results being from Eastern Finland, where nearly 70 per cent of adults have asbestos bodies in their lungs (Meurman, 1966). The frequency of such findings led critics to doubt whether the bodies had anything to do with asbestos, and the term 'ferruginous bodies' appeared in the literature (Gross and colleagues, 1968). Pooley and colleagues (1970) were able to confirm the presence of asbestos fibres by electron microscopy in a series of cases in which pathologists had reported asbestos bodies. Asbestos fibres are far more numerous in the lungs than the bodies, and although they were originally thought to be evidence of recent exposure, it is now accepted that uncoated fibres can remain in the lungs for at least 60 years after the last known exposure. A method of assessing the number of asbestos bodies and fibres in the lungs in various conditions is required, and the alkaline extraction method of Gold (1967) is being investigated.

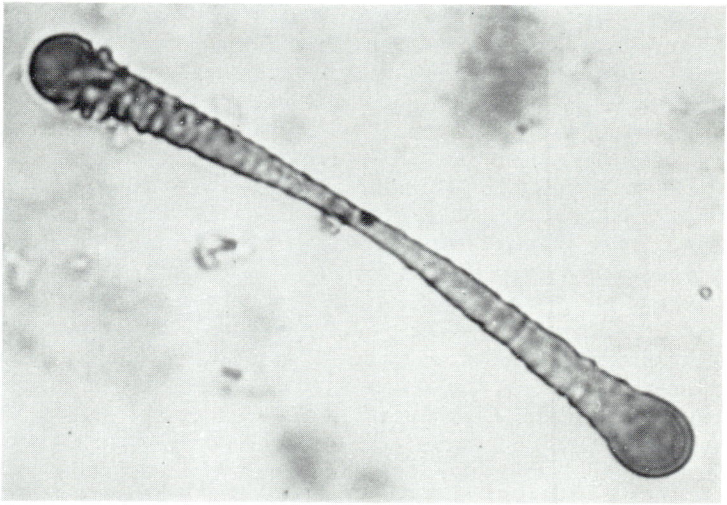

Figure 1. Typical asbestos body. Original magnification × 480, reduced to × 360

Pleural Plaques

Pleural fibrosis is a common feature in asbestosis, its severity not necessarily being similar to that of the underlying lung condition. This is most noticeable in the case of plaques. These dense cartilaginous-like lesions are observed bilaterally on the lower parietal pleura in cases of asbestosis. They occur particularly with environmental exposure to anthophyllite (Kiviluoto, 1960; Meurman, 1966). Diaphragmatic plaques are also commonly seen, some being as large as 10 cm in diameter. The surface may be smooth and glistening or may be covered in small nodules. Smaller linear plaques are seen which follow the line of the ribs. Only a minority of plaques are radio-opaque.

The plaques consist of dense hyaline acellular collagen fibres which have a laminated basket-weave appearance (Meurman, 1966). Calcium is deposited in these lesions, usually in foci of avascular necrosis. The radio-opacity of the plaque depends upon the amount of calcium present. Why the plaques should form on the parietal pleura and only infrequently on the visceral surface has not been explained. Asbestos fibres have been found in these lesions. The plaques do not produce symptoms.

Asbestosis

The suspicion that there was an association between exposure to asbestos dust and the development of pulmonary fibrosis, reported by Murray in 1907, was fully confirmed in the report of Merewether and Price (1930). The disease of asbestosis is now universally recognized. Asbestosis in scheduled occupations has been compensatable since 1931 in Great Britain.

The condition is now recognized as an insidious pulmonary fibrosis which may take up to 30 years to develop and is usually progressive after exposure has ceased. The fulminating pulmonary fibrosis which is frequently complicated by tuberculosis is no longer a feature of the disease in the United Kingdom. The symptoms are progressive breathlessness and a cough productive of a little mucoid sputum. Pain is not a common feature, and severe pain suggests some complication. Clubbing of the fingers occurs in some of the more severe cases, but is not necessarily a feature. Asbestos warts are commonly seen on the fingers and hands of miners and laggers. They are hyperkeratotic lesions surrounding asbestos fibres, and none has ever been recorded as having undergone malignant change.

The physical signs are essentially those of an interstitial pulmonary fibrosis with persistent coarse crepitations at the bases of the lungs. Cyanosis and signs of right heart failure are common in the more severe cases with a history of previous heavy exposure. The radiological features are those of a diffuse interstitial fibrosis with an irregular nodular pattern which progresses to severe honeycombing at the bases with loss of clear cardiac outline. There is a diffuse thickening of the visceral pleura and obliteration of the costophrenic angles. A new classification of the radiological features has been completed by the radiologists and physicians of the U.I.C.C. Committee and the United States Public Health Department at a recent meeting in Cincinnati (U.I.C.C., 1970).

Pathology

On macroscopic examination, the lungs at various stages of the disease show a progressive interstitial and pleural fibrosis, most severe at the bases of the lower lobes. The histological features are those of a peribronchiolar fibrosis starting in the alveoli, arising from the respiratory bronchioles and gradually spreading to enmesh whole lobules. Asbestos bodies and fibres are incorporated into the fibrous tissue or lie free in the distorted air spaces. This progressive involvement of the interstitial tissues distorts and occludes the pulmonary circulation, leading to right heart failure in the more severe cases.

Carcinoma of the Lung

The first cases of carcinoma of the lung in asbestos workers were reported by Lynch and Smith (1935) in the United States and by Gloyne (1935) in Britain. In 1947, Merewether (1949) analysed the deaths of those with asbestosis in Britain between 1924 and 1947 and showed that 17·2 per cent of male workers had died from pulmonary malignancy. By 1954 this figure had increased to 20 per cent, and in 1966 the report of the Chief Inspector of Factories on Industrial Health (Ministry of Labour, 1966) showed that over 60 per cent of deaths in which asbestosis was mentioned were accompanied by bronchial or pleural cancers. Doll (1955) reported on a survey of workers in scheduled occupations in an asbestos textile factory in Britain and showed that the incidence of pulmonary carcinoma was ten times greater than expected. This population has been followed up by Knox and colleagues (1968). The original and later reports show that there was a greater risk to workers in the scheduled occupations who were employed in industry before conditions were improved in 1931, while those who started in employment after this year were much less at risk.

Further cases of carcinoma of the lung in asbestos workers have been reported from Germany, the United States, Canada, Italy and Holland, and the association between asbestosis and bronchial carcinomas is now recognized in most countries.

Diffuse Mesotheliomas

The first large series of diffuse mesotheliomas of the pleura associated with exposure to asbestos dust was described by Wagner, Sleggs and Marchand (1960). They reported 33 cases of histologically diagnosed mesotheliomas in people who had been exposed to asbestos dust either in the vicinity of the Cape asbestos mines or in industry in South Africa. A further 60 cases were diagnosed by 1962.

The majority of the patients from the Cape asbestos fields had had only environmental exposure to the dust and had not been employed in the asbestos industry. Some had lived in the area for their whole lives, but others had either left at an early age or lived in the vicinity for less than ten years. One woman had been born there and left at the age of five. The average period between first exposure and development of the tumour was 44 years. Three patients stated that they had been in the region for only about three months. In the lungs of the majority of environmental cases coming to necropsy, no evidence of the pulmonary fibrosis of asbestosis was observed, only asbestos bodies and fibres being present as evidence of exposure to asbestos dust.

Although crocidolite, amosite and chrysotile are all mined in South Africa, the accepted cases were confined to the crocidolite mining area of the North West Cape. Intensive investigation of the populations of the other two mining areas has produced only one case with a possible pure amosite exposure (Webster, 1969—personal communication). In several other instances, patients from the amosite and chrysotile areas were found to have had previous exposure on the Cape asbestos fields.

On the available evidence, it was suggested that there was a link between exposure to crocidolite asbestos dust and the development of diffuse mesotheliomas of the pleura, unlike the association of the pulmonary carcinomas with the pulmonary fibrosis of asbestosis. It was decided to test this hypothesis in Great Britain, a country with a long-established asbestos industry. As previously mentioned, the association between carcinoma of the lung and asbestosis had been intensively investigated in Britain, but very few mesotheliomas had been reported. This was possibly due to the fact that the authorities had followed up the known cases of asbestosis and those working in scheduled occupations, but not those individuals who had received less exposure to the dust or had left the industry after a relatively short period.

It was decided, therefore, to investigate cases of diffuse mesotheliomas of the pleura and peritoneum which had been diagnosed in pathology departments in a number of hospitals in Great Britain. Within two years, more cases were found in the United Kingdom than had been diagnosed in South Africa. These tumours continue to occur, and more than 500 cases of mesothelioma have now been recorded in which an association with asbestos exposure has been established. The South African findings have been confirmed. In some of these cases, asbestos bodies and fibres were seen in the lung tissue but there was no evidence of pulmonary fibrosis; there was a long period between initial exposure and development of the tumour, and in some instances the actual period of exposure was six months or less. In addition, in a number of cases the exposure appears to have been domestic in nature, the patient either living in the vicinity of a factory or washing dust protective clothing used by another member of the family.

A feature of the British investigation was that peritoneal mesotheliomas constituted about 10 per cent of the cases. The existence of these tumours in asbestos workers had been suggested by Keal in 1960 and confirmed by Hourihane (1964) when he studied Keal's original cases and further material at the London Hospital. Although such tumours have been reported in small numbers from other regions in Britain, they appear to be more common in the London area.

Studies had been undertaken in the United States which showed that diffuse mesotheliomas were occurring among American insulators and asbestos factory workers. The papers of Mancuso and Coulter (1963) and Selikoff, Churg and Hammond (1964) produced evidence to suggest that these tumours occurred in workers exposed to chrysotile asbestos and that there was an increased incidence of gastro-intestinal tumours in the populations they had studied. A symposium on the biological effects of asbestos was organized by the New York Academy of Sciences in 1964 (Symposium, 1965) at which the current knowledge of the problem was discussed. It had been agreed that further investigations should be co-ordinated through the International Union against Cancer (U.I.C.C.).

Following the symposium, therefore, a U.I.C.C. (1965) working party met and recommended that it was essential to have correlated epidemiological surveys in areas where there was exposure to a single type of asbestos. The group also recommended the standardization of pathological criteria for the diagnosis of mesotheliomas and the preparation of standard reference samples of the main types of asbestos for experimental work. These recommendations are being carried out. A large-scale epidemiological investigation has nearly been completed in the Quebec asbestos fields in Canada, and an investigation has been conducted in Finland. A South African survey measuring the degree of general environmental pollution by asbestos fibres in mining and controlled areas has been completed. Long-term medical and environmental studies in several parts of the asbestos industry are progressing in the United Kingdom and the United States. Other studies have been initiated in the United States, Germany, Sweden, Italy, Australia, Cyprus, Canada and the

United Kingdom. The standardization of the pathological criteria for the diagnosis of mesotheliomas and asbestosis has been generally accepted. Pathology panels have been formed in the United Kingdom, South Africa, the United States and Canada. Radiologists and physicians from the United Kingdom, Germany, Canada, Finland, the United States and South Africa have produced a standardized classification of the radiological appearance of asbestosis.

Standard reference samples of asbestos are now available. The asbestos fibre was contributed by the asbestos producers in Canada, Finland, Rhodesia and South Africa under the supervision of the South African and Medical Research Council Pneumoconiosis Research Units. The physicists of these units are now characterizing the dusts which have been produced. This material is now available, and requests for it have been received from more than 100 laboratories throughout the world. The Ministry of Labour (1967) has published the report of its advisory panel on problems arising from the use of asbestos.

A second international conference on the biological effects of asbestos was held in Dresden in 1968 (Conference, 1968), the proceedings of which should be available in the near future.

Clinical Presentation

The clinical features of the diffuse mesotheliomas have been well described by Elmes (1966). The pleural cases usually present with a history of increasing breathlessness associated with a heavy feeling on the affected side of the chest. In a few instances the onset may be sudden, and these are usually associated with the development of a large pleural effusion. In most cases the pain in the early stages is described as dull and slight, while in a few it is severe from the start. Occasionally patients have presented with nodules of tumour on the chest wall. Usually the initial clinical and radiological features are those of a simple pleural effusion. It is only when the fluid is removed that nodules or lobulated masses can be seen on the pleural surface. In other cases there is only evidence of an irregular pleural thickening. In addition, particularly among those who have had occupational exposure to asbestos, there is radiological evidence of pulmonary fibrosis and calcified pleural plaques.

The presence of mesothelioma may be suspected on clinical grounds by exclusion of other possible causes, but the final diagnosis depends upon pleural biopsy and subsequent confirmation at necropsy. Cytological examination of the fluid has been shown to be helpful (Klempman, 1962; Naylor, 1963), but is still not generally accepted as conclusive. The presence of excess hyaluronic acid in the pleural fluid (Harington, Wagner and Smith, 1963) is still regarded by some as a diagnostic aid (Thompson, Bromberg and Amenta, 1969), but has been severely criticized by others. Needle biopsy is seldom successful. This is due to the variegated nature of the mesotheliomas, so that if tumour tissue is produced for examination it will usually be insufficient for a diagnosis. In addition, if the biopsy does not include tumour nodule, a non-specific histological picture may be seen. The correct diagnosis can usually be arrived at by open thoracotomy, in which there can be full examination and tissue can be produced from a number of separate sites. Unfortunately this procedure cannot be recommended as it appears to exacerbate the growth of the mesothelioma and tumour nodules frequently develop in the surgical scars.

Attempts at radical surgery and radiotherapy have not been successful and appear to encourage the growth of the tumour through the chest wall. There is a history of increasing pain and breathlessness as the tumour increases in size, with collapse of the completely compressed lung and mediastinal invasion with contralateral pleural effusion. The average survival period is nine months after the initial diagnosis.

Peritoneal cases usually present with persistent ascites, with rapid accumulation after paracentesis. This may be followed by acute obstruction of some site in the intestinal tract. The diagnosis is made from biopsy material taken at laparotomy. Following this investigation there is rapid progression of the tumour.

Mesothelioma in relation to asbestos exposure was prescribed as an industrial disease in the United Kingdom in 1966.

Pathological Features

Macroscopic Findings

The diffuse pleural mesotheliomas are included in the W.H.O. histological typing of lung tumours, type XII(2) (World Health Organization, 1967). They appear to originate as multicentric small nodules on the parietal and visceral pleura, with a predilection for the cardio-phrenic angle. The individual nodules rapidly coalesce and form a large nodular mass covering the parietal pleura of one hemithorax (*Figures 2* and *3*). Usually a thinner layer of tumour tissue covers the visceral pleura, spreading along the fissures and infiltrating into the intralobular septa. Frequently between these two layers there is an effusion of sticky fluid rich in hyaluronic acid. At a later stage the two layers fuse, leaving the lung compressed by a massive tumour. The commonest form of spread is by direct extension

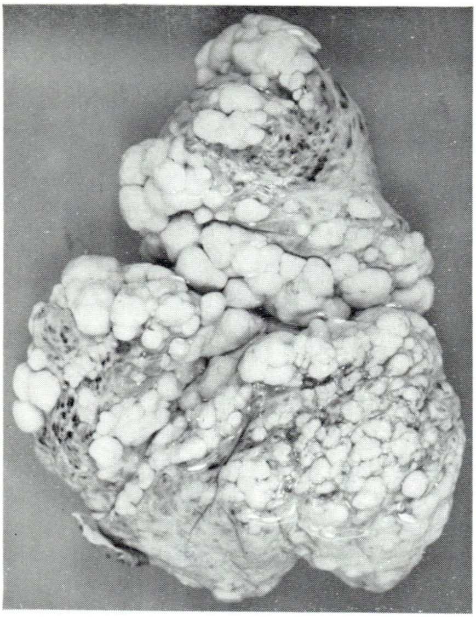

Figure 2 (*left*). *Diffuse mesothelioma on visceral pleura of a woman who had cobbed asbestos in N.W. Cape*

Figure 3 (*below*). *Mesothelioma. Whole lung section from an insulator in a British Naval dockyard*

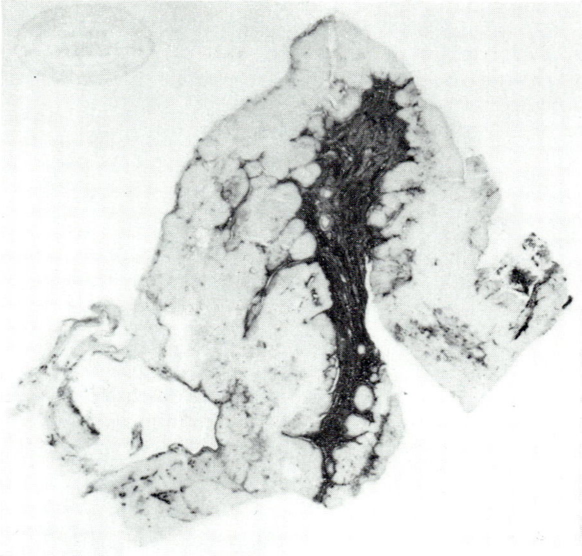

of the tumour mass to involve the pericardium, mediastinum and opposite lung. There may be infiltration of the diaphragm, followed by widespread seeding of the peritoneum. The underlying lung may be invaded with permeation of the lymphatics, and later intra-alveolar spread may occur. It was originally considered that these tumours spread only by direct extension, but metastases have now been recognized in most organs including the brain.

The peritoneal mesotheliomas are seldom as florid as those in the thorax. The usual appearance is that of a thin layer of tumour tissue invading the parietal peritoneum with spread to the serosal surface of most of the organs and marked infiltration of the omentum, the pancreas being frequently involved in the tumour mass. Large effusions are common. In a few cases, there is massive involvement of the pelvis with all the organs enveloped in dense tumour tissue. In both pleura and peritoneum, the consistency of the tumour may be either soft and gelatinous or dense and cartilaginous-like depending on the histological type and the hyaluronic acid content.

Histological Features

The microscopical appearances of diffuse mesotheliomas vary considerably because the mesothelial cell, when stimulated, can either proliferate in an epithelial-like manner or form spindle cells resembling fibroblasts. The epithelial type may (1) produce a complex tubulo-papillary structure, (2) appear as a single layer of cells lining clefts, or (3) appear as sheets of cells which on occasion contain foci of giant cells. The spindle-celled tumours vary from dense masses of cells resembling those of a low grade fibrosarcoma to lesions in which only occasional spindle cells are seen surrounded by a dense fibrous stroma. The most common form is the mixed type of tumour in which both elements can be seen, the histological pattern changing remarkably between adjoining sections. In other cases a large number of sections are required to discover that both elements are present. In general, the mitotic activity in these tumours is low and marked pleomorphism of either cell type is uncommon. Due to the complex histological patterns that can occur, a positive diagnosis of mesothelioma may be difficult unless all other possible primary sites of tumour origin have been excluded at necropsy. McCaughey (1965) reviewed criteria for diagnosis on biopsy material.

DISCUSSION

Over the years a number of controversial aspects have been discussed in relation to both carcinoma of the lung and the mesotheliomas. The British opinion that carcinoma of the lung occurs only with severe asbestosis has been challenged by Selikoff, Hammond and Churg (1968), who claim that in the New York insulation workers, carcinoma of the lung is associated with asbestos exposure and the risk is greatly increased among asbestos workers who smoke. There is no evidence as yet that the lung cancers are associated with exposure to any particular type of fibre. A more intensive study of the carcinoma cases is required to establish the site of the tumours and their cell type. There is a body of opinion that these carcinomas usually occur in the lower lobes and are multicentric in origin and squamous in type. Others consider that the sites of origin and the histological types vary, but that the peripheral adenocarcinomas are more common than expected.

In considering the diffuse mesotheliomas, it is agreed that these tumours do occur in cases in which there is no suggestion of asbestos exposure. However, it is generally accepted that in those cases in which asbestos is implicated the association is with exposure to the dust and not necessarily with the pulmonary fibrosis. It has not been possible to establish an association with a particular type of asbestos in the British cases since the majority of the workers, as in other industrial countries, have mostly been exposed to several types of fibre. However, Pooley and colleagues (1970) have developed a method by which individual fibres can be identified in tissue sections. This technique could be applied to a statistically selected sample of cases of mesothelioma from all parts of the world. The suggestion that gastro-intestinal tumours are related to asbestos exposure needs further investigation as the earlier findings have not been substantiated.

It can be appreciated that the association between asbestos and malignant neoplasms is both complex and a cause for concern. Unfortunately, with the increased amount of asbestos being used and the long latent period between exposure and tumour development, these problems will be with us for many years to come.

REFERENCES

Conference (1968). *Proceedings of 2nd International Conference on Biological Effects of Asbestos*, Dresden. In the Press.

Doll, R. (1955). *Br. J. ind. Med.* **12,** 81.

Elmes, P. C. (1966). *Postgrad. med. J.* **42,** 623.

Fahr, T. (1914). *Münch. med. Wschr.* **61,** 625.

Gloyne, S. R. (1932). *Lancet* **1,** 1351.

— (1935). *Tubercle, Lond.* **17,** 5.

Gold, C. (1967). *J. clin. Path.* **20,** 674.

Gross, P., de Treville, R. T. P., Cralley, L. J. and Davis, J. M. G. (1968). *Archs Path.* **85,** 539.

REFERENCES

Harington, J. S., Wagner, J. C. and Smith, M. (1963). *Br. J. exp. Path.* **44,** 81.

Hendry, N. W. (1965). *Ann. N.Y. Acad. Sci.* **132,** 12.

Hourihane, D. O'B. (1964). *Thorax* **19,** 268.

Keal, E. E. (1960). *Lancet* **2,** 1211.

Kiviluoto, R. (1960). *Acta radiol.*, Suppl. 194, 1.

Klempman, S. (1962). *Cancer, N.Y.* **15,** 691.

Knox, J. F., Holmes, S., Doll, R. and Hill, I. D. (1968). *Br. J. ind. Med.* **25,** 293.

Lynch, K. M. and Smith, W. A. (1935). *Am. J. Cancer* **24,** 56.

McCaughey, W. T. E. (1965). *Ann. N.Y. Acad. Sci.* **132,** 603.

McDonald, S. (1927). *Br. med. J.* **2,** 1025.

Mancuso, T. F. and Coulter, E. J. (1963). *Archs envir. Hlth* **6,** 210.

Merewether, E. R. A. (1949). *Annual Report of the Chief Inspector of Factories for the Year 1947.* London: H.M.S.O.

— and Price, C. W. (1930). *Report on Effects of Asbestos Dust on the Lungs and Dust Suppression in the Asbestos Industry.* London: H.M.S.O.

Meurman, L. (1966). *Acta path. microbiol. scand.*, Suppl. 181, 1.

Ministry of Labour (1966). *Annual Report of H.M. Chief Inspector of Factories on Industrial Health.* London: H.M.S.O.

— (1967). H.M. Factory Inspectorate. *Memorandum of the Senior Medical Inspector's Advisory Panel.* London: H.M.S.O.

Murray, H. M. (1907). *Report of the Departmental Committee on Compensation for Industrial Diseases.* London: H.M.S.O.

Naylor, B. (1963). *J. Path Bact.* **86,** 293.

Pooley, F. D., Oldham, P. D., Um, C. H. and Wagner, J. C. (1970). In *Pneumoconiosis: Proceedings of International Conference on Pneumoconiosis*, Johannesburg, 1969, p. 108. Ed. by H. A. Shapiro. Cape Town: Oxford University Press.

Selikoff, I. J., Churg, J. and Hammond, E. C. (1964). *J. Am. med. Ass.* **188,** 22.

— Hammond, E. C. and Churg, J. (1968). *J. Am. med. Ass.* **204,** 106.

Symposium (1965). Proceedings of Symposium on Biological Effects of Asbestos. *Ann. N.Y. Acad. Sci.* **132,** 5.

Thompson, M. E., Bromberg, P. A. and Amenta, J. S. (1969). *Am. J. clin. Path.* **52,** 335.

— (1970). *Chest* **58,** 57.

Thomson, J. G., Kaschula, R. O. C. and MacDonald, R. R. (1963). *S. Afr. med. J.* **27,** 77.

U.I.C.C. (1965). Report and Recommendations of the Working Group on Asbestos and Cancer. *Br. J. ind. Med.* **22,** 165.

Wagner, J. C., Sleggs, C. A. and Marchand, P. (1960). *Br. J. ind. Med.* **17,** 260.

World Health Organization (1967). *Histological Typing of Lung Tumours.* Geneva: W.H.O.

4—Methods of Obtaining Positive Histology and Cytology

I—Reliability of Cytological Diagnosis

William Umiker

Exfoliative cytology has now been acknowledged to be the most sensitive modality for the microscopic diagnosis of lung cancer. Cytologists no longer find it necessary to present supporting data to justify the inclusion of cytological studies in diagnostic regimens. Radiotherapists and others who are responsible for treating bronchogenic carcinomas may find the following questions more relevant to the current status of exfoliative cytology:

(1) How can maximal sensitivity be achieved within practical budgetary limits?

(2) How reliable are the cytological reports in any individual institution?

(3) How accurate is the microscopic typing of lung cancers by cytological smears?

(4) Is a positive cytological diagnosis likely to reveal a treatable neoplasm in the absence of radiographic evidence of a pulmonary lesion?

ACHIEVEMENT OF MAXIMAL CYTOLOGICAL SENSITIVITY

Every lung cancer suspect deserves a cytological study of at least three sputum specimens and one bronchial aspirate before being regarded as cytologically negative. The value of multiple specimens has been correctly emphasized, although the law of diminishing returns sets in rapidly after five specimens have been examined (Farber and colleagues, 1950; Philips, 1954). Equally important is the quality of the specimens. The patient must understand what sputum is and how he can produce it. Much time can be saved if sputum is obtained through the use of heated saline aerosol inhalations (Bickerman, Sproul and Barach, 1958), sulphur dioxide cough stimulation (Allan and Whittlesey, 1960) or related methods (Fontana and colleagues, 1962). The brush technique of Hattori and colleagues (1964) has been used with success by others (Valaitis and colleagues, 1969), and tracheal aspiration is recommended by Cahan and Farr 1950). Use of one of these techniques is mandatory for patients who have unproductive cough.

Most laboratories still rely upon the particle selection technique for the preparation of cytological smears. The most painstaking examination of smears cannot compensate for poor particle selection. This also pertains to smears which are too thick or too thin, and to specimens which are not processed promptly or not placed into fixatives.

The choice of stain is less important than the quality of the staining procedure. Many prefer the Papanicolaou stain, but (with the possible exception of the acridine orange stain) this stain when improperly utilized can produce the most inadequate smears. Fluorescence microscopy with acridine orange fluorochroming has not proved superior to light microscopy and has some distinct disadvantages (Umiker and Pickle, 1960).

Concentration techniques are worthy of trial, and different methods work better for different cytologists (Chang, Anken and Russell, 1962; Farber and colleagues, 1953; Saccomanno and colleagues, 1963; Umiker and Sourenne, 1961). It remains to be proved that the time spent on concentration methods might not be better devoted to the examination of additional material.

RELIABILITY OF CYTOLOGICAL REPORTS

Sensitivity

The sensitivity of cytological diagnosis of lung cancer reported by 28 different authors between the years 1935 and 1963 was found by Davies (1966) to range from 42·8 to 92·7 per cent. The experience of Koss, Melamed and Goodner (1964) probably represents that of many other investigators. They compared their results of 1952–53 with those of 1959–60 and found an increased sensitivity of over

10 per cent in their second series. This indicates the value of experience in collection, processing, screening and evaluation.

It should be emphasized that most reports are published by experienced workers and therefore represent optimal results. What is more important to the individual therapist is not what some internationally renowned expert can achieve, but rather the accuracy achieved by his own cytology service. This is no different from that of any other laboratory procedure. Modern laboratories determine the standard deviation and coefficient of error for their chemistry and haematology tests, but many do not determine (or report) the current accuracy of their cytology results.

The histological type, size and location of the neoplasms are also important factors in the accuracy of cytological results. Sputum from a patient with a peripheral lesion or with an adenocarcinoma is the least likely to contain malignant cells (Koss, Melamed and Goodner, 1964; Umiker, 1961b). Positivity seems to be directly proportional to the size of peripheral neoplasms, but inversely proportional to the size of hilar lesions (Umiker, 1961b).

Specificity

Even more important than sensitivity (percentage of false negatives) is specificity as indicated by the percentage of false positives. Poor results are sometimes concealed by reporting false positives in the percentage of total specimens or total patients examined, especially when the population being studied has a low prevalence of lung cancer. More meaningful, at least to the therapist, are the false positives in relation to the total number of positive reports. In other words, when a positive report is received, what are the odds that the patient does or does not have lung cancer? The incidence of false positives varies from 0 to 14·3 per cent of positive reports (Davies, 1966).

ACCURACY OF MICROSCOPIC TYPING BY CYTOLOGICAL SMEARS

Early investigators concentrated on the detection of malignant cells, with little or no attempt to identify the morphological type. It soon became apparent that the histological type could be predicted in most instances. The prognostic significance of histological type has been demonstrated (McDonald and colleagues, 1951).

The accuracy of such typing is remarkably similar in most reports (Table 1). It should be noted that the overall accuracy of cytological typing is about 80 per cent according to most reports. Equally evident is the lack of uniformity of results in the case of specific histological types of neoplasms, with the notable exception of epidermoid carcinoma. It is very likely that this variation is related, at least in part, to variations in the histological classification used by the histopathologists.

Prediction of histological type is most successful when an adequate number of malignant cells are present. Therefore when positive smears are obtained but the morphological type is in doubt, additional specimens should be examined unless a positive biopsy has been obtained.

TABLE 1
Accuracy of Microscopic Typing by Cytological Smears

Authors	*Histological type (per cent)*				
	Squamous	*Adenocarcinoma*	*Poorly differentiated*	*Undifferentiated*	*Total*
Foot (1952)	89·9	78·4	69·2	83·5	80·0
Spjut, Fier and Ackerman (1955)	89·2	39·3	—	76·2	79·3
Reid and Carr (1961)	85·5	40·0	80·0	—	79·5
Hastrup (1968)	88·0	87·5	82·1	51·1 (large) 84·6 (small)	84·3
Umiker (1961a)	85·7	44·4	87·5	75·0 (large) 100·0 (small)	80·9
Median	88·0	44·0	81·0	80·0	80·0

Epidermoid carcinoma cells are identified with ease when the neoplasm exfoliates cornified cells or cells with nuclei which are so hyperchromatic that they resemble pieces of coal. The major problem encountered with atypical squamous cells is the differentiation between malignant and bizarre metaplastic squamous cells.

Undifferentiated cells of 'oat cell' type present less difficulty in interpretation than in detection. Because of their small size, they may be overlooked despite the fact that they are usually present in large numbers. With experience, cytologists have little difficulty in differentiating these cells from lymphocytes or basal epithelial cells.

The latter are more likely to be encountered in bronchial aspirates, especially if the bronchoscopic examination has been traumatic.

Well-differentiated adenocarcinoma cells are often quite obvious with their characteristic pale vacuolated cytoplasm and giant nucleoli. However, more pleomorphic forms present a greater problem to the cytologist than to the histopathologist, since the latter has the advantage of visualizing in tissue sections glandular structures which are not usually preserved in the smears.

The cytological recognition of poorly differentiated carcinoma is based not only on the pleomorphism of the cells but also on the complete absence of features of squamous or glandular differentiation.

Although muco-epidermoid carcinomas, bronchiolar carcinomas, sarcomas and metastases may produce cells which suggest the histological nature of the neoplasm, such cells are usually more difficult to classify.

LIKELIHOOD OF REVEALING A TREATABLE NEOPLASM IN THE ABSENCE OF RADIOGRAPHIC EVIDENCE

The finding of malignant cells in a patient with negative radiological findings may elicit consternation (and often disbelief !) on the part of the clinician. Detection of increasing numbers of such cases can be predicted because of the more widespread cytological study of patients who are asymptomatic or whose physician is keen enough to suspect lung cancer despite negative x-ray findings. In such cases, additional specimens should be obtained to exclude laboratory error. Extrapulmonary sites such as the buccal cavity, pharynx, nasopharynx and larynx must be investigated. Attempts may be made to obtain differential bronchial secretions from each lung. If malignant cells are repeatedly recovered from only one lung, this indicates which lung is suspect. Hopefully, bronchoscopy or bronchograms will provide the necessary information. Melamed, Koss and Cliffton (1963) reported a series of 12 such cases, and in each instance the neoplasm was eventually localized by one or another of these methods or by the eventual appearance of radiological changes. We may therefore conclude that the finding of cancer cells in a radiographically negative patient is not of academic interest only.

REFERENCES

Allan, W. B. and Whittlesey, P. (1960). 'The results of the experimental use of sulfur dioxide in the production of material for cell studies in lung cancer.' *Ann. intern. Med.* **52,** 326.

REFERENCES

Bickerman, H. A., Sproul, E. E. and Barach, A. L. (1958). 'An aerosol method of producing bronchial secretions in human subjects.' *Dis. Chest* **33,** 347.

Cahan, W. G. and Farr, H. W. (1950). 'The tracheal aspiration—an additional method for the early diagnosis of carcinoma of the lung.' *Cancer, N.Y.* **3,** 475.

Chang, J. P., Anken, M. and Russell, W. O. (1962). 'Liquefaction and membrane filtration of sputum for the diagnosis of cancer.' *Am. J. clin. Path.* **37,** 584.

Davies, D. F. (1966). 'A review of detection methods for the early diagnosis of lung cancer.' *J. chron. Dis.* **19,** 819.

Farber, S. M., Pharr, S. L., Wood, D. A. and Gorman, R. D. (1953). 'The mucolytic and digestive action of trypsin in the preparation of sputum for cytologic study.' *Science, N.Y.* **117,** 687.

— Rosenthal, M., Alston, E. F., Benioff, M. A. and McGrath, A. K. Jnr. (1950). In *Cytologic Diagnosis of Lung Cancer*, p. 42. Springfield, Ill.: Thomas.

Fontana, R. S., Carr, D. T., Woolner, L. B. and Miller, F. K. (1962). 'An evaluation of methods of inducing sputum production in patients with suspected cancer of the lung.' *Proc. Staff Meet. Mayo Clin.* **37,** 113.

Foot, N. C. (1952). 'The identification of types of pulmonary cancer in cytologic smears.' *Am. J. Path.* **28,** 963.

Hastrup, J. (1968). In *Diagnostic Cytology and its Histopathologic Bases*, ed. by L. G. Koss, p. 378. Philadelphia: Lippincott.

Hattori, S., Matsuda, M., Sugiyama, T. and Matsuda, H. (1964). 'Cytologic diagnosis of early lung cancer: brushing method under x-ray television fluoroscopy.' *Dis. Chest* **45,** 129.

Koss, L. G., Melamed, M. R. and Goodner, J. T. (1964). 'Pulmonary cytology—a brief survey of diagnostic results.' *Acta cytol.* **8,** 104.

McDonald, J. R., McBurney, R. P., Carlisle, J. C. and Patton, M. M. (1951). 'The significance of cell types in bronchogenic carcinoma.' *J. thorac. Surg.* **22,** 62.

Melamed, M. R., Koss, L. G. and Cliffton, E. E. (1963). 'Roentgenologically occult lung cancer diagnosed by cytology: report of 12 cases.' *Cancer, N.Y.* **16,** 1537.

Philips, F. R. (1954). 'The identification of carcinoma cells in the sputum.' *Br. J. Cancer* **8,** 67.

Reid, J. D. and Carr, A. H. (1961). 'The validity and value of histological and cytological classifications of lung cancer.' *Cancer, N.Y.* **14,** 673.

Saccomanno, G., Saunders, R. P., Ellis, H., Archer, V. E., Wood, B. G. and Beckler, P. A. (1963). 'Concentration of carcinoma or atypical cells in sputum.' *Acta cytol.* **7,** 305.

Spjut, H. J., Fier, D. J. and Ackerman, L. V. (1955). 'Exfoliative cytology and pulmonary cancer: a histopathologic and cytologic correlation'. *J. thorac. Surg.* **30,** 90.

Umiker, W. (1961a). 'Typing of bronchogenic carcinoma.' *Archs Path.* **71,** 295.

— (1961b). 'The current role of exfoliative cytopathology in the routine diagnosis of bronchogenic carcinoma.' *Dis. Chest* **40,** 154.

— and Pickle, L. (1960). 'The cytologic diagnosis of lung cancer by fluorescence microscopy.' *Lab. Invest.* **9,** 613.

— and Sourenne, R. A. (1961). 'A simple method for concentrating carcinoma cells in sputum: use of an aqueous dissolution technic.' *Am. J. clin. Path.* **35,** 411.

Valaitis, J., McGrew, E. A., Chomet, B., Correll, N. and Head, J. (1969). 'Bronchogenic carcinoma-in-situ in asymptomatic high-risk population of smokers.' *J. thorac. cardiovasc. Surg.* **57,** 325.

II—TV Brushing Method for Early Diagnosis of Small Peripheral Lung Cancer

Shoji Hattori and Minoru Matsuda

INTRODUCTION

The value of cytology for the early diagnosis of lung cancer has been well established. Carcinoma *in situ* of the major bronchus is preoperatively detectable by cytological examination of the sputum or bronchial secretion as well as by bronchoscopy before the tumour shadow becomes demonstrable on the chest x-ray film. However, the positive rates of sputum cytology remain quite low for cancers situated in the peripheral zone of the lung. If malignant lesions in the lung periphery are less than 2 cm in diameter, the positive rate on sputum cytology is greatly decreased. Umiker (1961) was able to detect cancer cells in 84 per cent of hilar tumours and in only 66 per cent of peripheral tumours. Attar, Naib and Cowley (1961) detected 64 per cent of malignant tumours less than 4 cm in diameter and 79 per cent of all peripheral tumours by the cytological examination of the sputum. We have detected only 7 positive cases on sputum examination out of 21 confirmed peripheral lung cancers less than 3 cm in diameter (33·3 per cent) (Hattori and colleagues, 1965a).

It is generally accepted that an accurate diagnosis of small peripheral lung cancers (coin lesions less than 2 cm in diameter) has great value for early surgical treatment. To overcome the difficulties in establishing a cytological diagnosis of such small tumours, Motsch (1962) has used a catheter suction biopsy technique and Fridel (1961) has developed an irrigating technique through a radio-opaque catheter. Nordenström and Carlens (1965) and Nolting (1965) used a small alligator-type biopsy forceps, while Tsuboi (1959) and Tsuboi and colleagues (1967) employed a direct scrape-off technique through Métras' catheter under ordinary x-ray fluoroscopy for the collection of tumour cells from peripheral lung cancers. Fennessy (1966, 1967) has described a bronchial brushing technique in which selective catheterization of the appropriate segmental bronchus is done with a radio-opaque arterial catheter and small brushes are passed through the catheter into the region of the lesion. We have developed a TV brushing method for obtaining fresh tumour cells directly from the peripheral small tumour (Hattori and colleagues, 1964, 1965a, b). This method is a selective bronchial brushing technique under x-ray television fluoroscopy.

INSTRUMENTS FOR TV BRUSHING METHOD

TV Brushes (*Figure 1*)

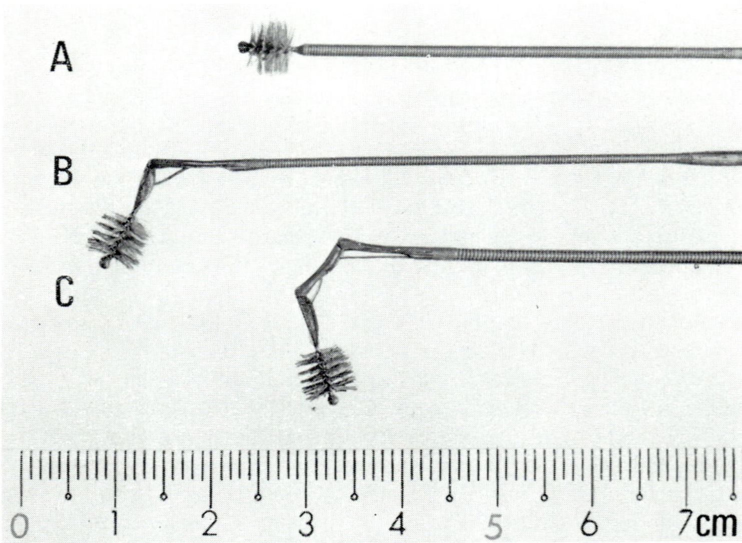

Figure 1. Brushes used for TV brushing method. A: straight brush. B: flexible brush. C: double flexible brush

Straight Brush

This consists of a tiny metal ball (1 mm in diameter) on the tip, a small nylon brush (5 mm in length) and a flexible stainless steel spiral wire SUS 27.

Flexible Brush

Two kinds of flexible brushes are used. One has an elbow-like joint near the tip. The other (double flexible brush) has two joints between the brush and the wire, enabling the operator to change its direction by manipulating an apparatus on the opposite end of the brush. The metal ball on the tip of the brush is 1 mm in diameter, the joint is 1·5 mm in diameter and the stainless steel spiral wire is 80 cm long.

Choice of Brush

Straight Brush

This brush is used for the following:

(1) Small subpleural lesions which communicate with a peripheral bronchus having only slightly angulated ramifications.

(2) Metastatic cancer where no direct bronchial communication is expected. In such cases the straight brush can sometimes be pushed into the tumour.

(3) Tumours situated in the major bronchus and accompanied by tumorous obstruction. The obstructed lesion can be penetrated by pushing the straight brush.

Flexible Brush

This brush can be bent or straightened as desired within the bronchus by manipulating an apparatus on the opposite end. It is applied to small peripheral lesions having a communication with sharply angulated bronchial ramifications.

Métras' Catheter

Métras' catheter (straight, slightly curved and fully curved types), manufactured by Willy Rusch Co., is used.

Sterilization of Instruments

Neutral liquid detergent is recommended as a disinfectant after washing the brush in tap water because boiling water and alcohol will damage the nylon brush.

PROCEDURE

Ascertainment of Bronchial Obstruction

Prior to the TV brushing, the obstructed area of the tumour-bearing bronchus must be determined by bronchography. Even when a peripheral cancer has a direct communication with the peripheral bronchus, it is not infrequent that the bronchus cannot be visualized by ordinary bronchography because the contrast medium fails to fill the bronchus completely. Moreover, it is sometimes difficult to differentiate bronchial changes due to functional abnormalities or mucous impaction from real organic obstruction. Selective bronchography should therefore be performed to eliminate possible technical difficulties in bronchography, and contrast material of optimal viscosity should be carefully selected. Our experience has shown that bronchi normally visualized on the bronchogram are as a rule devoid of malignancy, and so TV brushing must be performed in the non-visualized branches to the tumour.

TV Brushing Technique

Patients receive a subcutaneous injection of a small dose of atropine–morphine solution 20 minutes before the examination.

Métras' catheter is inserted into the trachea by an ordinary method as in selective bronchography. The catheter is then led to the involved bronchus under x-ray television fluoroscopy, and the lesion is brushed by a TV brush through Métras' catheter. The tip of the catheter is always checked through a monitor screen. A straight brush is convenient for brushing lesions located in the segments with only slightly angulated bronchial ramifications, and a flexible brush is used for the segments with sharply angulated ramifications.

Immediately after the brushing, the material obtained by the brush is directly smeared on 3–4 glass slides, fixed at once with ether–ethanol for 30 minutes and stained by Papanicolaou's method.

RESULTS

Results in Peripheral Lung Lesions

Three hundred and eighty-three peripheral lung lesions, especially coin lesions suggestive of lung cancer, were examined by the TV brushing method. The final diagnoses of examined cases are shown in Table 1. Of 171 confirmed primary lung cancers, 142 were

TABLE 1
Results of TV Brushing Method in Peripheral Lung Lesions

Final diagnosis	*Number of patients*	*Number with positive cytology by TV brushing technique*
Primary lung cancer	171	142 (83·04%)
Metastatic lung cancer	17	11 (64·7%)
Benign tumour	10	0
Tuberculosis	128	2
Pneumonia	17	0
Lung abscess	28	0
Silicosis	2	0
Sarcoidosis	1	0
Lung cyst	1	0
Bronchiectasis	1	0
Unspecified	7	0
Total	383	155

cytologically positive by this method (83·04 per cent), and 11 out of 17 cases of metastatic lung cancer were also positive. The smallest tumour was an epidermoid cell carcinoma having a maximum diameter of 6 mm (*Figure 2*), followed by an adenocarcinoma with a diameter of 14 mm (*Figure 3*). Two out of 128 cases of tuberculosis were false positive by this method. Although the cells obtained from the false positive cases had a fine, evenly distributed chromatin, some degree of anisokaryosis and amitotic change was observed (Hattori and colleagues, 1965b).

Comparison with Sputum Cytology in Diagnosis of the Same Cases

The efficiency of TV brushing was compared with that of sputum cytology in the diagnosis of 171 cases of confirmed primary lung cancer (Table 2). These cases proved positive in 83·0 per cent by the TV brushing method and in only 13·4 per cent by sputum cytology. Nine cases with coin lesions less than 2·0 cm in diameter proved positive in 77·7 per cent and the 49 cases with coin lesions less than 3·0 cm in diameter proved positive in 69·3 per cent by the TV brushing technique.

TABLE 2

Comparison of TV Brushing Method with Sputum Cytology in the Same Cases of Primary Lung Cancer

Technique	*Size of tumour (cm)**				*Total*
	1·0–2·0	*2·1–3·0*	*3·1–4·0*	*4·1 and over*	
TV brushing:					
Positive	7(77·7%)	27(67·5%)	39(90·7%)	69(87·3%)	142 (83·0%)
Negative	2	13	4	10	29
Sputum cytology:					
Positive	0(0%)	2(5·0%)	4(9·3%)	17(21·5%)	23 (13·4%)
Suspicious	0	1	1	2	4
Negative	7	25	28	42	102
Not examined†	2	12	10	18	42

* Maximum diameter of tumour was measured on plain postero-anterior chest x-ray.
† Patients did not raise sputum.

It must be pointed out that TV brushing was performed primarily on patients whose results were negative by sputum cytology or who did not produce any sputum. The positive rate of sputum cytology

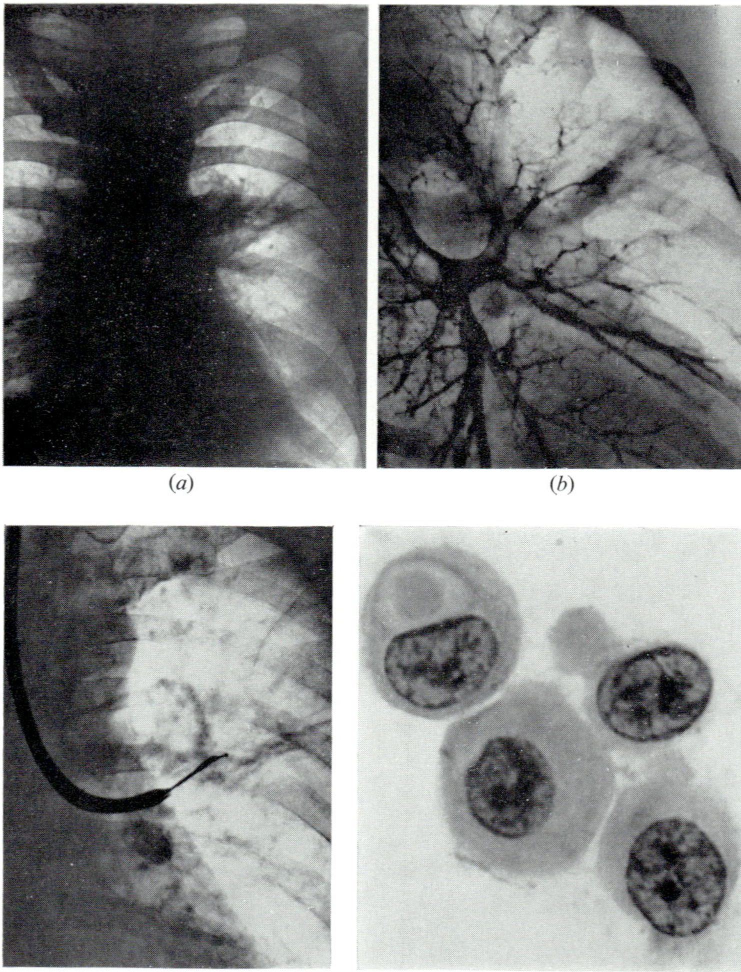

(a) (b) (c) (d)

Figure 2. Case 1. A 53-year-old man who complained of cough and sputum. (a) Chest x-ray reveals slight pneumonitis near left hilum. (b) Bronchogram of left oblique position shows obstruction of $B_{3a,b}$ and (c) a flexible brush was inserted into obstructed area. (d and e) Squamous cell carcinoma cells were obtained by TV brushing. (f) A small tumour (arrowed) is visible in $B_{3a,b}$. (g) Histological section of resected tumour shows no submucosal invasion by cancer. This is a case of very early lung cancer (maximum diameter of tumour is only 6 mm) diagnosed by the TV brushing method. P: pneumonitis. T: tumour in a bronchus. L: lymph node

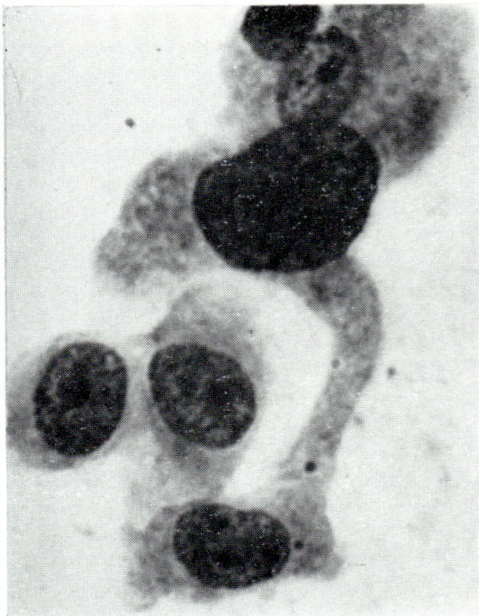

(*e*)

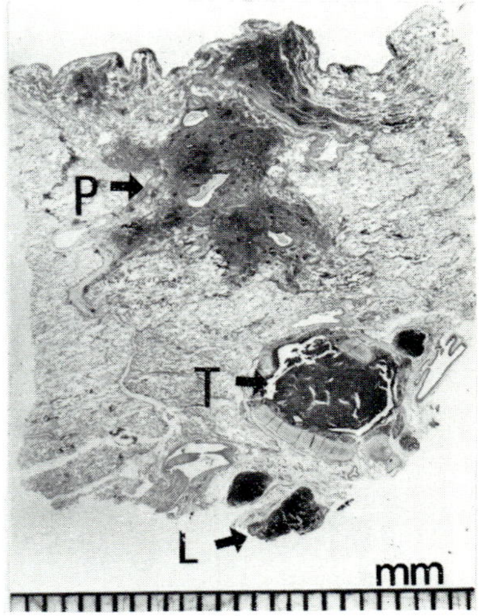

(*g*)

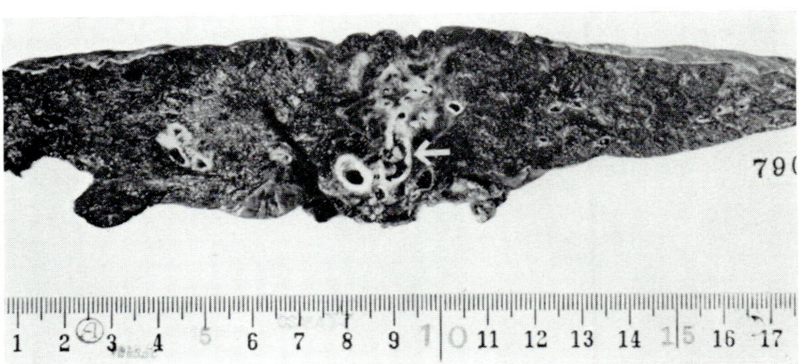

(*f*)

in our laboratory during the past five years was 70·7 per cent (435 positive cases out of 615 patients with confirmed primary lung cancer).

Positive Rate in Relation to Histology Type and Cytology

Surgery was performed in 87 out of 171 confirmed primary lung cancer cases, and the positive rate of the TV brushing method in relation to the histological type of resected tumours and their cytological classification was studied (Table 3).

(a) (b)

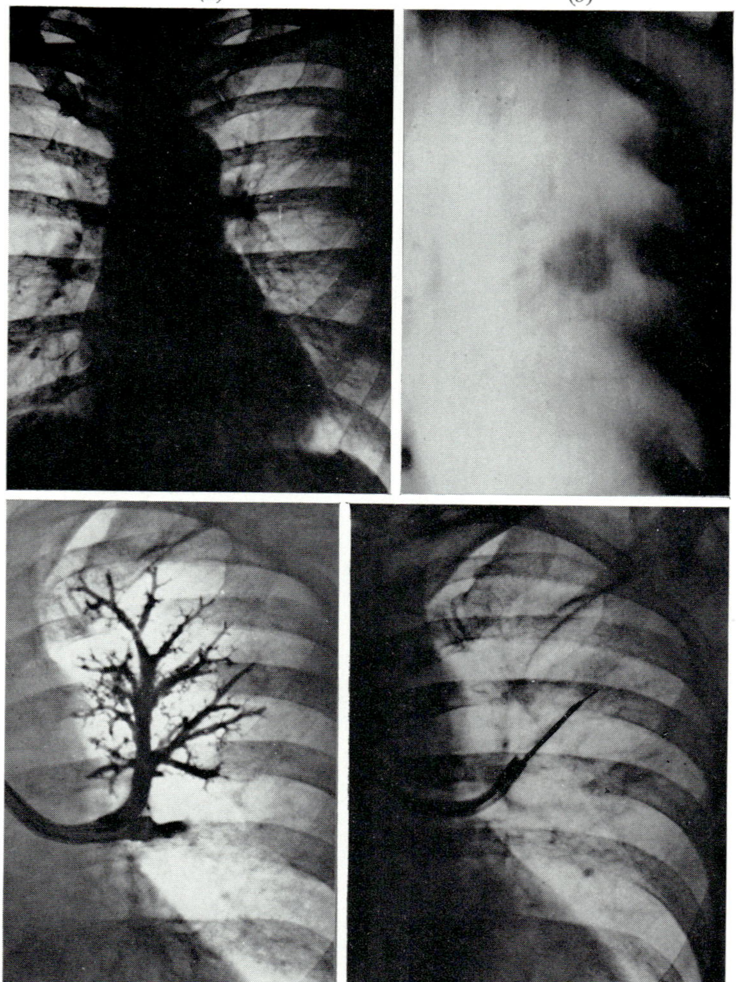

(c) (d)

Figure 3. Case 2. A 50-year-old housewife who had no subjective symptoms. (a) In mass survey, a small tumorous shadow was found in left second intercostal space. (b) Tomogram of this tumour. (c) Selective bronchogram reveals obstruction of B_{1+2b}. *(d) A flexible brush was inserted into obstructed area. (e) Adenocarcinoma cells were obtained by the brush. (f) Cut surface of resected lung shows a small tumour (maximum diameter 14 mm). (g) Histological section shows finely branched tumorous invasion all round the tumour and many small blood vessels penetrating it. These findings correspond to the typical x-ray of adenocarcinoma shown in Figure 3b*

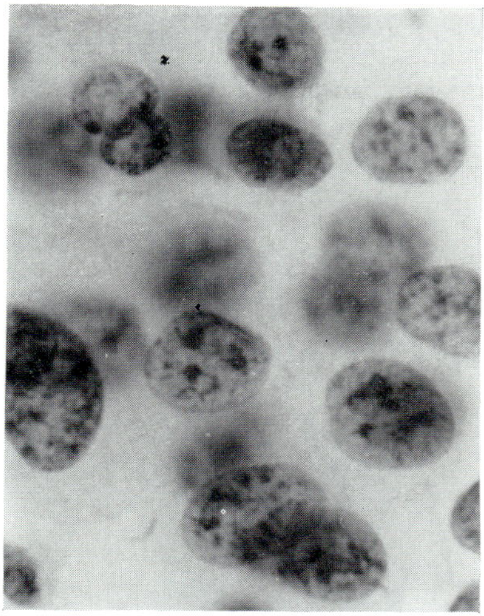

(*e*)

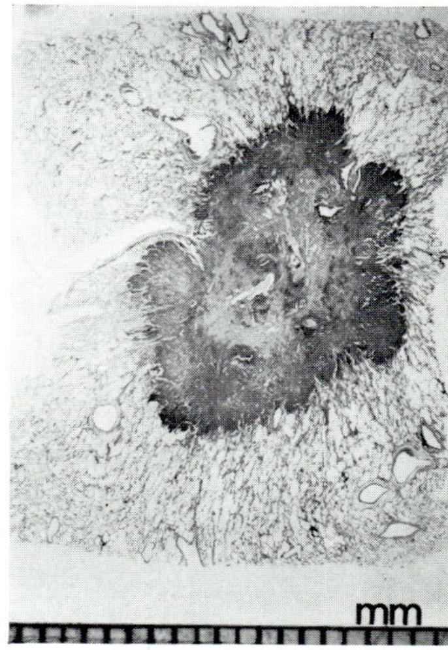

(*g*)

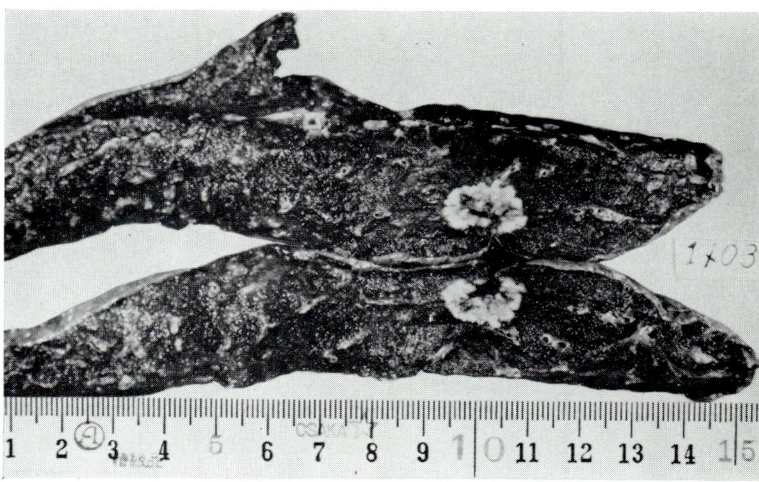

(*f*)

Cornified epidermoid carcinoma, alveolar cell carcinoma, undifferentiated cell carcinoma (small cell type) and mixed tumours yielded high positive rates of more than 90 per cent, whereas the positive rates in uncornified epidermoid carcinoma and adenocarcinoma were only 72·7 and 80·0 per cent respectively.

Adenoid cystic carcinoma and giant cell carcinoma could not be diagnosed by this method. There is general agreement that the former type of tumour originates in acini or ducts of bronchial mucous glands and tends to proliferate in two directions, that is, intrapulmonary and interluminal. We have recently discovered that giant cell carcinoma similarly originates in the bronchial mucous gland (Tateishi, Matsuda and Hattori, 1970). These tumours therefore have no communication with any bronchus during the earlier stage.

TABLE 3

Positive Rate of TV Brushing Method in Relation to Histological Type of Resected Tumour and Cytological Classification

Histological type of resected tumour	*Number of patients*	*Cytological diagnosis*		*Accuracy of cytological classification**
		Negative	*Positive*	
Cornified epidermoid carcinoma	12	1	11 (91·6%)	11 (100%)
Uncornified epidermoid carcinoma	22	6	16 (72·7%)	12 (75·0%)
Adenocarcinoma	25	5	20 (80·0%)	16 (80·0%)
Alveolar cell carcinoma	3	0	3 (100%)	3 (100%)
Adenoid cystic carcinoma	2	2	0	0
Giant cell carcinoma†	1	1	0	0
Undifferentiated cell carcinoma:				
Large cell type	11	1	10 (90·9%)	8 (80·0%)
Small cell type	5	0	5 (100%)	5 (100%)
Mixed type of carcinoma	6	0	6 (100%)	0
Total	87	16	71 (81·6%)	55 (77·4%)

* Rate of coincidence of cytological classification with histological typing.
† Giant cell carcinoma is considered to be of bronchial mucous gland origin.

Cornified epidermoid carcinoma, alveolar cell carcinoma and undifferentiated cell carcinoma (small cell type) yielded 100 per cent accurate cytological classification, whereas uncornified epidermoid carcinoma, adenocarcinoma and undifferentiated cell carcinoma (large cell type) yielded 75, 80 and 80 per cent accurate classification respectively.

Adenocarcinoma is occasionally misdiagnosed as uncornified epidermoid carcinoma or undifferentiated cell carcinoma (large cell type).

With regard to peripheral small lung cancers, when a tumour with a plexiform pattern without keratinization and with a small amount of cytoplasmic mucin is stained, histological classification is very difficult even for pathologists. In the cytological diagnosis of the TV brushed material, the distinction of adenocarcinoma from uncornified epidermoid carcinoma or undifferentiated cell carcinoma (large cell type) is easy only when the structure of the cell group can be observed: that is, a gland-like structure in the case of adenocarcinoma and a pavement structure in epidermoid carcinoma.

The mixed type of carcinoma was cytologically diagnosed as adenocarcinoma, epidermoid carcinoma or undifferentiated cell carcinoma depending on the site of brush insertion to the tumour.

Here it must be noted that the important purpose of the TV brushing method is not for histological typing but for diagnosing curable peripheral lung cancers.

Advantages of TV Brushing Method

The efficiency of the cytological diagnosis of lung cancers by this method depends wholly on accuracy in locating tumour shadows in the lung fields by fluoroscopy. The characteristic advantage of x-ray television fluoroscopy is its excellence in low-contrast detail perceptibility, which is of great merit for the detection of small densities (Hattori and colleagues, 1964; Matsuda and colleagues, 1961, 1963). TV brushing is greatly favoured by this advantage of the x-ray television unit and by the collaboration between patient and doctors in the illuminated examination room. The very small and flexible brush used in the procedure usually assures easy insertion into the subsegmental bronchus or the more peripheral bronchioles through Métras' catheter under x-ray television fluoroscopy. However, when the brush insertion is not easy, this collaboration is important because confirmation of the tumour-bearing bronchus by shifting the patient's posture or slightly changing the bronchial curvature by his taking a deep breath sometimes enables successful insertion of the brush into the tumour.

The cells obtained by TV brushing are very fresh and mostly in groups, enabling easy cytological diagnosis as in histological examination.

With this method, even when the brush is not successfully inserted into the small peripheral lesion, a few exfoliated malignant cells near the lesion can be obtained as cell clusters (*Figure 4*). So far 14 out of 142 cytologically positive cases of peripheral lung cancer were found to be positive, although the insertion of the brush was insufficient.

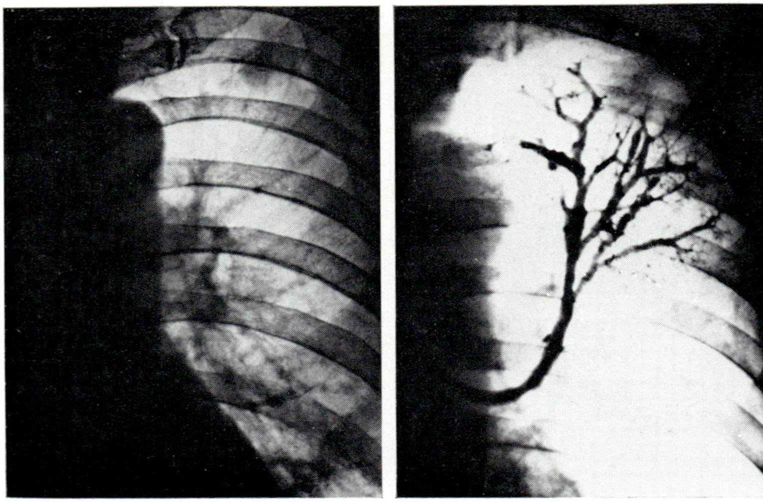

(*a*) (*b*)

Figure 4 (for legend see facing page)

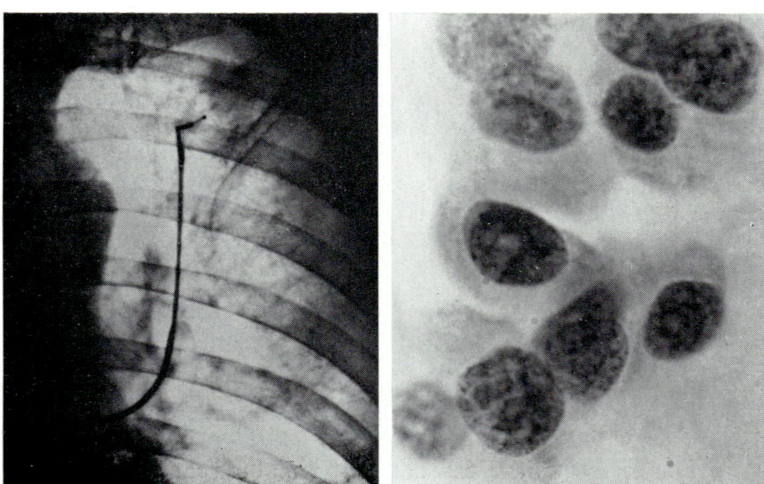

(*c*) (*d*)

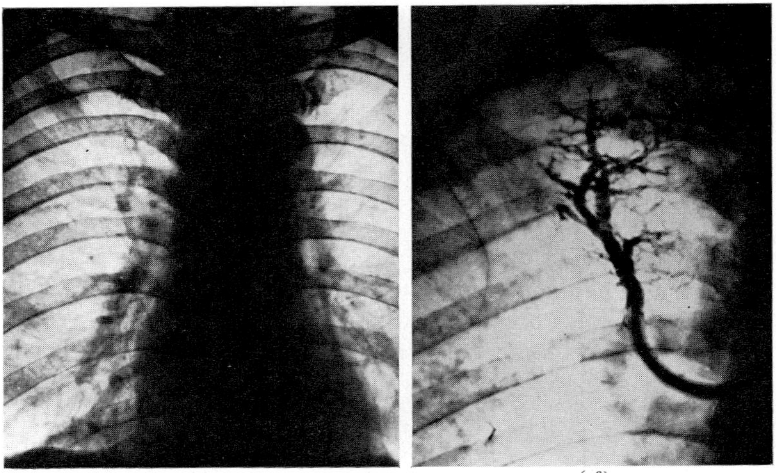

(e) (f)

Figure 4. Case 3. A 54-year-old man who had no subjective complaints. (*a*) *In mass survey, a tumorous shadow was found in left infraclavicular region.* (*b*) *Selective bronchogram reveals obstruction at ninth ramification of B_{1+2}.* (*c and d*) *A malignant cell cluster was obtained by a brush, though insertion of the brush was insufficient. Immediately, lobectomy of left upper lobe was performed.* (*e*) *One and half years after the first operation, another tumorous shadow was found in mass survey in the right upper field.* (*f and g*) *This lesion was diagnosed as adenocarcinoma by TV brushing method.* (*h*) *Cut surface of resected scar cancer. This is very rare case which was accurately diagnosed pre-operatively twice and was completely cured by surgery*

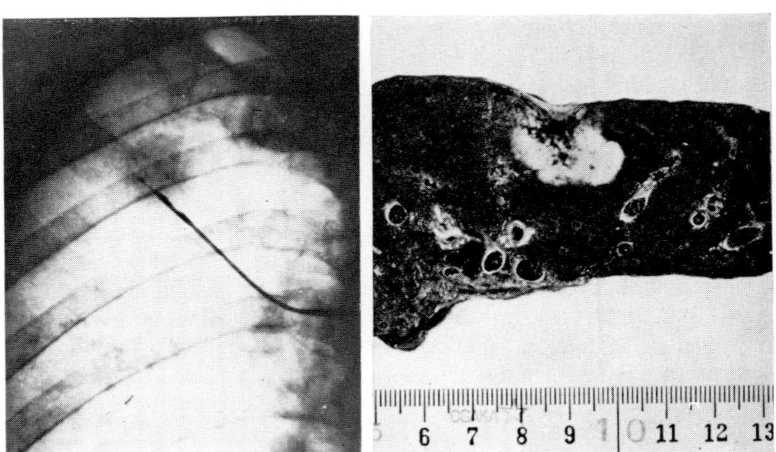

(g) (h)

The procedure, being neither tortuous nor time-consuming, can be performed easily on ambulatory patients without any hazards. Thus far, no side effect (haemoptysis, high fever or metastasis) has been experienced after TV brushing.

Suggestions for Obtaining Good Results

As described earlier, the obstructed area of the tumour-bearing bronchus must be determined by bronchography prior to TV brushing. It is recognized that bronchi well visualized in the bronchogram are as a rule devoid of malignancy and that TV brushing must be performed in the non-visualized branches.

Immediately after brushing, the material obtained must be smeared on glass slides and fixed at once with ether–ethanol solution. Air drying should be avoided.

In the cytological diagnosis of TV-brushed material from small peripheral lung cancers, morphological characteristics of malignancy such as hyperchromasia and irregularity in nuclear shape and thickness of nuclear border are not very remarkable when compared with sputum cytology, because such morphological changes of exfoliated cancer cells in the sputum are invariably exaggerated by the cellular degeneration in the bronchial airway. By the careful examination of fresh tumour cells obtained by TV brushing, a rather fine but unevenly distributed chromatin pattern, slight anisokaryosis and slight indentation of the nuclear membrane have been observed. Utmost care should therefore be exercised in the cytological diagnosis of TV-brushed material unless the tumour cells in question are observed as cell clusters.

When the material leads to a 'suspected' diagnosis, the procedure should be repeated one week later.

CONCLUSION

It is generally accepted that accurate diagnosis of small peripheral lung cancers (coin lesions less than 2·0 cm in diameter) has great value for early surgical treatment. However, cytological examination of the sputum or bronchial secretion has no value for early diagnosis of peripheral lung cancer, although it is very useful in detecting carcinoma *in situ* or early cancer of the major bronchus.

In order to overcome the difficulties of diagnosing small coin lesions in the lung periphery, the TV brushing method—selective bronchial brushing under x-ray television fluoroscopy—was introduced. This was performed on 383 cases suggestive of lung cancer, and positive cytological results were obtained in 142 out of 171 confirmed primary lung cancer cases and in 11 out of 17 metastatic lung cancer cases. TV brushing is a method of choice for accurate diagnosis of lung cancer, especially in its early stage.

REFERENCES

Attar, S., Naib, Z. M. and Cowley, R. A. (1961). 'Exfoliative cytology in solitary peripheral lesions of the lungs.' *J. thorac. cardiovasc. Surg.* **42,** 168.

Fennessy, J. J. (1966). 'Bronchial brushing in the diagnosis of peripheral lung lesions: a preliminary report.' *Am. J. Roentg.* **98,** 474.

— (1967). 'Transbronchial biopsy of peripheral lung lesions'. *Radiology* **88,** 878.

Fridel, H. (1961). *Die Katheterbiopsie des peripheren Lungenherdes.* Tuberculose Bibliothek No. 99. Leipzig: Barth.

Hattori, S., Matsuda, M., Sugiyama, T. and Matsuda, H. (1964). 'Cytologic diagnosis of early lung cancer: brushing method under x-ray television fluoroscopy.' *Dis. Chest* **45,** 129.

— — — Wada, A. and Terazawa, T. (1965a). 'Cytologic diagnosis of early lung cancer: an improved TV-brushing method and a review of negative results.' *Dis. Chest* **48,** 123.

— — — Terazawa, T. and Wada, A. (1965b). 'Some limitations of cytologic diagnosis of small peripheral lung cancers.' *Acta cytol.* **9,** 431.

Matsuda, H., Nagaoka, T., Takai, G. and Ninomiya, K. (1961). 'Medical applications of x-ray television.' *Am. J. Roentg.* **85,** 352.

— — Nakahori, T., Takai, G., Sohma, J., Nakai, A. and Ninomiya, K. (1963). 'X-ray examination with an improved x-ray television unit.' *Am. J. Roentg.* **89,** 432.

Motsch, H. (1962). 'Die morphologischen Befunde der Katheterbiopsie. Ein Beitrag zur Frühdiagnose des peripheren Bronchialkarzinoms.' *Münch. Med. Wschr.* **8,** 349.

Nolting, H. (1965). Personal communication.

Nordenström, B. and Carlens, E. (1965). 'Bronchial biopsy in connection with bronchography.' *Acta radiol.* **3,** 37.

Tateishi, R., Matsuda, M. and Hattori, S. (1970). 'Electron microscopic studies on giant cell carcinoma of the lung in reference to its histogenesis.' *A. Rep. Cent. Adult Dis., Osaka* **10,** 1.

Tsuboi, E. (1959). 'Studies on an early diagnosis of lung cancer—Especially cytological diagnosis of bronchial cells obtained by a direct scrape-off method.' *Nippon Acta radiol.* **19,** 133.

— Ikeda, S., Tajima, M., Shimosato, Y. and Ishikawa, S. (1967). 'Transbronchial biopsy smear for diagnosis of peripheral pulmonary carcinomas.' *Cancer, N.Y.* **20,** 687.

Umiker, W. O. (1961). 'The current role of exfoliative cytopathology in the routine diagnosis of bronchogenic carcinoma.' *Dis. Chest* **40,** 154.

III—The Value of Drill and Aspiration Biopsy

S. J. Steel

The growing public awareness of the dangers of cigarette smoking and the general availability of mass miniature radiography have increased the number of patients presenting with doubtful radiographic shadows. When the lesion is situated peripherally out of the range of bronchoscopic vision, sputum examination is inconclusive and there are no special indications for scalene node biopsy or mediastinoscopy, an attempt must be made to obtain histological material from the lung itself. This usually entails thoracotomy, and in those cases where there is a presumptive diagnosis of an operable bronchial carcinoma this is the logical course to follow. However, there are other patients likely to prove inoperable due to bilateral disease or to their age or general condition, and also those who present problems of differential diagnosis. In such cases the hazards of thoracotomy can usually be avoided by using one of the techniques of percutaneous biopsy.

PERCUTANEOUS LUNG BIOPSY

Liver and renal biopsy have now become standard medical practice, but although percutaneous lung biopsy was attempted as long ago as 1883, when Leyden aspirated organisms from a case of pneumonia, it is only comparatively recently that a satisfactory method has been evolved and has gained general acceptance.

The various methods of percutaneous biopsy can be divided into (1) aspiration biopsy, (2) biopsy with needles or punches incorporating a cutting mechanism, and (3) drill biopsy.

Aspiration Biopsy

Aspiration biopsy for cytological examination was described by Martin and Ellis (1930). Craver and Binkley (1939) performed aspiration biopsy in 92 cases of suspected primary cancer of the lung, but Ochsner, De Bakey and Dixon (1947) criticized this procedure, citing three cases in which tumour tissue had been implanted along the needle track. However, Lauby and colleagues (1965) found no clinical evidence of implantation after 648 biopsies in patients with pulmonary tumours and concluded that the theoretical danger was greatly exaggerated. Dahlgren and Nordenström (1966) improved the technique of aspiration biopsy, using image-intensified fluoroscopy to locate small isolated lesions, and reported that they found no instance of local spread or implantation of tumour tissue in their series of 900 biopsies. The only complications they encountered were pneumothorax in 15–20 per cent of the biopsies, blood-streaking of the sputum in some cases, local bleeding occasionally at the site of the biopsy, and one instance of pleurisy. One patient died of a coronary occlusion shortly after the biopsy, but this appeared fortuitous.

The limitation of aspiration biopsy is that it usually produces a very small quantity of tissue, sometimes only a few cells, which are most conveniently studied by making a smear preparation for cytological examination.

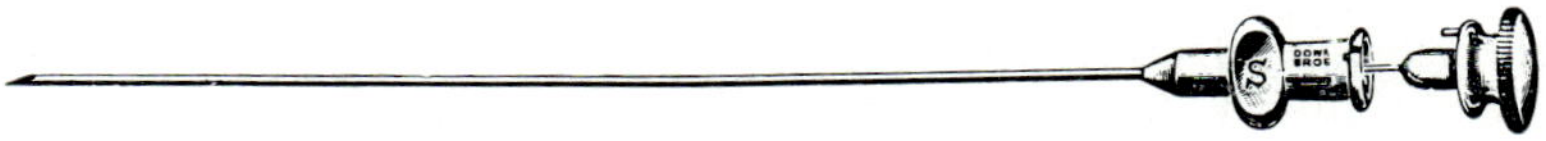

Figure 1. Aspiration biopsy needle. External diameter 1 mm (19 s.w.g.). The point is obliquely ground with sharp edges. The ground-in stylet is shown partly withdrawn. (Reproduced by courtesy of Down Bros. and Mayer & Phelps Ltd., London)

Aspiration Biopsy Technique

Apparatus (Figure 1)

This consists of an ordinary 10 ml syringe and a biopsy needle measuring about 1 mm in external diameter and sufficiently long to reach the tumour. The point is obliquely ground with sharp edges and the needle is fitted with a ground-in stylet.

Procedure

(1) The lesion is accurately located with radiographs and a marker placed over a suitable intercostal space. If the lesion is small, the biopsy can be performed under visual control with image-intensified fluoroscopy.

(2) The skin and tissue down to the parietal pleura are infiltrated with local anaesthetic, and premedication is not usually necessary.

(3) A small stab incision is made with a scalpel through the skin.

(4) The biopsy needle, with the stylet in position, is introduced and pushed into the tumour, which can usually be felt by the increased resistance as the needle enters it.

(5) While the patient holds his breath, the stylet is removed and the syringe is attached to the needle.

(6) Rotating movements are made to loosen tumour tissue, which is retained in the needle by continuous suction applied with the syringe.

(7) The suction is then gradually released and the needle withdrawn from the chest.

(8) The cell material is blown out on to a glass slide and a smear preparation is made.

Cutting Needle and Punch Biopsy

In order to obtain a larger specimen for histological examination, special needles incorporating a cutting mechanism have been used. Tripoli and Holland (1940) gave an account of lung biopsy with a Vim–Silverman needle in a patient with bronchial carcinoma, and Sarin and Bhatnagar (1959) used the same procedure in 9 patients. Manfredi and colleagues (1960) described experimental lung biopsy using this needle in dogs. Sabour and colleagues (1960) reported a series of 137 biopsies with the Vim–Silverman needle in patients of whom 113 were suffering from bronchial carcinoma. Complications were few, but included one severe haemoptysis and one case of surgical emphysema. A similar series which included cases of neoplasm and acute bacterial pneumonia was published by Avasthi, Chakravarty and Gupta (1962).

Manfredi, Rosenbaum and Behnke (1963) and Krumholz and Weg (1966), using the Franklin–Silverman needle, extended the technique to diffuse lesions, although the tissue obtained in such cases often consisted of fragments less than 2 mm in diameter. Krumholz and colleagues (1966) published their combined experience of 126 biopsies in which tissue was obtained in 86 per cent and contributed to the diagnosis in 66 per cent. Complications included pneumothorax 16·6 per cent, minor haemoptysis 30 per cent and 3 larger haemoptyses.

Smith (1964a) published a series of 61 patients who had needle biopsy of the lung, 39 with a Vim–Silverman and 22 with a Jack needle, which was a specially designed punch. In an addendum, further experience with the Jack needle was mentioned, but the incidence of pneumothorax was 41 per cent, and Smith (1964b) subsequently recorded a fatal pulmonary haemorrhage and recommended that the procedure should be performed in an operating theatre with a thoracic surgeon at hand.

Vim–Silverman or Franklin–Silverman Biopsy Technique

Apparatus (*Figure 2*)

The Vim–Silverman needle consists of an outer sheath with bevelled point, fitted with a ground-in stylet. A split hollow cutting needle fits inside the outer sheath so that the ends protrude and

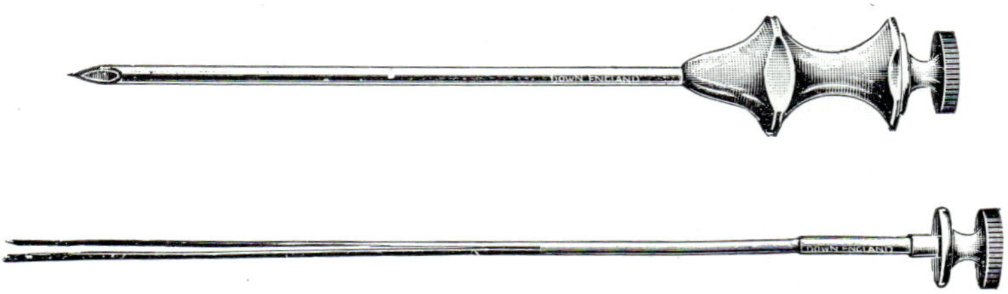

(*a*)

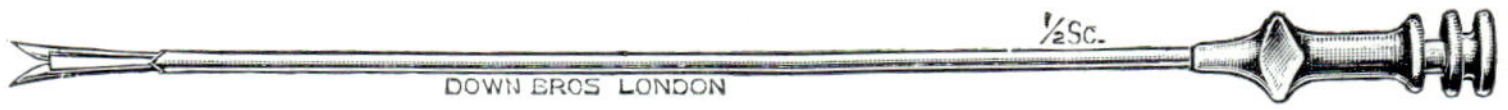

(*b*)

Figure 2. (*a*) *Vim–Silverman and* (*b*) *Franklin–Silverman needles. The latter differs in that the guttering of the split cutting needle is blocked at the tip.* (*Reproduced by courtesy of Down Bros. and Mayer & Phelps Ltd., London*)

separate when pushed fully home but close when withdrawn. The Franklin–Silverman needle differs in that the guttering of the split cutting needle is blocked at the tip to retain the specimen.

Procedure

(1), (2) and (3) The procedure is the same as for aspiration biopsy.

(4) The Silverman needle outer sheath, with the stylet in position, is introduced as far as the tumour.

(5) While the patient holds his breath, the stylet is replaced by the split cutting needle, which is pushed into the tumour.

(6) The outer sheath is then slid forward to compress the blades of the split needle.

(7) Both needles are rotated 180 degrees and withdrawn together.

(8) The biopsy material is removed from the split needle and placed in formol saline.

Drill Biopsy

Drill biopsy of various tissues, using an electric dental drill and cylindrical rotating cutting needle, was described by Kirschner (1935). The method was modified by Christiansen (1940), and further results were reported by Ellis (1947). Morrison and Deeley (1955) introduced the high-speed air drill, and Deeley (1960) produced good biopsy specimens from peripheral lung tumours with a trephine of 1·5 mm bore. In order to obtain bigger specimens and extend the technique to diffuse pulmonary lesions, a larger trephine with special features was designed by the author, and a report of the first 100 biopsies of lung and pleura was published by Steel and Winstanley (1967).

Indications and Contra-indications

Indications include diffuse as well as localized lesions of the lung or pleura where a definitive diagnosis is needed for the purpose of treatment or prognosis. There are no specific contra-indications other than bullae, cysts or vascular tumours, but it is wise not to attempt biopsy in patients with a bleeding diathesis or with insufficient respiratory reserve to risk a pneumothorax. Some upper lobe lesions may prove inaccessible, and those adjacent to the mediastinum are best avoided.

Advantages

The procedure can be performed at the bedside under local anaesthesia without occupying operating theatre time, although thoracic surgical cover should be available. It is rapid and painless, and breath-holding is unnecessary. It can be repeated if an adequate specimen is not obtained.

Experimental Evidence

In order to find out whether drill biopsy caused dissemination of cancer, Burn, Deeley and Malakar (1968) carried out experimental biopsies from a series of solid Walker 256 tumours growing in the flanks of adult Wistar rats. Compared with a control series, they found no shortening of the length of survival and no increase in the incidence of circulating tumour cells, distant metastases or recurrent tumours after local excision.

The ideal biopsy must be large enough to include several alveoli and must not be torn, crushed or twisted. The high-speed air drill, rotating at 15,000 revolutions per minute, imparts a speed of 1·6 metres per second to the cutting edge of the trephine, which slices cleanly through the lung and cuts out a core of tissue approximately 2 mm in diameter and up to 30 mm long. This compares favourably with the average size of specimen obtained with the Franklin–Silverman or Jack needle.

Hausser (1965) asserted that the lung would wrap itself round a rotating needle and sustain damage, but this was not borne out in personal experiments with the high-speed air drill. In fact there is virtually no trauma to the specimen or to surrounding tissue.

Results

Recent results (Table 1) reported by Steel and Winstanley (1969) show that 111 out of 119 (93 per cent) consecutive lung biopsies were successful in producing specimens of lung tissue for histological

TABLE 1

Histological Analysis of 119 Consecutive Lung Biopsies

Histological findings	*Number of biopsies*
Adenocarcinoma	9
Squamous carcinoma	2
Alveolar cell carcinoma	3
Oat cell carcinoma	1
Undifferentiated carcinoma	5
Lymphangitis carcinomatosa	1
Lymphatic lymphoma	1
Lymphosarcoma	1
Organizing pneumonia	9
Tuberculosis	4
Sarcoidosis	12
Polyarteritis nodosa	3
Berylliosis	2
Asbestosis	4
Diffuse interstitial pulmonary fibrosis	18
Miscellaneous conditions, e.g. alveolar proteinosis, rheumatoid lung, idiopathic haemosiderosis, oil granuloma, bird-fancier's lung	26
Total diagnostically significant	101 (85%)
Normal lung—despite abnormal radiograph	10
Total successful biopsies	111 (93%)

examination from a variety of different conditions, and 101 (85 per cent) of these biopsies were diagnostically significant. The relatively high incidence of adenocarcinoma in this series is attributable to the peripheral situation of the tumours.

Complications

Complications were not serious. Pneumothorax, which occurred in 26 per cent of the lung biopsies, was usually shallow and asymptomatic, and only a quarter required insertion of an intercostal tube. Haemoptysis (12 per cent) consisted of transient staining, except for one instance when it amounted to 50 ml, and there was only one minor occurrence of local bleeding intrapleurally. No instance of air embolism or local spread of neoplasm or infection occurred.

Drill (Trephine) Biopsy Technique

Apparatus (*Figure 3*)

A small Desoutter air drill, easily held in the hand, is driven by compressed air from a cylinder fitted with a reducing valve. A speed of up to 15,000 revolutions per minute at a pressure of 100 pounds per square inch (7 kg/cm^2) is controlled by a trigger. The spindle of the drill is connected by a Luer fitting to a hollow trephine 7·5 cm long, 3 mm in external diameter and 2·1 mm in bore, with a right-angled smooth cutting edge. The trephine is rifled internally for 5 mm behind the cutting edge to guide the specimen into its lumen, and fitted with a sharp-pointed keyed stylet projecting 2·5 mm beyond the end.

The whistling noise produced by the air drill should be demonstrated beforehand to the patient. He should be instructed not to move, cough or breathe deeply during the drilling process, but breath-holding is not necessary.

The air drill is not sterilized and a no-touch technique is used at the bedside. The trephine is sterilized by autoclaving.

Procedure

(1), (2) and (3) The procedure is the same as for aspiration biopsy, except that a 1·5 cm skin incision is made to allow free rotation of the trephine.

(4) The trephine is flushed with 3·8 per cent sodium citrate to minimize clotting within the lumen, and about 5 ml of the citrate is left in a 20 ml syringe. Then, with the pointed stylet in position, the trephine is introduced just above the lower rib to avoid damage

to the intercostal bundle and, unless a specimen of pleura is required, the point is firmly pushed through the parietal pleura.

(5) The stylet is removed and the drill attached to the trephine, using the gloved thumb to prevent any outside air entering during this manoeuvre.

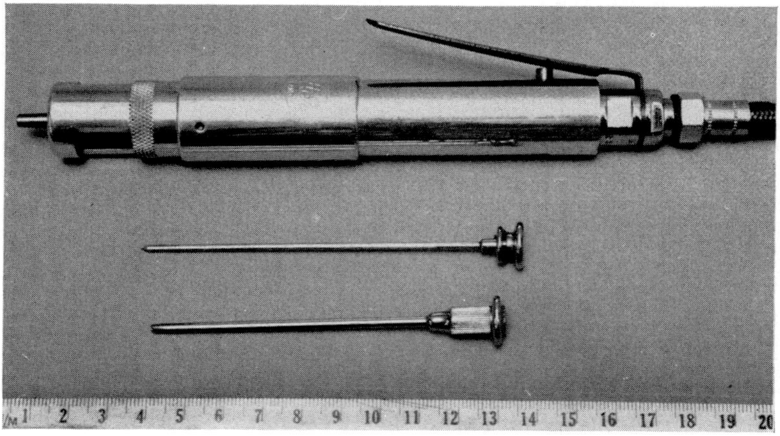

(*a*)

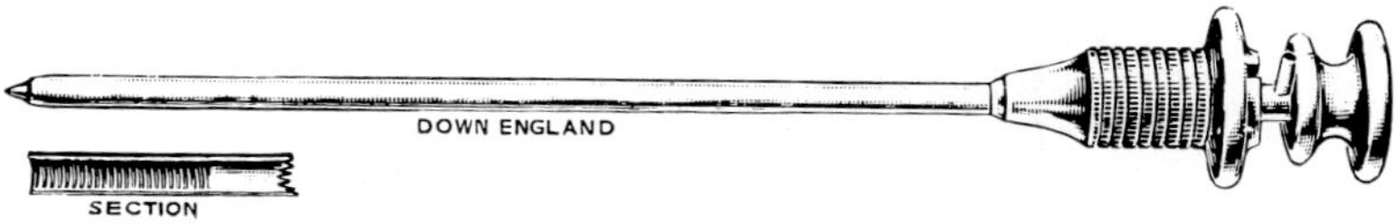

(*b*)

Figure 3. (*a*) *High-speed air drill, stylet and trephine.* (*b*) *Lung biopsy trephine in detail. Length 7·5 cm. External diameter 3 mm. Bore 2·1 mm. Internal rifling for 5 mm at the end. Sharp-pointed keyed stylet fitted.* (*Reproduced by courtesy of Down Bros. and Mayer & Phelps Ltd., London*)

(6) The patient is told to keep still. The trigger is pressed and the trephine, revolving at maximum speed, is steadily pushed into the tumour to an estimated depth of 2–3 cm; this should take about three seconds.

(7) The drill is detached from the trephine and replaced by the 20 ml syringe, which is used to provide suction to retain the specimen while the trephine is withdrawn.

(8) The specimen is ejected into filter paper in a funnel and the liquid allowed to run through before transferring it into fixative.

Illustrative Cases

Case 1. A 63-year-old salesman was recalled following mass miniature radiography. He was well and free from symptoms. He smoked 20 cigarettes a day. There were no abnormal physical signs. The chest radiograph (*Figure 4*) showed a rounded opacity in the left lower lobe and a mass at the left hilum. Lateral tomography showed a circumscribed 2 cm opacity lying posteriorly, and a hilar mass surrounding

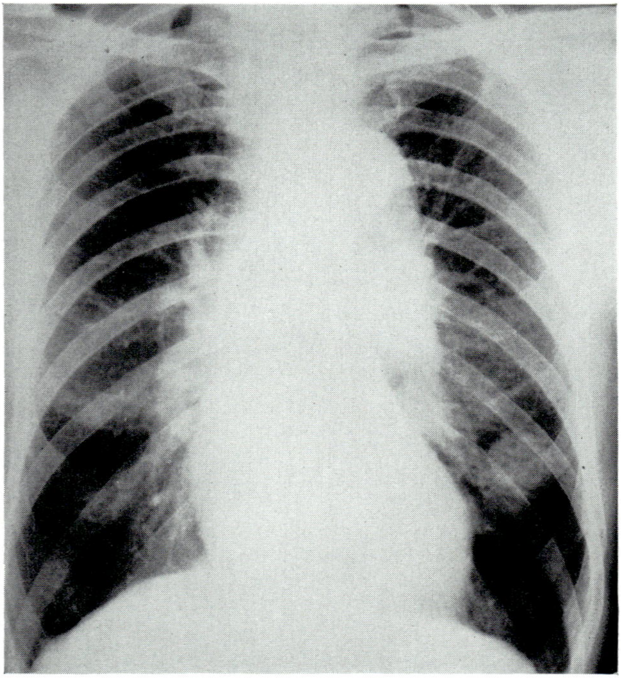

Figure 4. Case 1. Rounded opacity in left lower lobe and a mass at left hilum

the left pulmonary artery and narrowing the descending and apical bronchi of the left lower lobe. Bronchoscopy and sputum examination were negative. The appearances suggested an inoperable bronchial carcinoma, and it was considered that lung biopsy was indicated to confirm the diagnosis. Trephine biopsy of the left lower lobe opacity was performed under image-intensified fluoroscopic control and a specimen obtained (*Figure 5*). The histology showed the lung parenchyma to be invaded by oat cell carcinoma (*Figure 6*). A shallow pneumothorax resulting from the biopsy absorbed uneventfully and he was referred for treatment with radiotherapy.

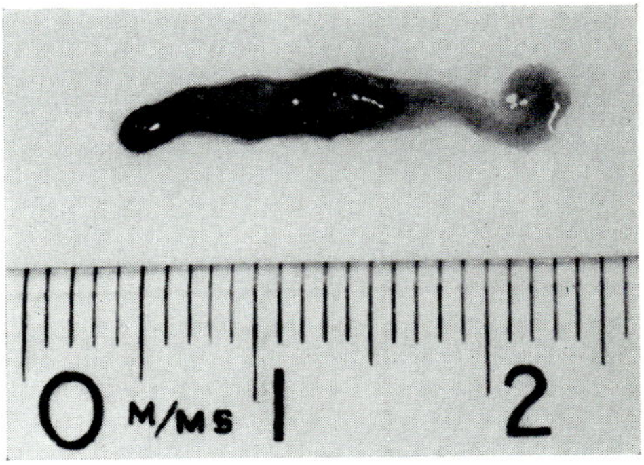

Figure 5. Case 1. Specimen obtained by trephine biopsy

Figure 6 (below). Case 1. Oat cell carcinoma (H and E × 107)

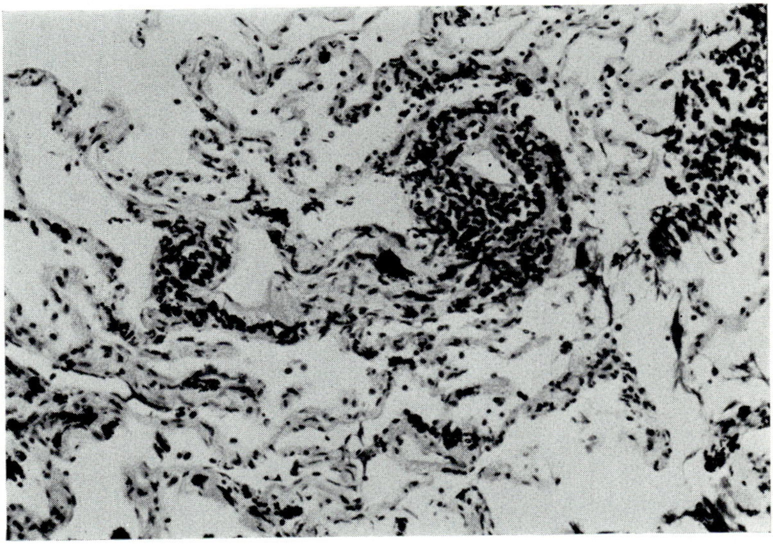

Case 2. A 53-year-old housewife had an upper respiratory infection followed two weeks later by cough, watery sputum and dyspnoea on exertion. She smoked 20 cigarettes a day. There were physical signs of bilateral basal pneumonia, which failed to respond to treatment with ampicillin. The chest radiograph (*Figure 7*) showed a dense opacity

in the region of the right middle lobe and confluent nodular shadowing in the lower two-thirds of both lungs. Sputum examination was negative. At bronchoscopy, frothy secretions were found in the bronchial tree but neoplastic cells were not identified. It was decided that lung biopsy

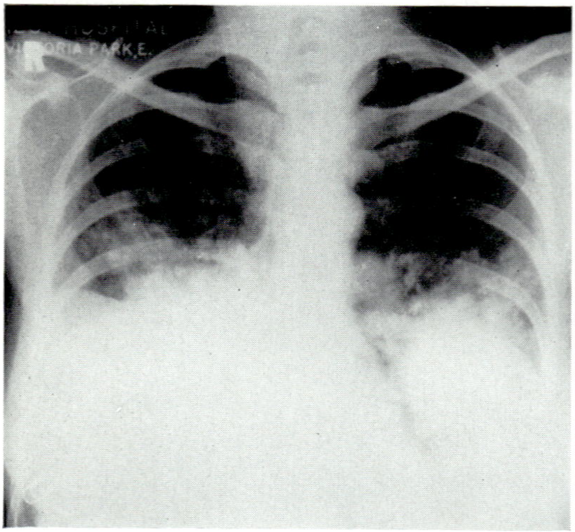

Figure 7. Case 2. Dense opacity in region of right middle lobe and confluent nodular shadowing in lower two-thirds of both lungs

Figure 8 (*below*). *Case 2. Alveolar cell carcinoma* (*H and E* × *107*)

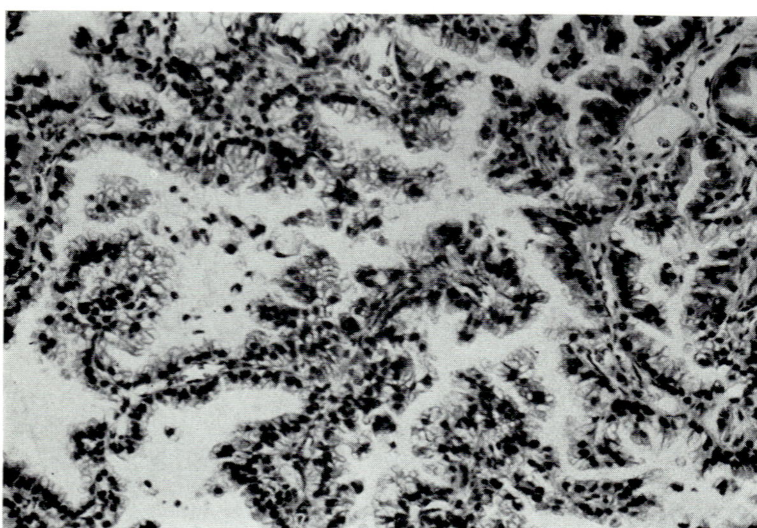

was indicated to establish a diagnosis. Trephine biopsy of the right lung was performed at the position indicated by a marker placed at the base. Histology showed the alveolar spaces lined by a layer of mucus-secreting columnar cells, the appearance being typical of alveolar cell carcinoma (*Figure 8*). Treatment was symptomatic and she died at home three months later.

PLEURAL BIOPSY

When the parietal pleura is thickened by neoplastic invasion or chronic inflammation, biopsy can be successfully performed with the Vim–Silverman or Franklin–Silverman needle or with the high-speed air drill and trephine. Steel and Winstanley (1969) reported that 18 out of 21 consecutive pleural trephine biopsies produced good specimens, including two adenocarcinomas, one oat cell carcinoma and one undifferentiated carcinoma.

However, when there is an effusion without much pleural thickening, the above techniques seldom produce a sufficiently large specimen of pleura and the Abrams punch gives better results. At the same time pleural fluid can be aspirated for cytological examination.

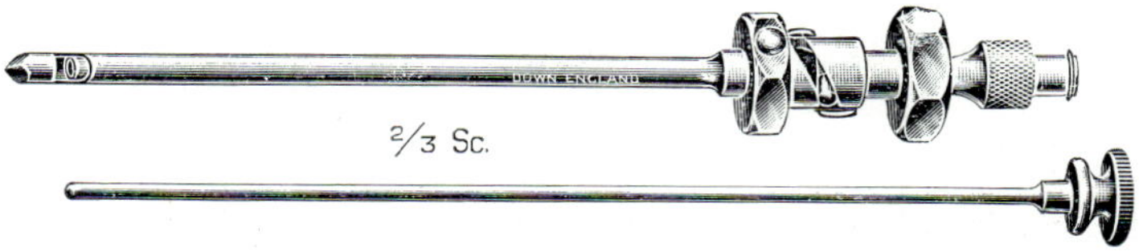

Figure 9. Abrams punch for pleural biopsy. The blunt stylet is used for clearing the lumen. (Reproduced by courtesy of Down Bros. and Mayer & Phelps Ltd., London)

Abrams Punch Technique

Apparatus (Figure 9)

The punch consists of two concentric tubes. Behind the point of the outer tube is a deep notch which can be closed by twisting the grip of the inner cutting cylinder clockwise along an oblique groove. This cuts off and retains any tissue engaged by the notch of the outer tube, the position of which is indicated by a knob on the mounting.

Procedure

(1), (2) and (3) The procedure is the same as for aspiration biopsy.
(4) The punch is introduced with the notch closed.

(5) A syringe large enough for aspiration is attached. The notch is opened by twisting the grip of the inner cylinder anti-clockwise and aspiration is carried out.

(6) The notch is directed along the intercostal space and the punch is slowly withdrawn, maintaining lateral pressure until the notch is felt to engage the parietal pleura.

(7) While holding the notch in position, the grip of the inner cylinder is twisted sharply clockwise and the punch is withdrawn.

(8) The tissue, which is found in the hollow point or in the end of the cutting cylinder, is placed in fixative.

CONCLUSIONS

Aspiration biopsy has a place when used in combination with image-intensified fluoroscopy for the location of small isolated pulmonary lesions. For the lung, cutting needle techniques are less effective than trephine biopsy with the high-speed air drill, which produces much larger specimens without increasing the risk of complications. Trephine biopsy or cutting needles are suitable for obtaining specimens from thickened pleura, but the Abrams punch is preferable when a pleural effusion is present.

REFERENCES

Avasthi, P. S., Chakravarty, S. N. and Gupta, S. P. (1962). 'Needle biopsy of the lung.' *J. Indian med. Ass.* **39,** 289.

Burn, J. I., Deeley, T. J. and Malakar, K. (1968). 'Drill biopsy and the dissemination of cancer.' *Br. J. Surg.* **55,** 628.

Christiansen, H. (1940). 'Aspiration trepan for tissue biopsy.' *Acta Radiol.* **21,** 349.

Craver, L. F. and Binkley, J. S. (1939). 'Aspiration biopsy of tumours of the lung.' *J. thorac. Surg.* **8,** 436.

Dahlgren, S. and Nordenström, B. (1966). *Transthoracic Needle Biopsy.* Stockholm: Almqvist & Wiksell.

Deeley, T. J. (1960). 'Drill biopsy results with a high-speed pneumatic drill.' *Acta Un. int. Cancr.* **16,** 338.

Ellis, F. (1947). 'Needle biopsy in the clinical diagnosis of tumours.' *Br. J. Surg.* **34,** 240.

Hausser, R. (1965). 'Über die diagnostische gezielte Gewebspunktion bei unklaren Lungen- Pleura- und Mediastinalprozessen.' *Dt. med. Wschr.* **90,** 1809.

Kirschner (1935). 'Die Probebohrung.' *Schweiz. med. Wschr.* **65,** 28.

Krumholz, R. A. and Weg, J. G. (1966). 'Percutaneous needle biopsy of the lung—a valuable diagnostic procedure.' *J. Am. med. Ass.* **195,** 38.

— Manfredi, F., Weg, J. G. and Rosenbaum, D. (1966). 'Needle biopsy of the lung.' *Ann. intern. Med.* **65,** 293.

REFERENCES

Lauby, V. W., Burnett, W. E., Rosemond, G. P. and Tyson, R. R. (1965). 'Value and risk of biopsy of pulmonary lesions by needle aspiration.' *J. thorac. cardiovasc. Surg.* **49,** 159.

Leyden (1883). 'Ueber infectiöse Pneumonie.' *Dt. med. Wschr.* **9,** 52.

Manfredi, F., Rosenbaum, D. and Behnke, R. H. (1963). 'Percutaneous needle biopsy of the lung in diffuse pulmonary diseases.' *Ann. intern. Med.* **58,** 773.

— Buckley, C. E. III, Patrick, R. L., Barry, W. F. and Sieker, H. O. (1960). 'Lung needle biopsy in the evaluation of diffuse pulmonary disease.' *Am. Rev. resp. Dis.* **82,** 800.

Martin, H. E. and Ellis, E. B. (1930). 'Biopsy by needle puncture and aspiration.' *Ann. Surg.* **92,** 169.

Morrison, R. and Deeley, T. J. (1955). 'Drill biopsy; a technique using a high-speed drill.' *J. Fac. Radiol.* **6,** 287.

Ochsner, A., De Bakey, M. and Dixon, J. L. (1947). 'Primary cancer of the lung.' *J. Am. med. Ass.* **135,** 321.

Sabour, M. S., Osman, L. M., LeGolvan, P. C. and Ishak, K. G. (1960). 'Needle biopsy of the lung.' *Lancet* **2,** 182.

Sarin, L. R. and Bhatnagar, L. (1959). 'Needle biopsy of the lung.' *Indian J. med. Sci.* **13,** 901.

Smith, W. G. (1964a). 'Needle biopsy of the lung.' *Thorax* **19,** 68.

— (1964b). Letter. *Lancet* **2,** 318.

Steel, S. J. and Winstanley, D. P. (1967). 'Trephine biopsy for diffuse lung lesions.' *Br. med. J.* **3,** 30.

— — (1969). 'Trephine biopsy of the lung and pleura.' *Thorax* **24,** 576.

Tripoli, C. J. and Holland, L. F. (1940). 'Carcinoma of lung; analysis of 195 cases with special note on needle puncture biopsy.' *Sth. med. J., Birmingham (Ala.)* **33,** 559.

M.R.C.B.—7

IV—Scalene Node Biopsy and Mediastinoscopy

H. C. Nohl-Oser

Many of the pathological processes inside the chest involve the lymph nodes, and this applies especially to malignant disease. The lymphatic drainage of the lungs passes from the broncho-pulmonary nodes to those in the hilum of the lung and from there mainly upwards to the tracheo-bronchial nodes. It then proceeds upwards to the scalene nodes via the paratracheal lymph nodes.

The description of the lymphatic pathways from the lungs is peculiarly sparse in the textbooks of anatomy, and the reader is referred for greater detail to the more recent work by Cordier, Papamiltiades and Cedard (1958), Nohl (1962), Baird (1965) and Maassen (1967).

There is still considerable controversy about the principal pathways from each lung to the superior mediastinum, especially whether the upward lymphatic spread from a carcinoma in the left lung occurs on the ipsilateral or the contralateral side. There is no doubt that contralateral spread does take place from either lung and that bilateral involvement is frequently seen in advanced cases. Maassen (1967), however, found on mediastinoscopic examination of 675 patients with bronchogenic carcinoma that contralateral spread rarely occurs from a primary in the right lung (9 per cent), while it happens frequently with lesions in the left lung (23 per cent), depending on the situation of the growth; thus the left lower lobe tumours show a greater tendency to contralateral spread (37 per cent) than those situated in the left upper lobe (22 per cent).

SCALENE NODE BIOPSY

Daniels (1949) showed that the lymph nodes enmeshed in the deep cervical pad of fat overlying the scalenus anterior muscle often reflected pathological changes inside the thorax, and that a biopsy of these nodes could be of considerable diagnostic value. Many papers on scalene node biopsy have since been written (Shefts, Terrill and Swindell, 1953; Connar, 1955; Nohl, 1958; Maloney and colleagues, 1964).

Operative Technique

The technique is well described by Connar (1955) and is carried out best under general anaesthesia. Through an incision 1·5 cm above and parallel to the inner third of the clavicle, an area bounded by the internal jugular vein medially, by the subclavian vein below, by the brachial plexus laterally and by the omohyoid muscle above is laid bare down to the scalenus anterior muscle by removing all fat and the enmeshed lymph nodes. The phrenic nerve crossing this muscle must be preserved.

The operation requires care and operative skill. Particular caution is needed in the presence of superior vena caval obstruction. Serious complications such as haemorrhage from the great veins, air embolism and injury to the thoracic duct are not unknown (Berger, Boyd and Strieder, 1963). The percentage of positive results depends on the extent and thoroughness of the exploration (Maloney and colleagues, 1964).

Results

Experience indicates that a positive diagnosis can be made in approximately 30 per cent of cases, depending on the selection of patients. Thus the incidence of positive findings is very high in sarcoidosis, approaching 60–80 per cent (Carstensen, 1954; Scott, 1957), while the positive yield in bronchial carcinoma in the absence of palpable nodes is low. In 705 cases of bronchial carcinoma collected from the literature by Reynders (1963), 136 (19·3 per cent) had a positive biopsy when nodes were impalpable. Harken and colleagues (1954) therefore suggested an extension of the procedure which they termed cervico-mediastinal exploration, in which the upper mediastinum is explored through Daniel's incision with a laryngoscope. By this means they obtained a positive biopsy in the cervical or mediastinal nodes in 31 out of 78 cases of bronchogenic carcinoma (39·8 per cent). In view of the uncertainty of the lymphatic drainage and the occurrence of contralateral spread, one of the disadvantages of this procedure, in the absence of palpable nodes, is that it is a unilateral exploration. Denk and Wurnig (1957) therefore carried out bilateral scalene node biopsy in 100 patients without palpable nodes and yet obtained a positive result in only 5 cases.

The limitations of scalene node biopsy have further been expressed by Morgan and Scott (1962), who state: 'In our experience, scalene fat pad biopsy revealed extrapulmonary extension in approximately 12 per cent of the cases of bronchogenic carcinoma, but a negative scalene fat pad biopsy did not indicate that the lesion was resectable . . . The indications for scalene node biopsy are palpable supraclavicular lymph nodes, bronchogenic carcinoma, diagnosed or suspected and clinically suspected sarcoidosis. In those patients not meeting the above criteria for scalene node biopsy, there was an incidence of positive nodes of only 1 per cent.'

MEDIASTINOSCOPY

Carlens (1959) described the method of mediastinoscopy. The technique is the logical sequel to scalene node biopsy and is in many respects easier to perform. It has, in the author's opinion, completely superseded scalene node biopsy in all patients with impalpable nodes. The operation is carried out under general anaesthesia.

Operative Technique

A 5 cm incision is made in the suprasternal notch as for a low tracheostomy. The dissection is carried down to the pretracheal fascia, which is incised. With blunt finger dissection a tunnel is made downwards into the mediastinum, keeping the dorsum of the finger all the time in contact with the anterior surface of the trachea. The plane of dissection is depicted by an arrow in the diagram (*Figure 1*) and lies behind the large vessels in the superior mediastinum. Consequently anterior mediastinal tumours are not really accessible by this method.

The origin of each main bronchus can be palpated by feeling for the superior tracheo-bronchial angle. The following lymph node stations can be reached: the right and left paratracheal nodes alongside the trachea, the right superior tracheo-bronchial nodes lying in close relation to the arch of the vena azygos, the left superior tracheo-bronchial nodes under the arch of the aorta, and finally the inferior tracheo-bronchial nodes at the bifurcation of the trachea.

Much information can be obtained by this palpation alone. The mobility or fixity of the tissues can be assessed, and carcinomatous involvement of the bronchus at its origin by peribronchial lymphatic spread can be discovered. It has also been valuable in the pre-operative assessment of Pancoast tumours, since invasion of the vertebrae can readily be appreciated by palpation. The next step, breaking gently with the palpating finger through the pretracheal fascia lower down, precedes the introduction of a laryngoscope into the prepared tunnel. The lymph nodes lie outside this layer of fascia. Sometimes a whole node can safely be removed with crocodile dissecting forceps, while at other times only a small biopsy is possible.

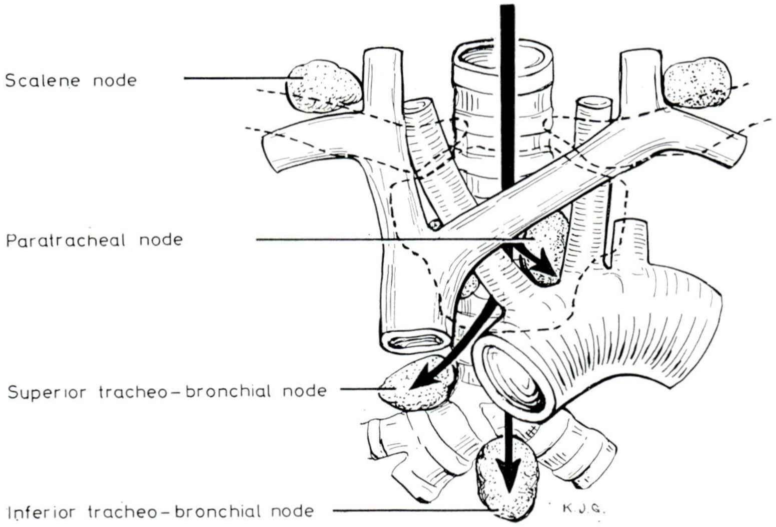

Figure 1

Complications

Table 1 indicates the complications which have been encountered in three large series of mediastinoscopic examinations. In the author's series, major haemorrhage occurred on three occasions in the first 35 cases and required thoracotomy after packing the mediastinum. One of these patients died. The risk of haemorrhage in this procedure cannot be denied, but in all three instances considerable traction was used while taking the biopsy, and this is now carefully avoided. In Maassen's series the mortality was 0·19 per cent, while the author records a mortality of 0·25 per cent in 400 mediastinoscopies.

Indications

The value of this diagnostic procedure is manifold. Table 2 gives the diagnosis in the 400 patients subjected to this examination. Its special merit lies chiefly in the investigation of any case of mediastinal lymphadenopathy.

Results

Table 3 gives the results of the investigation of 300 cases of bronchogenic carcinoma by the author.

The following observations are worth recording. The mediastinal nodes showed invasion in 43·3 per cent of all cases: the lowest rate of invasion (32·4 per cent) was shown by the squamous cell growths, while mediastinal involvement could be demonstrated in 66 per cent of the oat cell variety. These figures conform very much with an earlier observation by the author (Nohl, 1962), when 211 surgical

TABLE 1

Complications of Mediastinoscopy Encountered in Three Series

Complication	*Reynders (1963): 164 mediastinoscopies*	*Maassen (1967): 1,625 mediastinoscopies*	*Nohl-Oser: 400 mediastinoscopies*
Major haemorrhage	2	6	3
Recurrent laryngeal palsy	3	3	3
Pneumothorax	1	—	—
Metastases in scar	1	—	1
Wound infection or mediastinitis	2	2	—

TABLE 2

Diagnosis and Positive Results in 400 Patients Subjected to Mediastinoscopy

Diagnosis	*Number of patients*	*Positive mediastinal biopsy*
Primary bronchogenic carcinoma	296	126
Secondary extrathoracic carcinoma (breast, prostate, etc.)	9	4
Carcinoid tumour of bronchus	1	—
Intrathoracic malignant tumours of non-pulmonary origin	11	1
Sarcoidosis (clinically suspected)	31	24
Hodgkin's disease	12	10
Tuberculous lymphadenopathy	14	9
Inflammatory and infective conditions of lung	13	—
Miscellaneous (silicosis, cysts, etc.)	13	2
Total	400	176

specimens were examined for lymph node invasion. The other significant result from the mediastinoscopy series is that in 63 cases this investigation was the only means by which histological evidence could be obtained.

It has been the author's practice for the last three years to carry out a mediastinoscopy as part of the pre-operative assessment in all cases of bronchogenic carcinoma, because the earlier investigations (Nohl, 1962) had shown that the four-year survival of patients with

TABLE 3

Results of Mediastinoscopy in 300 Cases of Bronchogenic Carcinoma

Diagnosis	*Number of patients*	*Mediastinal and bronchial biopsy both positive*	*Mediastinal biopsy only positive*	*Bronchial biopsy only positive*	*Mediastinal and bronchial biopsy both negative*	*Percentage of positive mediastinal biopsies*
Squamous cell carcinoma	145	27	20	67	31	32·4
Adeno-carcinoma	29	3	13	3	10	55
Oat cell carcinoma	90	34	26	22	8	66
Undifferen-tiated carcinoma	17	3	4	6	4	41
Unidentified histology	19	—	—	—	19	—
Total	300	67	63	98	72	43·3

mediastinal lymph node invasion following surgery was only 9·7 per cent after an initial operative mortality of 10·4 per cent. No patient with mediastinal lymph node invasion has since been subjected to surgery. Of the 300 patients with bronchial carcinoma, 120 with negative mediastinoscopy findings were submitted after taking all factors concerning operability into account—for example, general condition and respiratory reserve—to thoracotomy. In only 7 cases was it found impossible to resect the tumour. It is noteworthy that mediastinal node involvement was found in only 9 instances in the resected cases. The other outcome of this policy has therefore been a considerable reduction in the number of patients in whom resection is not possible at thoracotomy. Reynders (1963), in a review of the literature, described the range of non-resectability to be between 20 and 50 per cent, with an associated operative mortality of 7–16 per cent. Since the introduction of mediastinoscopy, the author's non-resectability rate has been reduced to 6 per cent (7 out of 120).

The majority of patients with mediastinal node involvement were referred to the radiotherapist.

SUMMARY

Scalene node biopsy is indicated only in the presence of palpable nodes. In other cases it has been superseded by mediastinoscopy. The advantages of the latter method over the former are as follows:

(1) Both sides of the mediastinum can be explored through the same incision.

(2) Biopsies can be obtained from lymph nodes much nearer to the lung root. Hence the positive diagnostic yield is very much higher.

(3) Mediastinoscopy gives a definite indication of resectability in cases of bronchogenic carcinoma; scalene node biopsy does not.

REFERENCES

Baird, J. A. (1965). 'The pathways of lymphatic spread of carcinoma of the lung.' *Br. J. Surg.* **52,** 868.

Berger, R. L., Boyd, T. F. and Strieder, J. W. (1963). 'Complications of scalene lymph node biopsy.' *J. thorac. cardiovasc. Surg.* **45,** 307.

Carlens, E. (1959). 'Mediastinoscopy: a method for inspection and tissue biopsy in the superior mediastinum.' *Dis. Chest* **36,** 343.

Carstensen, B. (1954). 'Experiences with retroclavian lymph node biopsy in the diagnosis of certain intrathoracic diseases.' *Dis. Chest* **25,** 443.

Connar, R. G. (1955). 'Prescalene and deep cervical lymph node biopsy.' *Surgery Gynec. Obstet.* **101,** 733.

Cordier, G., Papamiltiades, M. and Cedard, C. (1958). 'Les lymphatiques des bronches et des segments pulmonaires.' *Bronches* **8,** 8.

Daniels, A. C. (1949). 'A method of biopsy useful in diagnosing certain intrathoracic diseases.' *Dis. Chest* **16,** 360.

Denk, H. and Wurnig, P. (1957). 'Die supraklavikuläre Probeexcision der Lymphdrüsen der oberen Thoraxapertur zur Feststellung der Operäbilitat des Bronchus Karzinoms.' *Thoraxchirurgie* **4,** 504.

Harken, D. E., Black, H., Clauss, R. and Farrand, R. E. (1954). 'A simple cervicomediastinal exploration for tissue diagnosis of intrathoracic disease.' *New Engl. J. Med.* **251,** 1041.

Maassen, W. (1967). 'Ergebnisse und Bedeutung der Mediastinoskopie und anderer thoraxbioptischer Verfahren.' In *Die Tuberkulose und ihre Grenzgebiete in Einzeldarstellungen*, Vol. 19. Berlin, Heidelberg, New York: Springer.

Maloney, J. V., Franks, R., Makoff, D. and Sherman, P. H. (1964). 'Biopsy of the scalene lymph nodes and the right thoracic duct lymph node for the diagnosis of pulmonary disease.' *J. thorac. cardiovasc. Surg.* **47,** 438.

Morgan, W. S. and Scott, S. M. (1962). 'A critical reappraisal of scalene fat pad biopsies.' *J. thorac. cardiovasc. Surg.* **43,** 548.

REFERENCES

Nohl, H. C. (1958). 'The value of scalene node biopsy in intrathoracic disease.' *Br. J. Tuberc. Dis. Chest* **52,** 286.

— (1962). *The Spread of Carçinoma of the Bronchus.* London: Lloyd-Luke.

Reynders, H. (1963). *Mediastinoscopie.* Academisch Proefschrift, Universitat Amsterdam.

Scott, S. M. (1957). 'A critical review of one hundred and sixty consecutive scalene node biopsies.' *Am. Rev. Tuberc. pulm. Dis.* **76,** 1002.

Shefts, L. M., Terrill, A. A. and Swindell, H. (1953). 'Scalene node biopsy.' *Am. Rev. Tuberc. pulm. Dis.* **68,** 505.

5—*Diagnostic Radiology in Localization of Lung Cancer*

G. Simon

In lung cancer, exact localization of the neoplasm is obviously of value to the radiotherapist, and it would appear that diagnostic radiology can often help in this respect

In *Figures 1* and *2* a circular shadow, roughly 8 cm, is seen on the left side anteriorly. Although bronchoscopy was negative, the presence of oat cells in the sputum would justify the assumption that the shadow defined a neoplasm.

DEFINING SITE AND EXTENT OF NEOPLASM

Unfortunately there are numerous pitfalls in trying to define the anatomical site and the extent of the tumour from the x-ray shadows.

Anatomical Site

If the growth is large as in *Figures 1* and *2*, the spatial and to some extent the anatomical site will be well enough defined by routine anterior and lateral view radiographs. If, however, the neoplasm is only 1–2 cm in size and a relatively small therapy field is contemplated, some care may be needed with the x-ray technique.

It is probably wise in such a case to take the radiographs with the patient in the position in which he will lie when the radiotherapy is given. This usually means that he should be supine with a pillow under his head. The shadow can then be localized in relation to the ribs, to its distance from the midline and to its depth below the sternum in the lateral view. Localizing radiographs are best taken during quiet respiration and not in full inspiration as is usually done. If the patient has a moderate kyphosis, special care must be taken to position him in regard to any lateral rotation which he may assume in order to lie comfortably.

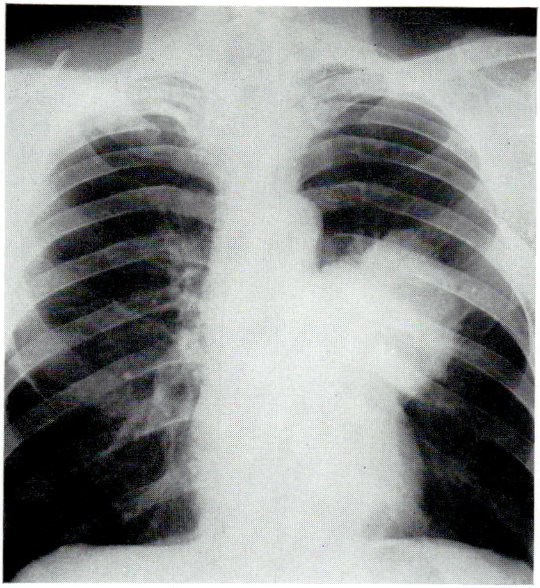

Figure 1 (above). Squamous carcinoma, size 8 cm, in left upper lobe. Male aged 51 years. Pain in left chest. Lobectomy

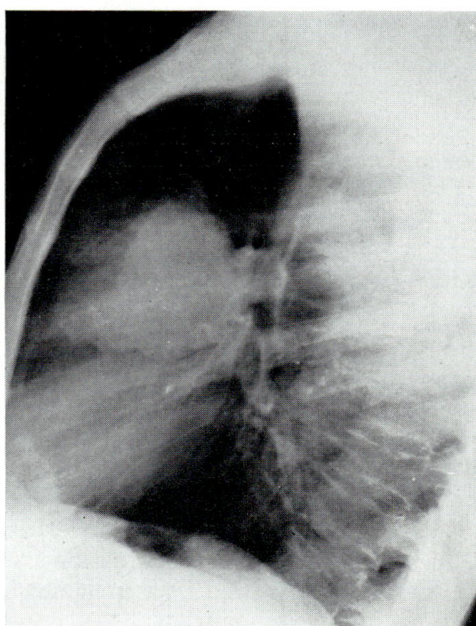

Figure 2 (right). Same case as in Figure 1 to show depth of lesion in lateral view

If the neoplasm involves a main or lobar bronchus and is visible only on bronchoscopy and not in the plain radiographs, its position beneath a chest wall marker or rib can be fixed if the proximal large bronchi are shown in a high penetration radiograph or in a tomogram (*Figure 3*). In the latter case a multisection box can be used in which the tomograms are all in the same plane, and the rib layer can be superimposed on the layer showing the main bronchi and the tumour. If a small arc of swing is used so that the layer of visible shadows is relatively thick, this will aid identification of the appropriate structures.

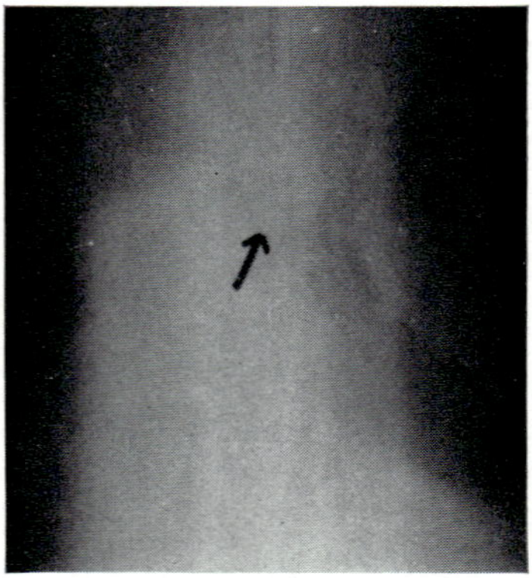

Figure 3. Tomogram showing defects in both main bronchi. Plain radiograph was normal. Oat cell carcinoma. Bronchial biopsy

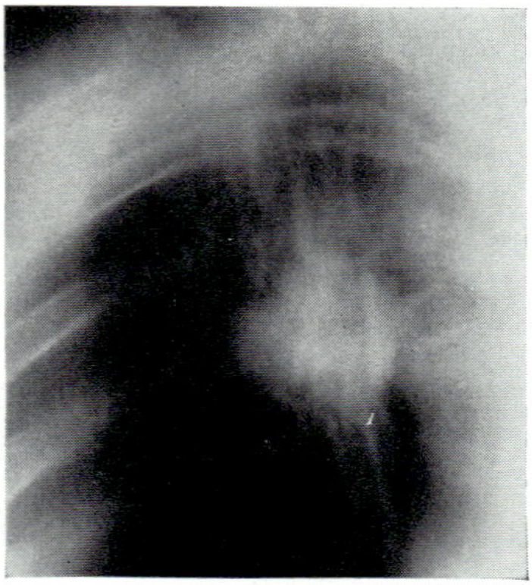

Figure 4. Shadow, 2 cm, with line shadows radiating from it. Squamous carcinoma

Limitations of Radiograph in Assessing Extent of Lesion

It is very uncommon to see a primary neoplasm smaller than 1·5 cm or an isolated secondary deposit smaller than 8 mm. This is partly due to the relatively large size of the focal spot of the x-ray tube, the 2 mm focal spot being in common use. It is thus apparent that small satellite neoplastic masses near the main shadow will often not be detected, nor will lymphatic or other lines of permeation be seen unless they are gross.

Figure 4 shows numerous line shadows radiating from a large tumour. Pathological examination has revealed many mechanisms causing these line shadows. In some cases neoplastic cells were seen permeating a lymphatic, while in others they were blocking it and causing perilymphatic fibrosis. In yet other cases the lines were identified as neoplastic cells growing along arteries, veins, connective tissue septa, or even smaller bronchi. Finally, any of these structures may be blocked by the main mass of the neoplasm, and their distension or reaction to the occlusion may be the cause of the line. Often several causes are found in one specimen, and when the line is due to local spread of the cancer cells, only the grosser lesions will result in a radiologically visible line shadow, while spread with a smaller volume of cells or a less intense fibrotic reaction or local small bronchus distension may be invisible in the radiograph.

Another difficulty arises when the neoplasm gives rise to a reaction in the lung distal to it which may also be the cause of a shadow and the extent of the neoplasm may thus be over-estimated. Quite a small tumour in a lobar or segmental bronchus near the hilum may occlude a bronchus or a vessel either partially or completely, and thus result in a lesion in the lung distal to it which will not contain neoplastic tissue but which nevertheless may cast a shadow in the radiograph.

Four types of lung lesion may be found in this situation, and the radiological features may indicate in many cases which is the predominant abnormality.

Atelectasis

Occlusion of a lobar bronchus by the neoplasm commonly results in atelectasis of the lobe distal to it. In *Figure 5* a large shadow is seen. The neoplasm of the upper lobe bronchus lay near the hilum and was no more than 1·5 cm. The larger part of the shadow was the atelectatic lobe, with oedema and mucus-distended bronchi and some pre-existing chronic pneumonia. Quite a small therapy field directed on the upper lobe bronchus would suffice in many such cases. In the example shown, the radiotherapy relieved the obstruction, and the lobe became re-aerated and the radiograph normal (*Figure 6*). The patient died from a cerebral metastasis and at autopsy there was no evidence of any residual neoplasm in the thorax.

In the case of an atelectatic lobe, a high penetration film or a tomogram (*see Figure 8*) is often useful to show at least the position of the lobar bronchus and thus the proximal extent of the neoplasm.

If atelectasis occurs without pre-existing inflammation, the lobe will shrink to a very small size, but if there is much distal pneumonia before the bronchial occlusion becomes complete, this will to some extent prevent great shrinkage of the lobe as in *Figure 5*. Occasionally the neoplasm itself grows to a considerable size before causing

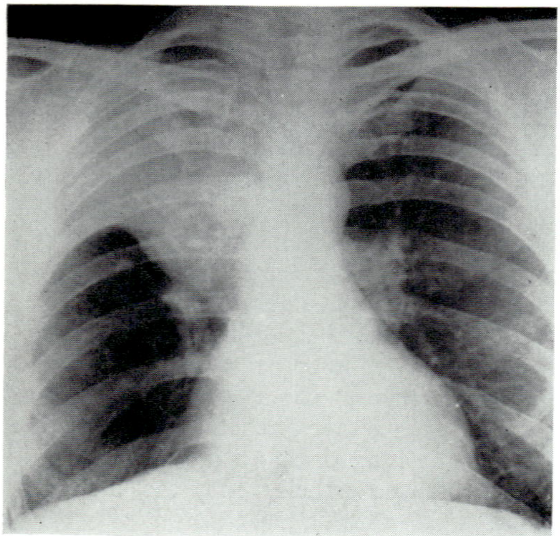

Figure 5. Shadow in right upper zone with concave inferior margin representing horizontal fissure elevated from shrinkage and atelectasis of right upper lobe due to oat cell carcinoma of upper lobe bronchus

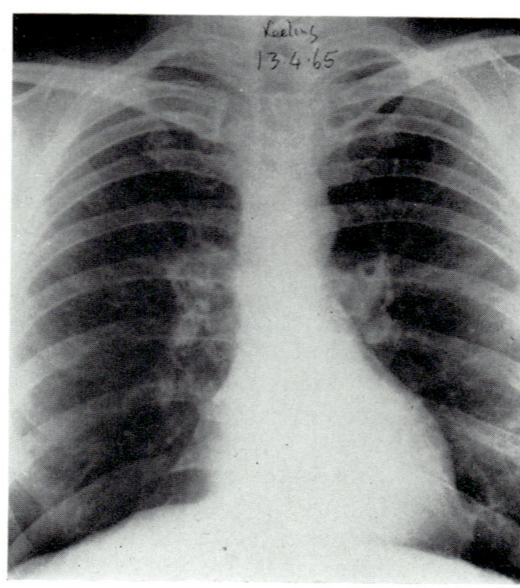

Figure 6. Same case as in Figure 5 after radiotherapy (5,000 rads). Right upper lobe re-aerated. Chest normal. Died from cerebral secondary. No intrathoracic neoplasm remained

collapse, and this will also result in an opaque lobe with comparatively little shrinkage. This course of events is in fact not very common and could well be ignored in planning the field size.

Inflammatory

Consolidation

Another common change is partial obstruction of a lobar bronchus with distal inflammatory changes in the lobe beyond. In *Figure 7*, the extensive patchy clouding towards the axilla was due to distal pneumonia, and again the neoplasm around the right upper lobe

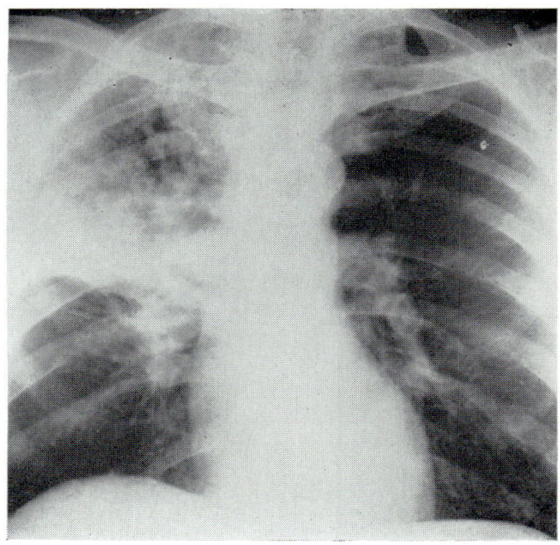

Figure 7. Shadows in right upper lobe due to inflammation distal to a 2 cm carcinoma narrowing the upper lobe bronchus. Confirmed on lobectomy

bronchus was quite small. The inflammation may progress to form a lung abscess. It is obviously necessary to try and determine whether the abscess is distal to a tumour, which will then be seen on bronchoscopy, or represents a breaking-down neoplasm, in which case it will not be seen on bronchoscopy although the presence of malignant cells in the sputum (if any) may indicate the diagnosis. The thickness or thinness of the cavity wall is not an accurate guide to solving this problem.

Distal Bronchiectasis

Tubular, band-like or ring shadows will suggest bronchiectasis, or if the lobe is also consolidated, only the central circular translucent zone within the ring may be visible (*Figure 8*). Such a bronchiectasis may be the result of partial occlusion of the lobar or segmental bronchus by a neoplasm. Again the therapy field should not include the bronchiectatic area.

Distal Vascular Lesions

In some 10 per cent of bronchial carcinomas there is an area of pulmonary infarction distal to the neoplasm. The shadow from this is frequently lost in that of the distal atelectasis or pneumonia, but sometimes it is the predominant shadow (*Figure 9*). Often it is roughly triangular and reaches the pleura, and if a small proximal shadow (of the carcinoma) can be seen, an infarct should be strongly suspected and the therapy field should avoid this area. The infarct may be due to a carcinoma of a lobar or segmental bronchus extending outward and pressing on the segmental artery or vein, or it may occur without any obvious local mechanical cause. An infarct may be seen even in a different lobe from the neoplasm, in which case the shadow of the infarct will be mistaken for a secondary deposit from the tumour or even for a second primary carcinoma.

Pleural Effusion

The presence of a pleural effusion will suggest that the neoplasm extends to involve the pleura, but sometimes this presumption is not correct, the effusion being secondary to distal inflammatory changes or to a distal infarct.

SECONDARY DEPOSITS

Glandular Secondary Deposits

Radiology has proved disappointing in the demonstration or exclusion of glandular secondary deposits of bronchial carcinoma. In fairness to the radiologists it must be said that the glandular deposits which are found at surgery and which cause such consternation are often only 1 cm or even less in size and thus would not be shown in the radiographs, but somewhat larger deposits also may pass undetected even in tomograms.

Hilar Gland Enlargement

Hilar gland enlargement can be detected in posterior view tomograms better than in the plain radiographs. Actually hilar glands more than 1 cm in size are not all that common in bronchial carcinoma.

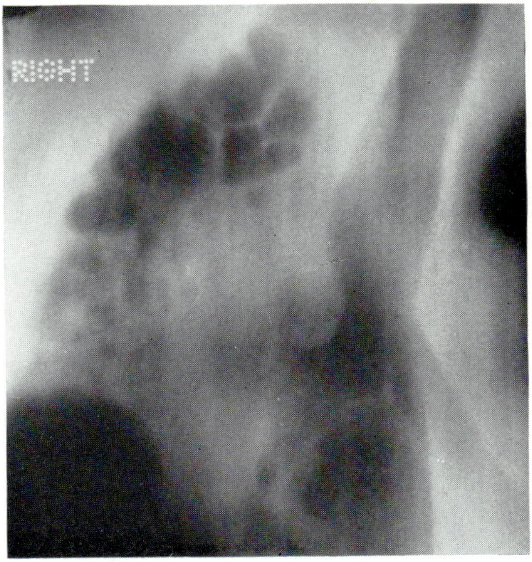

Figure 8. Translucent areas in opaque right upper lobe due to bronchiectases distal to occlusion of the bronchus seen in this tomogram and caused by a 2 cm carcinoma

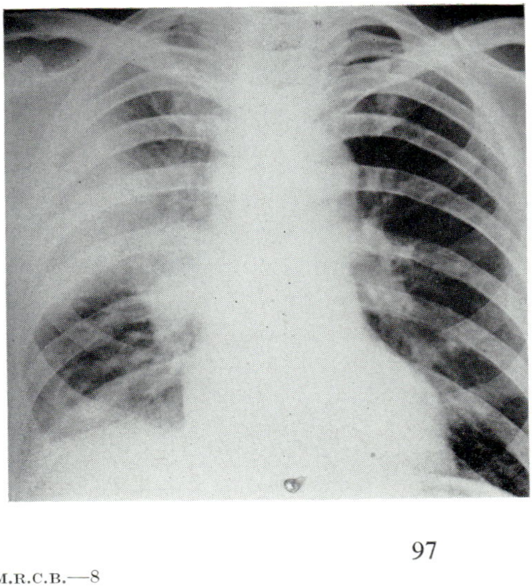

Figure 9. Shadow close to hilum is a squamous carcinoma of the anterior bronchus; large (8 × 7 cm) shadow reaching axilla is a distal infarct. Pneumonectomy

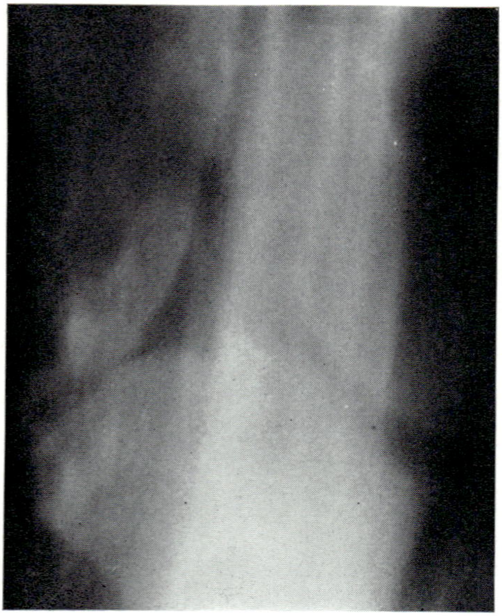

Figure 10. Tomogram showing narrowing of both main bronchi from a lower lobe carcinoma with enlarged subcarinal glands. Greatly improved on radiotherapy

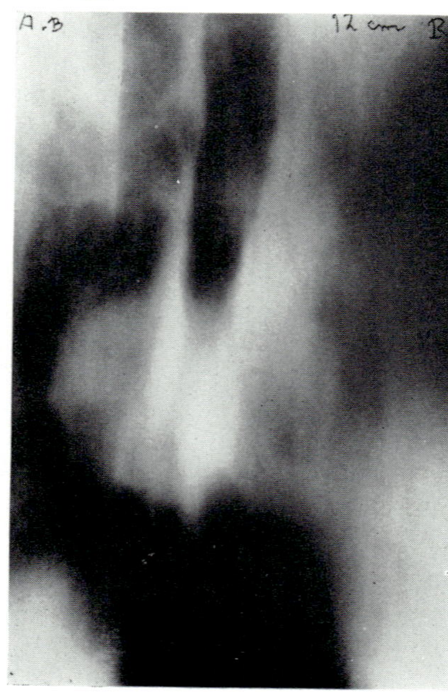

Figure 11. Oval shadow, 3 cm, below tracheal translucency is a large subcarinal gland. Lateral view tomogram near midline

Subcarinal Gland Enlargement

Enlargement of the subcarinal glands must be considerable before it can be detected in a radiograph. It is rarely seen in the plain film, but can be demonstrated in posterior view tomograms taken with sufficient exposure to outline the lower trachea and the main bronchi (*Figure 10*). It may cause splaying out of the carina, or it may indent the lumen of either or both main bronchi. Such changes

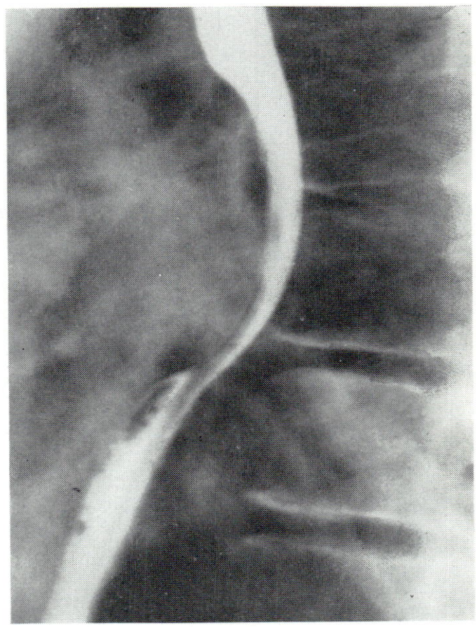

Figure 12. Narrowing and displacement of oesophagus by enlarged subcarinal gland. Left anterior oblique view

can of course be seen on bronchoscopy, but the tomograms are of value if the bronchoscopic findings are inconclusive or if, after the initial bronchoscopy, a subsequent examination is not considered kind to the patient. If the bronchial narrowing is gross, it may be wise to proceed with caution lest too rapid a dose gives rise to oedema leading to further narrowing and consequent respiratory obstruction. The lower extent of the glandular shadow may be shown in the posterior view tomograms or may be best seen in midline lateral view tomograms, when the shadow will be visible starting just below the tracheal translucency (*Figure 11*).

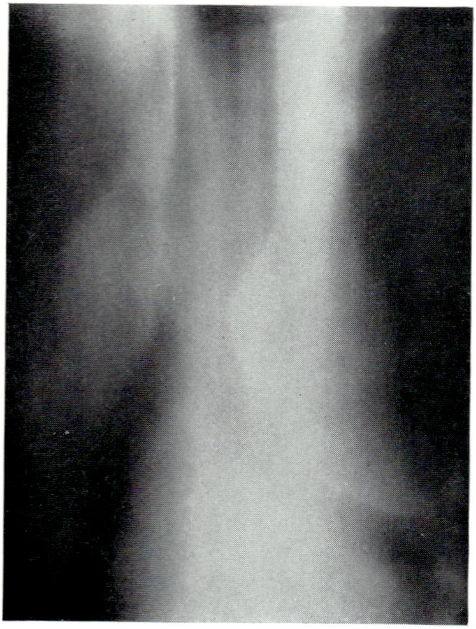

Figure 13. Enlarged paratracheal glands from secondary deposits. Oat cell carcinoma in right upper lobe. Large hilar gland below narrowed upper lobe bronchus and paratracheal gland above it

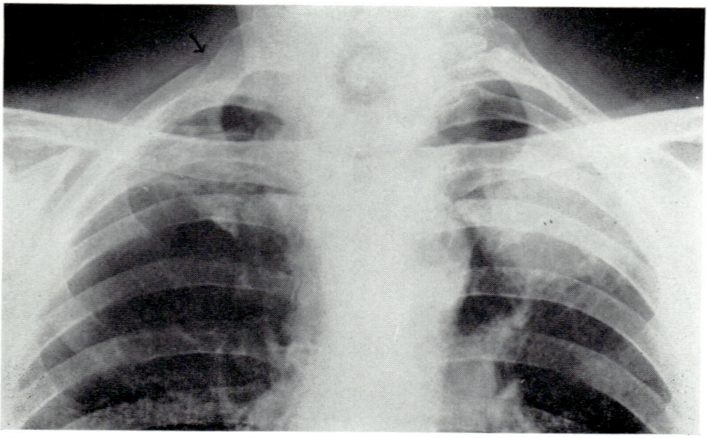

Figure 14. Carcinoma of left upper lobe. Secondary deposit in the right second rib

The evidence is inconclusive that glandular enlargement can be shown by transaxial tomography which cannot be demonstrated in the posterior and lateral view tomograms.

A barium swallow is sometimes useful, since large subcarinal glands may press on and indent the oesophagus. These are frequently best demonstrated in a left anterior oblique view with only about 20 degrees rotation (*Figure 12*). In cases of bronchial carcinoma considered sufficiently confined for surgery, the routine use of a barium swallow is not very profitable, but in late cases such as those often referred for radiotherapy it might be used with advantage as a routine.

In a large right lower lobe neoplasm, oesophageal displacement may be of no significance since it may be caused by the primary neoplasm itself, which may be entirely in the lung and invading neither the pleura nor the pericardium.

Should subcarinal glands be demonstrated by any method, this may be an indication for taking the radiotherapy field low enough to include this region, which will unfortunately also include some of the heart.

Paratracheal Gland Enlargement

Paratracheal glandular enlargements can be seen only when they are gross and at least 2 cm in size. They can sometimes be shown in tomograms (*Figure 13*) even when they are not clearly visible in the plain radiographs, but may pass undetected by either method. Unfortunately thoracic lymphangiography has so far been impracticable. Pneumomediastinum and tomography can show retrosternal gland masses, but have been less helpful in the demonstration of paratracheal gland masses.

Other Secondary Deposits

A careful scrutiny of the chest radiograph may reveal abnormalities which may influence treatment. It may show shadows in the other lung suggestive of secondary deposits, although this is relatively uncommon. It may show rib erosions as in *Figure 14*, indicating a secondary deposit. This may modify the radiotherapeutic policy. For instance, a smaller dose may be given to the primary or, if pain is present from the rib lesion, radiotherapy may be concentrated on this with a view at least to pain relief.

BRONCHOGRAPHY

Bronchography has not been used to define the extent of the neoplasm, but in the absence of any noticeable distal shadow, the presence of a blocked bronchus with malignant cells in the sputum will indicate the site of the neoplasm which cannot be shown by any other means. This is a relatively rare finding, and in most cases of this nature the tumour is resected. If for some reason this is not done, then bronchography is the only way to localize the tumour for the radiotherapist.

ANGIOGRAPHY

Some authors (Amundsen and Sorensen, 1956; Dotter, Steinberg and Holman, 1950; Engelman and Higgins, 1969; Greenspan and Capps, 1963) recommend angiography almost as a routine to decide whether a bronchial carcinoma is operable or not, but this policy is not generally accepted in the United Kingdom. Of course distortion, encroachment on the lumen or blockage of arteries or veins may be found, but these are generally important only when they are seen in the proximal vessels in the hilum or deep in the mediastinum. Usually by the time such changes are present the disease is far advanced and this is obvious clinically, so that radical treatment is not considered. The comparative rarity of proximal vessel involvement in less advanced cases means doing a great many angiograms before finding a patient in whom the positive findings from this method will assist the radiotherapist. With the relatively limited resources in equipment and personnel, the investigation is not worth while as a routine. It may, however, be indicated in specific instances. One is when the neoplasm encroaches on a main pulmonary trunk sufficiently to cause a turbulent systolic murmur. Another is when a shadow is suspicious of mediastinal gland enlargement, but there is uncertainty. In *Figure 15* the displaced aorta indicates a mediastinal mass.

Finally there is an indication for venography in some cases of superior vena caval obstruction, particularly if the plain radiograph does not show a large shadow to account for it. A subclavian venogram is simple and painless and can be done with routine radiographic equipment. It may show the site of the obstruction, and if some filling to the right atrium can be obtained it will show any displacement of the vein and the degree of encroachment on the lumen, which in its turn will help to indicate the extent of the neoplasm (*Figure 16*) and thus aid the radiotherapist. Care should be taken to flush out the contrast medium with normal saline to avoid the risk of thrombosis, particularly if the obstruction is almost complete.

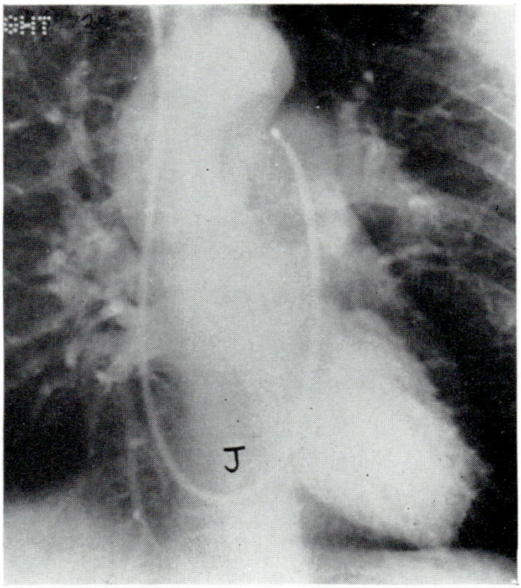

Figure 15 (above). Angiogram showing aorta displaced to the right. Displacement was by mediastinal secondary deposits from carcinoma of left lung

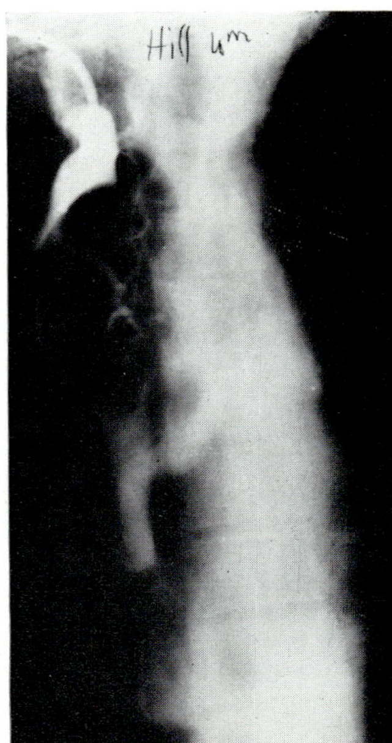

Figure 16 (right). Venogram showing obstruction of superior vena cava, which is also displaced to the right and shows an intraluminal mass due to a tumour

RESPONSE OF NEOPLASM TO RADIOTHERAPY

Disappearance of the shadow, whether it represents the neoplasm or a distal atelectasis, is a favourable sign. Shrinkage of the shadow of the neoplasm without total resolution of the shadow does not necessarily mean failure to kill the neoplastic cells. In *Figure 17* the residual shadow with a hazy margin and linear shadows radiating from it is the result of scarring from destruction of the neoplasm and of radiation damage to the lung nearby, and when the patient was examined at a later period, no residual neoplastic tissue was found in the thorax.

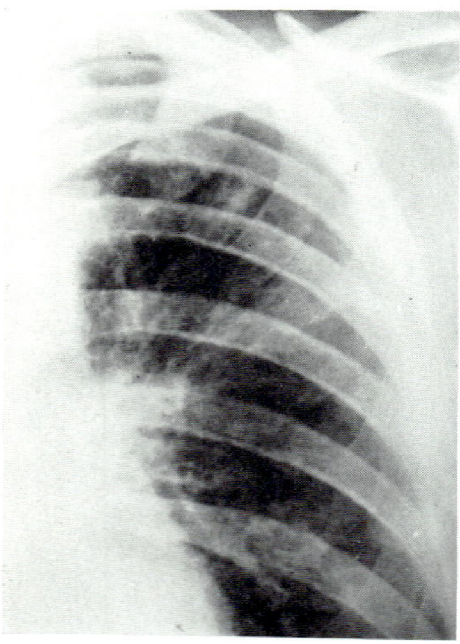

Figure 17. Carcinoma of left upper lobe after radiotherapy. Residual shadow is due to radiation damage and healing after eradication of tumour. No residual intrathoracic neoplasm seen on autopsy; cerebral secondary

REFERENCES

Amundsen, P. and Sorensen, E. (1956). *Acta radiol.* **45,** 185.

Dotter, C. T., Steinberg, I. and Holman, C. W. (1950). *Am. J. Roentg.* **64,** 222.

Engelman, R. M. and Higgins, G. A. (1969). *J. thorac. cardiovasc. Surg.* **57,** 356.

Greenspan, R. H. and Capps, J. H. (1963). *Radiol. Clin. N. Am.* **1,** 315.

Steinberg, I. and Finby, N. (1959). *Am. J. Roentg.* **81,** 807.

6—Bronchoscopic Examination

Peter Stradling

The bronchoscope has wide diagnostic and therapeutic uses, many of which are outside the scope of this volume. Here discussion will be restricted to those features of bronchoscopy relevant to bronchial carcinoma.

INDICATIONS

So much information may be obtained bronchoscopically in cases of bronchial carcinoma that this examination should be carried out in all patients who present with the slightest suspicion of the disease. The advantages of reaching a definitive diagnosis and of assessing suitability for thoracotomy or radiotherapy, both so often possible bronchoscopically, make the investigation imperative and justifiable in the overwhelming majority of patients; even negative findings can be of the utmost value in assessing treatment possibilities. With modern apparatus and anaesthetic techniques the procedure becomes remarkably safe and the patient must be gravely ill, or have quite gross reduction in his respiratory reserve, before bronchoscopy becomes dangerous. Clearly in the immediately hopeless case investigation would be both unkind and an impertinence. A similar argument applies to great age and frailty. Certain patients with advanced superior vena caval obstruction and urgently needing radiotherapy can, with advantage, have their bronchoscopy delayed until after treatment has started and there has been some subsidence of the neck swelling. Bronchoscopy before radiation in such circumstances can sometimes be troublesome due to post-operative laryngeal oedema or excessive bleeding when a biopsy is taken. Bronchoscopists would also be wise to hesitate in cases where aneurysm comes into the differential diagnosis; if there is real doubt, aortography should be performed before the investigation is undertaken.

Suspicion of bronchial carcinoma may be found in the history, the physical signs, the radiological picture, and the results of laboratory procedures such as sputum cytology or blood biochemistry. A history of heavy cigarette smoking must always add to the index of suspicion. Clinical pictures which should lead to further investigation, including bronchoscopy, are thus protean and manifold. A full discussion is beyond the scope of this book, but certain points are worth stressing; the bronchoscopist could often have helped earlier if pointers in the clinical picture had led to more prompt action.

Of particular importance are a change in cough habit, which is frequently missed in chronic bronchitics who may already have a long history of cough and sputum; onset and persistence of wheeze, particularly associated with a unilateral rhonchus which will not cough away or, if it does, always returns to the same place; a central aching pain in the chest which has been impossible to explain by other investigations, and persistent small haemoptyses. Such symptoms are potentially sinister even if no other sign or radiological change is present; it is not appreciated as often as it should be that a tumour can be present in a large airway without producing any physical signs or radiological change, but making its presence known by symptoms alone.

Any clinical picture suggesting bronchial obstruction should clearly lead to further investigation: elucidation of the cause at bronchoscopy is frequently possible. Particularly suggestive are repeated infections in the same pulmonary segment, and pneumonia that does not clear rapidly with antibiotic treatment.

Various other manifestations, if otherwise unexplained and even if lone signs, should all lead to bronchoscopy which may reveal a carcinoma as the primary source of the changes seen. Such signs are lymph node enlargement in the neck, axillae, mediastinum or pulmonary hila; vena caval obstruction; finger clubbing; neuromuscular dystrophies; certain changes in blood chemistry, and gynaecomastia.

Two conditions deserve special mention: pleural effusions and peripheral pulmonary shadows found radiologically. A pleural effusion is a common accompaniment of bronchial carcinoma and may be the presenting feature of the case; if an effusion is not clearly due to another cause, bronchoscopy is imperative. Patients with peripheral radiographic shadows are commonly considered not worth bronchoscoping because the causal lesions will not be seen bronchoscopically. This, however, is a specious argument, for much information can be obtained bronchoscopically without a view of the tumour itself: the segmental bronchus involved can be inspected for secondary invasion, secretions may be obtained for cytology and, furthermore, it may become evident that there is local node enlargement, indicating metastatic involvement which was not visible radiologically. Finally, negative findings are themselves of value in weighing up treatment alternatives.

It is thus clear that indications for bronchoscopy may be many and varied. A tumour may be discoverable in no other way, although giving a definite hint of its presence to those who are prepared to react to minor pointers in the history or the clinical examination. Bronchoscopy, in skilled hands and with the best anaesthesia, is a safe procedure and should be undertaken at the first suspicion of bronchial carcinoma.

TECHNIQUE

Modern ventilating bronchoscopes, and the light anaesthesia possible with a combination of intravenous barbiturates and muscle relaxant drugs, make general anaesthesia so safe that local analgesia need no longer be insisted upon to avoid hypoxaemia and CO_2 retention with their attendant risks of cardiac arrhythmias and arrest. Although it is still chosen by some operators, in my opinion it is doubtful whether local analgesia is any safer than general anaesthesia in skilled hands. It is certainly more unpleasant for the patient. It would seem reasonable to reserve this technique for physiological studies where spontaneous respiration is essential.

The advantages of modern apparatus, with its greater convenience and the excellent lighting possible, are very great. Now that glass fibre light guides are available to provide cold light at the tip of the bronchoscope sheath and within the telescope assembly itself, there is no excuse for the dim and unreliable lighting inherent in the use of the small tungsten filament lamps of older types of apparatus. Confident diagnosis is rarely possible without good lighting.

Although bronchoscopic technique can be learned only by experience in the theatre with the help of fully illustrated texts (Stradling, 1968), certain pointers to successful and safe diagnosis, together with a few practical points for those working with bronchoscopists, will not be out of place here.

The importance of the utmost gentleness in all manipulations must be stressed. The slightest misuse of the sucker tube, for instance, can lead to sufficient haemorrhage and mucosal blushing to preclude full appreciation of a lesion. The time provided by safe general anaesthesia, and the knowledge that the patient is insensible, both allow an unhurried, gentle technique not always otherwise possible.

Nevertheless, because slight trauma is inevitable and may confuse the issue, adherence to a strict sequential examination is of great importance: all bronchial orifices must be examined *seriatim* to the limit of visibility and of the apparatus available. Furthermore, both sides of the bronchial tree must be examined; most experienced bronchoscopists will have discovered the second, unexpected primary carcinoma or secondary node involvement on the contralateral side, which may completely alter the prognosis and the form of treatment chosen.

Recent chest radiographs, both postero-anterior and a lateral view on the side of the lesion, together with tomograms and bronchograms where appropriate, should be provided in the theatre for inspection before commencing the operation. The fuller the appreciation of the clinical and anatomical situation, particularly relating to pulmonary segmental distribution, the more complete will be the information obtained at bronchoscopy.

Finally, apart from the obvious precaution of removing dentures before transportation to the theatre, it is important that the patient should know what to expect when recovering from the anaesthetic. Certainly he will be coughing more than usual; if a biopsy has been taken there may be a small amount of haemoptysis; the throat and mouth may be a little uncomfortable, but with good technique this should never be obtrusive; later, some muscle aching may follow the use of the relaxant drug. Forewarned, the patients seldom seem distressed or complain about these minor symptoms.

FINDINGS IN BRONCHIAL CARCINOMA

It is rare that the histological type of a bronchial carcinoma can be appreciated bronchoscopically, for all varieties have similar well-defined and repeatedly recurring patterns of behaviour which can be recognized bronchoscopically. First it must be realized that little more than half of the carcinomas diagnosed prove visible bronchoscopically. Of those seen, the primary lesions may present in two main ways: (1) tumour involvement of the bronchial wall only, with perhaps local extension submucosally, and (2) intraluminal eruption of the tumour following breach of the bronchial mucosa. A special type in the second class is the polypoidal tumour presenting its free end to the bronchoscopist.

A secondary effect of mural or intraluminal growth is often partial or complete closure of the affected bronchus, ultimately leading to collapse of the associated pulmonary segment and displacement of the bronchial tree. Secondary bacterial infection is then frequent, often making diagnosis difficult. It is this phenomenon of bronchial block and infection which so frequently generates the presenting symptoms.

The conformation, texture and surface of tumours varies considerably. Mural growths may have only reddened, swollen mucosa overlying them, or may present as more clearly infiltrated yellow tissue with a delineated edge indicating the visible limit of the creeping tumour (*Plate 1*). The local tissues are often less pliable and are frequently rigidly fixed, indicating wider surrounding infiltration than can be seen bronchoscopically: this may suggest malignancy even when mucosal changes are less diagnostic. Normal mural features such as cartilage outlines and mucosal corrugations may be obscured or distorted.

Breach of the mucosa allows an intraluminal tumour to develop as an irregular projection of abnormal tissue which may appear in many forms, varying in size according to the stage at diagnosis: firm, fleshy and smooth or lobulated; soft and haemorrhagic, often with overlying vessel engorgement; crumbling and necrotic (*Plate 2*); difficult to identify because of gross associated infection and mucosal swelling; sometimes presenting in polypoidal fashion more proximally than its point of origin.

Even if the tumour itself is not visible bronchoscopically, certain features can support the diagnosis suspected on clinical grounds. The appropriate segmental bronchial orifice may be exuding blood or pus, compatible with a bleeding tumour or associated local secondary infection. Such secretions may be valuable material from which a cytological diagnosis can be made. Most importantly, lymph node enlargement, due to tumour involvement, may be distorting the bronchial tree: this is more fully described in the next section.

ASSESSING SUITABILITY FOR TREATMENT

Assessment of suitability for surgery or radiotherapy in a case of bronchogenic carcinoma will depend on a complete appraisal of many factors: general clinical condition including age, frailty, cardiac and renal states, respiratory reserve, and severity of associated bronchitis; evidence of extrathoracic metastases, particularly lymphatic, bony, hepatic and cerebral; radiological indications of the intrathoracic extent of the disease; the cause of any pleural fluid present; and, often decisively, the bronchoscopic findings. Only the last will be discussed here.

Metastatic involvement of vital intrathoracic structures commonly precludes successful surgical removal; bronchoscopic appearances can often give some indication of the situation, so saving the patient from a fruitless thoracotomy and helping to plan the field for radiotherapy. Apart from increased rigidity of the bronchial tree, bronchoscopic evidence of tumour spread may be found in the tracheo-bronchial, mediastinal and paratracheal lymph nodes. Commonly the first nodes involved are those lying just beneath the bronchial bifurcation nearest to the tumour. This leads to a widening or 'blunting' of this usually knife-like structure. The change is usually well seen at the bifurcation of the left main bronchus into upper and lower bronchi. If widening of a peripheral bifurcation is the only obvious distortion and the main carina and lower trachea are normal, thoracotomy with a view to lobectomy or pneumonectomy may be considered.

Further proximal progression of the growth may follow the lymph channels to involve mediastinal and/or paratracheal lymph nodes. This is often clearly seen bronchoscopically as lateral displacement of the medial wall of either main bronchus, widening of the carina, or distortion and narrowing of the lower trachea (*Plate 3*). Clearly, any one or any combination of such anatomical findings makes successful thoracotomy most unlikely and radiotherapy usually becomes the treatment of choice.

In even more advanced cases, there may be fungation of the tumour through the mucosa overlying the nodes. In this way huge areas of the visible bronchial tree may be involved in growth. Even if the mucosa overlying enlarged nodes appears normal, it is worth obtaining biopsies from these areas because a surprising number reveal that invasion has proceeded further than expected. Needle biopsies through the carina may also give unexpected information or confirm the presence of tumour in the subcarinal nodes.

In the majority of cases the choice between surgery, radiotherapy and palliation is clear, and in many the bronchoscopist plays a leading role in this choice. If, however, the bronchoscopy reveals only normal tissues and thus no contra-indication to surgery, the actual treatment will then be decided entirely on other factors.

DIFFERENTIAL DIAGNOSIS

In many cases the diagnosis of a tumour is obvious, particularly when there is no serious secondary infection to obscure the issue, as may be the case when a growth has not yet obstructed the bronchus. Here it is clear that tumour tissue is present and the only question is whether it is carcinomatous. Usually, at bronchoscopy, this is a relatively unimportant matter and the diagnosis is soon made clear from biopsy tissue. Some tumours, however, have clear characteristics which make it possible to suspect their true nature immediately: typical adenomas are smooth and cherry red, bleeding readily on biopsy, while benign tumours produce relatively little secondary infection and the mucosa overlying them is usually pale and normal.

In most cases, however, secondary infection is present and it is here that the main problem in differential diagnosis lies, for exactly similar inflammatory changes can be produced by other causes. For example, although uncommonly met with in adult practice, a foreign body can be completely lost in the inflammatory reaction to its presence. If it is radiolucent and there has been no clinical indication of aspiration, it may be only on attempting to take a biopsy that the foreign body can be suspected. Even simple local infections can be confusing and, in particular, aspiration of infected material from the upper respiratory tract, or blocking of a bronchus by a mucous plug, can produce changes remarkably similar to those of carcinoma. Biopsy and examination of removed inflammatory material, or of the plug itself, will often help in the diagnosis.

Tuberculosis, sarcoidosis and other diseases affecting lymph nodes within the thorax can also confuse the issue by producing widened carinas and other distortions of the bronchial tree. Benign lymph node enlargements and lymphomas, however, can often lead to similar bronchial distortions but without the overlying mucosal inflammatory changes usual in malignancy. Such normal mucosa suggests a benign condition but is not, of course, diagnostic.

Tuberculosis can also imitate carcinoma involving the bronchial wall. Local endobronchial tuberculosis can produce gross inflammatory changes in the mucosa with swelling and distortion of the bronchial wall, while granulations or caseation can suggest intraluminal carcinoma. Although one can usually have intelligent suspicions as to the pathological nature of endobronchial findings, surprises in biopsy reports are not very rare.

COLLECTING SPECIMENS

It will be clear from previous sections that specimens removed from the bronchial tree at bronchoscopy can be of supreme diagnostic value. Secretions and inflammatory exudates should be removed by sucking and retained for subsequent examination. Both malignant cells and bacteria, particularly tubercle bacilli, should be looked for in appropriate cases. Material obtained by gently abrading the bronchial walls, particularly beyond the reach of biopsy forceps, such as can be obtained by swabs on flexible wires, can sometimes be valuable in yielding malignant cells. Direct biopsy from visible lesions is naturally of the greatest value and should be obtained wherever possible. It is my practice to do this under telescopic vision; not only can the instrument be more accurately placed on the lesion, but smaller forceps can be used to obtain an adequate sample, so providing a safe technique. Finally, in cases where distortion of the bronchial tree has been produced by node enlargement or where node enlargement is suspected even without gross distortion, needle biopsies can be obtained—again best under telescopic vision—from the subcarinal areas and examined for malignant cells and tubercle bacilli.

Bronchoscopy does not, however, end with the diagnosis. The therapeutic possibilities of removing tumour material from the bronchial tree are very real, particularly in cases where an intraluminal tumour has grown proximally in polypoid fashion. In its passage upwards the tumour may have obstructed a bronchial side-branch without actually invading the mucosa; with care and patience, much of the tumour tissue may be removed, allowing re-aeration of areas of lung which collapsed following the bronchial obstruction. This can produce marked symptomatic improvement and also helps to determine the site of origin of a tumour which will have proved to be less invasive and extensive than at first thought. Clearly, with such additional knowledge available, surgery might now be contemplated or much more accurate radiotherapy planned.

BRONCHOSCOPY IN FOLLOW-UP

The bronchoscopist can still help the bronchial carcinoma patient and his clinician even when the diagnosis has been confirmed and radiotherapy or surgery completed. Most obviously, immediate repeat bronchoscopy is of use in reassessing the situation in a patient who presents new or recrudescent symptoms some time after treatment has been completed. A recrudescence of growth may be found, but symptoms by no means always prove to be related to tumour spread. Persistent cough can be associated with bronchial distortion or stenosis, perhaps with added secondary infection, following the treatment itself; bleeding may occur from granulation tissue around a stitch in a bronchial stump or from telangiectasia

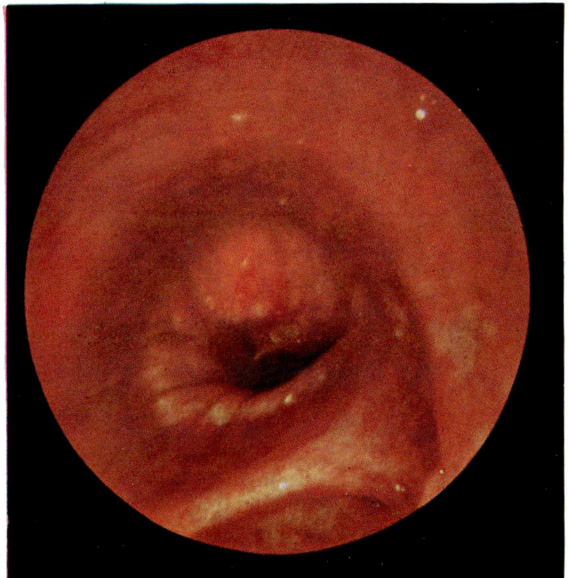

Plate 1

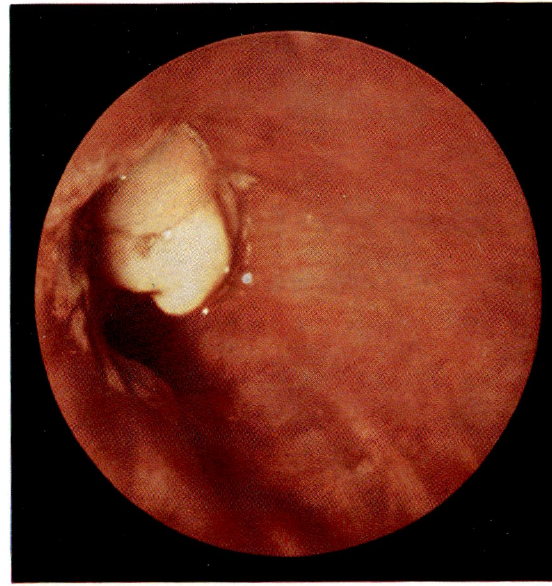

Plate 2

Plate 1. Carcinoma of left lower bronchus. The mucosa is generally reddened. In the foreground can be seen the inferior margin of the apical lower bronchial orifice. Beyond this a tumour has involved the bronchial wall, spreading in annular fashion, to raise the longitudinal elastic bundles into prominence. The macroscopic proximal edge of the tumour is thus clearly delineated. The point of maximal growth is seen anteriorly, and here a little blood and a yellow nodule indicate an early breach in the mucosa. Biopsy: squamous-celled carcinoma

Plate 2. Carcinoma of left main bronchus. Purulent secretion has already been removed. The mucosa is generally reddened. Mucosal corrugation is seen on the posterior wall and some secretion adheres to the lateral wall. The medial bronchial wall is thrust laterally by lymph nodes enlarged by metastastic carcinoma. Erupting from the upper bronchus and largely occluding the main bronchial lumen is a large, yellow, fungating, necrotic tumour. Biopsy: oat-celled carcinoma

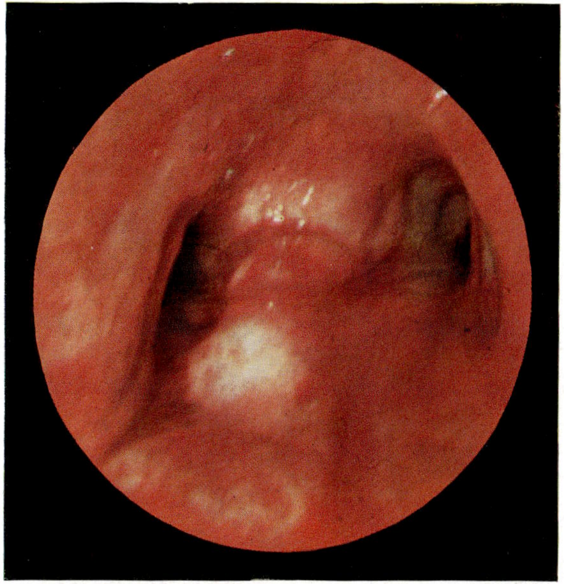

Plate 3

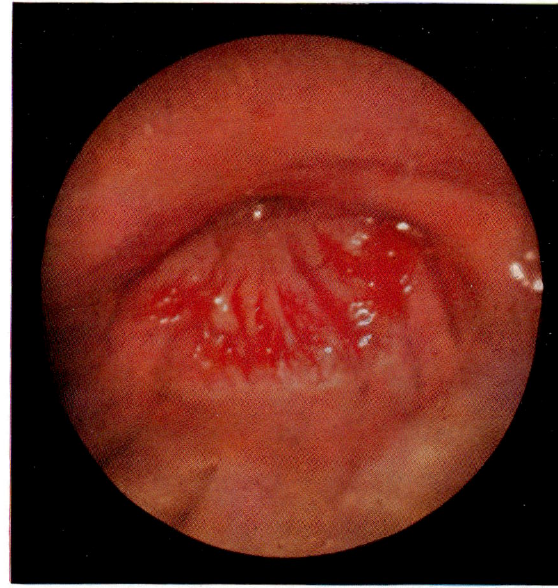

Plate 4

Plate 3. Carcinoma of lower trachea and carina. There is considerable metastatic involvement of tracheo-bronchial lymph nodes from a primary tumour in the right lower bronchus. Superior vena caval obstruction is present. The lower trachea is compressed from the left and from behind. The posterior node involvement has gone beyond simple compression: the carcinoma has involved the mucosa and a bilobed tumour is encroaching on the tracheal lumen. A large subcarinal node has greatly widened the carina and produced some narrowing of the main bronchi. The mucosa is markedly reddened and swollen and some bleeding is seen. Biopsy: poorly differentiated squamous-celled carcinoma

Plate 4. Carcinoma of right main bronchus. A tongue-like submucosal carcinoma is creeping up the posterior wall of the main bronchus just beyond the upper orifice. The overlying mucosa is invaded by exuberant interlacing leashes of vessels which bled freely on biopsy (anaplastic carcinoma). The posterior mucosal corrugations have been almost obliterated in the tumour area and the bronchial lumen has been reduced to a slit

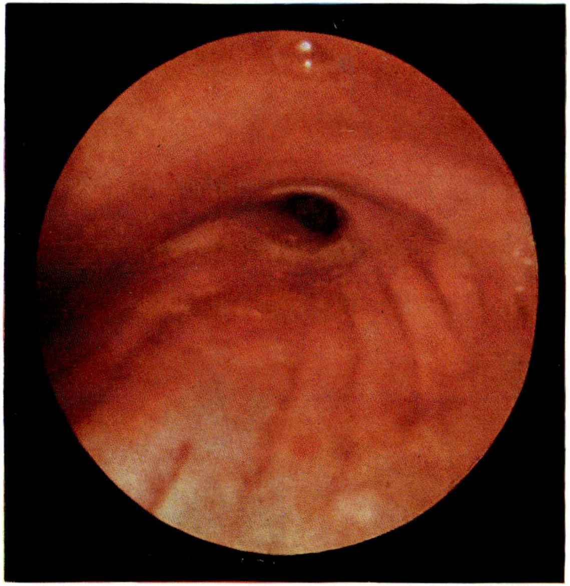

Plate 5

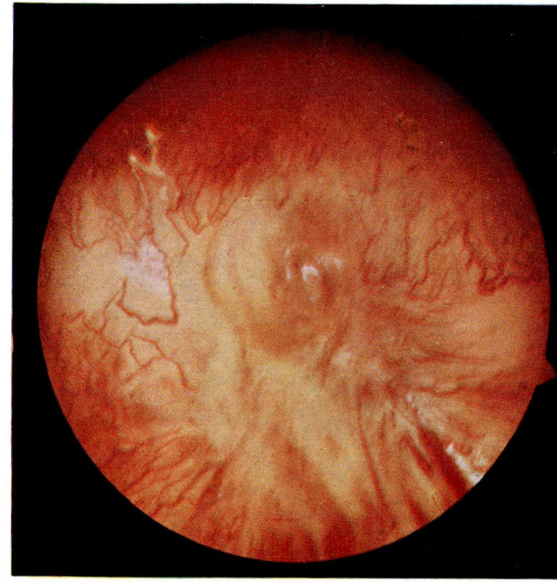

Plate 6

Plate 5. The same patient as in Plate 4, six weeks after finishing a radical course of radiotherapy. The tumour has largely disappeared, although some submucosal thickening remains to make the upper limit of the original tumour still discernible. The posterior mucosal corrugations are more visible, and the lumen has increased, the exuberant vessels have disappeared, but the mucosa remains very red

Plate 6. Effect of radiotherapy in right upper bronchial carcinoma. The photograph was taken one year after completing a course of radiotherapy. The changes are typical of those following irradiation of carcinoma: pale mucosa over fibrous scarring, surrounded by intense telangiectasia. The picture was unchanged another year later

following radiotherapy. Such conditions can be assessed most accurately if there is experience gained from bronchoscopy carried out as a routine follow-up measure to assess progress in treated cases of bronchial carcinoma. Of particular interest here are the changes found following irradiation.

Irradiation Changes

These follow a regular pattern, and early changes may be dramatic. Radiosensitive tumours shrink or disappear quite rapidly, usually within weeks of the treatment. Bronchial obstruction may thus be relieved, either by contraction of enlarged lymph nodes which had been distorting the bronchus or by shrinkage of an intraluminal tumour (*Plates 4 and 5*). At the same time there is a transitory local mucosal inflammatory reaction to the radiation itself. This is subsequently replaced by local pallor of the mucosa and frequently by contractive scarring, particularly if the area was previously infiltrated by the growth. Such scarring can be very marked, leading to gross distortion and rigidity of the bronchial tree. This does not necessarily mean that further growth has taken place, but probably that it was extensive originally. Such a condition may remain unchanged for many months, or even years, following irradiation.

Appearing many months later than the other changes is telangiectasia. Often delicate but sometimes very florid, the dilated vessels are found most commonly around pale scarred areas but may occur anywhere in the area of irradiation (*Plate 6*). The extent of this change appears to be related to the dose of radiation itself.

CONCLUSION

It will be seen that the bronchoscope is an indispensable diagnostic tool, extremely useful in follow-up and occasionally of great help as a therapeutic weapon in the management of bronchial carcinoma. Maximal usefulness is only obtained, however, with first-class anaesthesia so that the most careful and meticulous investigation can be made together with the removal of adequate specimens for histology and cytology.

It is equally important that the radiotherapist, if he is the doctor responsible for the follow-up of carcinoma patients, should have a full understanding of the potentialities of bronchoscopy so that referral for diagnosis and further assessment during the follow-up period may be as prompt as possible. Perhaps the most satisfactory and satisfying arrangement is found in those hospitals where joint clinics are held for the assessment and follow-up of bronchial carcinoma patients: here the greatest co-operation, for the patient's benefit, is attained between the radiotherapist and the (physician or surgeon) bronchoscopist.

REFERENCE

Stradling, P. (1968). *Diagnostic Bronchoscopy*. Edinburgh: Livingstone.

7—Associated Changes with Lung Cancer

I—Endocrine Syndromes

Gerald Anderson

In lung cancer, endocrine abnormalities may occur without tumour involvement of endocrine glands. These endocrinopathies cause unpleasant symptoms and may shorten life. Effective treatment may be available if the nature of the disorder is recognized.

The endocrine syndromes are due to tumour production of substances with hormonal activity. These substances are chemically and immunologically indistinguishable from naturally occurring hormones, but final proof of their identity has not been obtained.

HYPERCALCAEMIA

Hypercalcaemia without evidence of bone metastases is the commonest endocrine disorder in the lung and is present in about 6 per cent of cases (Locke, 1962; Carey, 1966), almost all of which are of squamous cell type. It also occurs in other tumours, especially renal carcinoma.

The condition may be asymptomatic. Thirst and polyuria are common, with varying combinations of malaise, anorexia, nausea, vomiting, abdominal pain, constipation, headache, drowsiness and psychosis. Unlike that of hyperparathyroidism, the onset is acute and without ectopic calcification, renal stones or radiological changes in bone.

Albright and Riefenstein (1948) first described hypercalcaemia in a renal carcinoma and postulated tumour production of a parathormone-like compound. The finding that tumour resection abolished hypercalcaemia (Connor, Thomas and Howard, 1956) supported this hypothesis. Many reports subsequently claimed to demonstrate such a substance in the serum in malignant hypercalcaemia. The assay techniques used probably gave false positive results, but an immunoassay method has now shown that the tumour and the plasma contain a substance indistinguishable from parathyroid hormone (Munson, Tashjian and Levine, 1965).

The serum calcium may rise above 20 mg/100 ml with a normal or low serum phosphate and normal alkaline phosphatase. Hypercalciuria is present, and the tubular reabsorption of phosphate is decreased with a raised phosphate clearance. Hypercalcaemia may result in renal failure due to tubular damage. The syndrome is biochemically indistinguishable from hyperparathyroidism.

Treatment (Marsden, 1965) is by restriction of dietary calcium to less than 200 mg and hydration with about 5 litres of fluid daily. Corticosteroids reduce the serum calcium in about 50 per cent of cases, but the response may be incomplete or absent (Grimes and colleagues, 1967). They probably act by reducing tubular reabsorption of calcium. Prednisone 100 mg or hydrocortisone 400 mg daily is given initially, reducing to a maintenance dose. Hypercalcaemia responds to oral sodium phosphates (Thalassinos and Joplin, 1968). Intravenous sodium phosphate is effective, but may cause extensive ectopic calcification. Intravenous sodium sulphate can result in dangerous hypernatraemia. Tumour resection and radiotherapy cause a rapid fall in serum calcium (Connor, Thomas and Howard, 1956; Turkington and colleagues, 1966). This may rise again with tumour regrowth or metastases, but cure of hypercalcaemia may be permanent, since metastases often lack the ability to produce hypercalcaemia.

THE ECTOPIC–ACTH SYNDROME

In 1928 Brown described Cushing's syndrome due to bilateral adrenocortical hyperplasia in a patient with an oat cell bronchial carcinoma. This form of Cushing's syndrome occurs in about 2 per cent of cases of lung cancer and is associated with oat cell tumours. It is also found with bronchial carcinoids and adenomas and with malignant non-pulmonary tumours, and is due to release of an adrenocorticotrophic substance by the tumour.

The prominent clinical features of the ectopic–ACTH syndrome are oedema, skin pigmentation, diabetes mellitus, psychosis and the clinical manifestations of hypokalaemia. The patients do not live long enough to develop the typical body fat distribution and striae of Cushing's syndrome, so that the clinical features lag behind the biochemical disturbances.

Meador and colleagues (1962) demonstrated high levels of ACTH-like activity in tumour, metastases and plasma in this condition. Comparison of pituitary ACTH with tumour adrenocorticotrophin gave parallel dose–response curves and similar assays for steroid production and adrenal weight-maintaining factor (Liddle and colleagues, 1963). They are also indistinguishable immunologically (Jarrett, Lacey and Kipnis, 1964).

The striking biochemical abnormality is hypokalaemic alkalosis (Bagshawe, 1960), which distinguishes the ectopic–ACTH syndrome from other forms of Cushing's disease. The serum cortisol level is raised, with loss of diurnal rhythm and a raised cortisol secretion rate. Urinary excretion of oxogenic steroids is raised with normal oxosteroids. Administration of exogenous ACTH does not result in a further rise in serum cortisol, since the adrenal response is already maximal. Cortisol output has escaped from pituitary control and is not suppressed by dexamethasone. In bronchial carcinoma the serum cortisol is elevated in about 70 per cent of cases (Hatch, Segaloff and Ochsner, 1965), but only a few of these have the ectopic–ACTH syndrome. In the majority the raised serum cortisol is not accompanied by hypokalaemia, is suppressed by dexamethasone, and rises further with injection of exogenous ACTH. This common type of raised cortisol is probably a non-specific effect of illness and occurs in other diseases such as heart failure.

The ectopic–ACTH syndrome is a medical emergency, since the mean life-span after the first attendance is about 24 days. The poor prognosis is probably due to a combination of hypokalaemia, diabetes mellitus and a very malignant tumour. Where the associated tumour is a bronchial carcinoid, its removal abolishes the Cushing's syndrome, but in bronchial carcinoma the patient is either too ill or the tumour too widespread for successful resection. Bilateral total adrenalectomy is effective (Bagshawe, 1960), but is a formidable undertaking in a patient who will soon die of lung cancer. Radiotherapy is very effective and is the treatment of choice, since all therapy is palliative and this procedure involves least discomfort to the patient. Drug treatment has been widely used, but with inconstant effect. Metapyrone inhibits the 11β-hydroxylase system responsible for the final stage in cortisol synthesis. In the ectopic–ACTH syndrome it produces little benefit (Pfohl and Doe, 1963). Disappointing results have usually been obtained with the drug O′p-DDD, which produces adrenal necrosis and atrophy in dogs. The diuretic triamterene causes potassium retention and is useful for relieving hypokalaemia (Meador and colleagues, 1962).

HYPONATRAEMIA

Hyponatraemia in lung cancer was first described by Winkler and Crankshaw (1938). It is uncommon and occurs with undifferentiated and oat cell tumours.

This syndrome may be asymptomatic, but the symptoms of water intoxication are usually present if the serum sodium falls below 115 mEq/litre. These are lethargy, weakness, irritability, drowsiness, confusion and nausea. Oedema does not occur.

The biochemical findings are a marked fall in serum sodium and, to a lesser extent, in serum potassium and chloride. The blood urea and haematocrit are low, with a hypotonic serum and hypervolaemia. The urine is hyperosmolar to the plasma. These biochemical abnormalities can be reproduced by giving antidiuretic hormone (ADH) and water to normal subjects. Normally ADH secretion is reduced in the presence of a hypotonic plasma, so that its continued secretion is 'inappropriate' (Schwartz and colleagues, 1957). In the hyponatraemic syndrome, the plasma and tumour contain ADH-like activity (Amatruda and colleagues, 1963; Lee, Long and Barraclough, 1964; Uttiger, 1966). If the substance secreted is assumed to be arginine vasopressin, the total daily secretion is about 8 times the normal pituitary output (Thorn and Transbøl, 1964). ADH secretion results in hyponatraemia by two mechanisms. Hypervolaemia causes increased renal blood flow with a natriuresis and depletional hyponatraemia. It also results in reduced aldosterone secretion with a dilutional hyponatraemia.

Hyponatraemia responds to fluid restriction and to 9-fluorocortisone, a potent sodium-retaining steroid which may also act by reducing ADH secretion by the pituitary and possibly by the tumour. Treatment of the tumour by irradiation (Schwartz, Tassel and Bartter, 1960) or by cytotoxic drugs (Linton and Hutton, 1965) also relieves the hyponatraemia.

The hyponatraemic syndrome is uncommonly associated with a proximal tubular defect of unknown cause (Rees, Rosalki and Maclean, 1960; Daly, Nelson and Rose, 1963; Ross, 1963). There are aminoaciduria, glycosuria and inability to acidify the urine.

THE CARCINOID SYNDROME

The commonest lung tumour associated with this condition is the bronchial carcinoid, but it occasionally occurs with oat cell carcinomas (Montgomery and colleagues, 1957; Williams and Azzopardi, 1960).

The clinical findings are flushing, wheezing, diarrhoea, cardiac lesions and sometimes psychosis. The flushes are dusky red and usually last a few minutes. They may be precipitated by anaesthetics, adrenalin, alcohol, emotion, food, or handling of the tumour at operation. The cardiac lesions are usually right-sided, but in lung tumours may involve the mitral valve. The valves are deformed by fibrin plaques. Unexplained high-output cardiac failure may develop. The diarrhoea varies in severity and is accompanied by increased peristalsis. Wheezing is often absent.

Normally 99 per cent of dietary trytophane is converted to protein or nicotinic acid, while 1 per cent enters a cycle in which it is first converted to 5-hydroxytrytrophane (5-HTP). This is decarboxylated to 5-hydroxytryptamine (5-HT serotonin), which is excreted in the urine as 5-hydroxyindoleacetic acid (5-H IAA). In the carcinoid syndrome, as much as 60 per cent of dietary trytrophane enters the serotonin cycle. Insufficient protein and nicotinic acid synthesis may cayse hypoproteinaemia and pellagra. Carcinoid tumours contain 5-HT (Lembeck, 1953), and the urinary excretion of 5-H IAA is raised. Foregut carcinoid tumours such as lung tumours often lack the ability to convert 5-HTP to 5-HT, so that 5-HTP may also be present in the urine. Hyperserotoninaemia does not explain all the manifestations of the carcinoid syndrome, and a normal plasma serotonin may be present with continuous flushing. Oates and colleagues (1964) reproduced the flush in a patient with the carcinoid syndrome by intravenous injection of bradykinin, and the hepatic vein blood during a spontaneous flush contained a high level of a kinin peptide. Tumour secretion of such a peptide may be responsible for many features of this disorder.

In bronchial carcinoid tumour, resection has relieved this syndrome. Radiotherapy is not helpful in management. Methyldopa inhibits decarboxylation of 5-HTP to 5-HT, but the clinical benefit is inconstant. Chlorpromazine is useful in the control of diarrhoea, possibly due to its activity as a kinin antagonist. Corticosteroids may control flushing (Melmon, Sjoerdsma and Mason, 1965) by an unknown mechanism.

GYNAECOMASTIA

Gynaecomastia in lung cancer was first described by Locke (1915) and is present in about 0·4 per cent of cases (Bariéty, Coury and Rullière, 1964). About 10–15 per cent of patients with hypertrophic osteoarthropathy due to bronchial carcinoma develop gynaecomastia.

The condition is usually bilateral and is not accompanied by galactorrhoea. Histological examination of the breasts reveals simple hypertrophy, and testicular atrophy may be present. Rarely gynaecomastia precedes radiological appearance of the tumour.

Fusco and Rosen (1966) demonstrated raised urinary gonadotrophin excretion in four patients with gynaecomastia due to bronchial carcinoma. In three cases where tumour tissue was available, this contained gonadotrophin. Removal of the tumour (Fischl, 1950) or radiotherapy (del Castillo, de la Balze and Reforzo Membrives, 1941) abolishes the gynaecomastia.

HYPERGLYCAEMIA

Freund (1885) detected hyperglycaemia in 62 out of 70 cancer patients, and the association has been described frequently. Glicksman and Rawson (1956) found diabetic oral glucose tolerance tests in 9·3 per cent of control subjects and in 36·7 per cent of a large series of cancer patients. Of those with lung cancer, 41 per cent had diabetic curves. Weisenfeld, Hecht and Goldner (1962) found a similar incidence of diabetic glucose tolerance tests in cancer subjects, but claimed that this finding was present in 37 per cent of a control series. The high control incidence may have been due to a deficient carbohydrate intake before the test or to ill-health of the controls, since diabetic curves are found in many diseases including tuberculosis, multiple sclerosis and schizophrenia.

A diabetic glucose tolerance test does not indicate that the patient has diabetes and may only show an inability to cope with an abnormal glucose load. The cause of cancer hyperglycaemia is unknown, but there is a decreased sensitivity to insulin (Bishop and Marks, 1959). The high serum cortisol of cancer may possibly cause hyperglycaemia by peripheral opposition to the action of insulin.

THYROTOXICOSIS

Thyrotoxicosis may occur in choriocarcinoma or hydatidiform mole (Tisné, Barzalatto and Stevenson, 1955; Odell and colleagues, 1963). Usually there were no clinical features of thyrotoxicosis and the diagnosis was based on abnormal tests of thyroid function. The plasma level of thyroid-stimulating hormone (TSH) was raised and TSH was present in tumour extracts. De Gennes, Briccaire and Lepratt (1962) described 40 patients with other types of malignancy and thyrotoxicosis, and 6 of these had bronchial carcinoma. A further case with lung cancer was described by Pisapia (1965). De Gennes, Briccaire and Lepratt distinguished this form of thyrotoxicosis from a chance association of malignancy and Graves disease by the late onset, higher male incidence, and absence of goitre and eye signs. Hennen (1967) isolated a TSH-like substance from a bronchial carcinoma which had not been associated with thyrotoxicosis during life. Higher doses of TSH are required to produce a goitre than to release thyroxine, and this may explain the absence of eye signs in this type of thyrotoxicosis.

MELANOCYTE-STIMULATING HORMONE (MSH) SECRETION

Skin pigmentation is a prominent feature of the ectopic–ACTH syndrome and was attributed to the MSH-like action of ACTH. Abe and colleagues (1967), using a specific immunoassay technique, showed that the plasma in the ectopic–ACTH syndrome contained MSH or a closely related substance which was separable from the ACTH content. It seems probable that the production of MSH and ACTH is governed by a common mechanism, since they occur together in tumours and in the pituitary.

GROWTH HORMONE

The similarity between acromegaly and hypertrophic osteoarthropathy has often been noted. Steiner, Dahlbach and Waldenstrom (1968), in a single case of hypertrophic osteoarthropathy in lung cancer, found a raised serum level of growth hormone which fell to normal after tumour resection. This interesting observation has not yet been confirmed.

The production of hormones by tumours suggests that some malignant cells either regain their primitive totipotent abilities or lose the normal suppressor mechanisms. One point of clinical importance is that ignorance of the underlying malignant nature of an endocrinopathy may distract attention from the causative tumour, while awareness will focus attention on it.

REFERENCES

Abe, K., Wendell, E. N., Liddle, G. W., Island, O. P. and Orth, D. N. (1967). 'Radioimmunoassay of β MSH in human plasma and tissues.' *J. clin. Invest.* **45,** 1609.

Albright, F. and Riefenstein, E. C. (1948). *The Parathyroid Gland and Metabolic Bone Disease.* Baltimore: Williams & Wilkins.

Amatruda, T. T. Jnr., Mulrow, P. J., Gallagher, J. C. and Sawyer, W. H. (1963). 'Carcinoma of the lung with inappropriate diuresis.' *New Engl. J. Med.* **269,** 544.

Bagshawe, K. D. (1960). 'Hypokalaemia, carcinoma and Cushing's syndrome.' *Lancet* **2,** 284.

Bariéty, M., Coury, C. and Rulliere, R. (1964). 'Les syndromes paranéoplastiques dans le cancer broncho-pulmonaire primitif.' *J. fr. Méd. Chir. thorac.* **18,** 19.

Bishop, J. S. and Marks, P. A. (1959). 'Studies in carbohydrate metabolism in patients with neoplastic disease. II. Response to insulin administration.' *J. clin. Invest.* **38,** 668.

Brown, W. H. (1928). 'A case of pluriglandular syndrome and diabetes in a bearded woman.' *Lancet* **2,** 1022.

Carey, V. C. (1966). 'The incidence of hypercalcaemia in association with bronchogenic carcinoma.' *Am. Rev. resp. Dis.* **93,** 584.

Connor, T. B., Thomas, W. C. and Howard, J. E. (1956). 'Etiology of hypercalcaemia associated with lung carcinoma.' *J. clin. Invest.* **35,** 697.

Daly, J. J., Nelson, M. A. and Rose, D. P. (1963). 'Hyponatraemia with carcinoma of bronchus.' *Postgrad. med. J.* **39,** 158.

de Gennes, L., Briccaire, H. and Lepratt, J. (1962). 'Paraneoplastic endocrine syndromes. II. Hyperthyroidism and various endocrinopathies.' *Presse méd.* **70,** 2137.

del Castillo, E. B., de la Balze, F. A. and Reforzo Membrives, J. (1941). 'Ginecomastia y cancer del pulmón.' *Semana méd.* **48,** 1419.

Fischl, J. R. (1950). 'Severe hypertrophic pulmonary osteoarthropathy: report of a case due to carcinoma of lung with operation and recovery.' *Am. J. Roentg.* **64,** 42.

Freund, E. (1885). 'Zu Diagnose des Carcinoms.' *Wein. med. Bl.* **8,** 268.

Fusco, F. D. and Rosen, S. W. (1966). 'Gonadotropin-producing anaplastic large cell carcinomas of the lung.' *New Engl. J. Med.* **275,** 507.

Glicksman, A. S. and Rawson, R. W. (1956). 'Diabetes and altered carbohydrate metabolism in patients with cancer.' *Cancer, N.Y.* **9,** 1127.

Grimes, B. J., Fisher, B., Finn, F. and Danowski, T. S. (1967). 'Steroid-resistant hypercalcaemia and parathyroid hyperplasia in non-osseous cancer.' *Acta endocr., Copenh.* **56,** 510.

Hatch, H. B., Segaloff, A. and Ochsner, A. (1965). 'Adrenocortical function in bronchogenic carcinoma: study of 100 patients.' *Ann. Surg.* **161,** 645.

Hennen, G. (1967). 'Characterization of a thyroid-stimulating factor in a human cancer tissue.' *J. clin. Endocr. Metab.* **27,** 610.

Jarrett, L., Lacey, P. E. and Kipnis, D. M. (1964). 'Characterization by immunofluorescence of an ACTH-like substance in non-pituitary tumours from patients with hyperadrenocorticism.' *J. clin. Endocr. Metab.* **24,** 543.

Lee, J., Long, J. J. and Barraclough, M. A. (1964). ''Inappropriate secretion of vasopressin.' *Lancet* **2,** 792.

Lembeck, F. (1953). '5-Hydroxytryptamine in a carcinoid tumour.' *Nature, Lond.* **172,** 910.

Liddle, G. W., Island, D. P., Ney, R. L., Nicholson, W. E. and Shimizu, N. (1963). 'Non-pituitary neoplasms and Cushing's syndrome.' *Archs intern. Med.* **111,** 471.

Linton, A. L. and Hutton, I. (1965). 'Hyponatraemia and bronchial carcinoma. Therapy with nitrogen mustard.' *Br. med. J.* **2,** 277.

Locke, E. A. (1915). 'Secondary hypertrophic osteoarthropathy and its relation to simple club fingers.' *Archs intern. Med.* **15,** 659.

Locke, M. O. (1962). 'Incidence of hypercalcemia in patients with proved carcinoma of lung.' *J. Lancet, Minneap.* **82,** 165.

Marsden, J. A. (1965). 'The management of hypercalcaemia in malignant disease.' *Med. J. Aust.* **2,** 411.

Meador, C. K., Liddle, G. W., Island, D. P., Nicholson, W. E., Lucas, C. P., Nuckton, J. C. and Leutscher, J. A. (1962). 'Cause of Cushing's syndrome in patients with tumours arising from non-endocrine tissue.' *J. clin. Endocr. Metab.* **22,** 693

Melmon, L. Sjoersdma, A. and Mason, D. T. (1965). 'Distinctive clinical and therapeutic aspects of the syndrome associated with bronchial carcinoid tumours.' *Am. J. Med.* **39,** 568.

Montgomery, D. A. D., Ramsey, A. S., Robertson, J. H. and Welbourn, R. B. (1957). 'Cushing's syndrome with carcinoma of bronchus and with features suggesting carcinoid tumour.' *Lancet* **1,** 23.

Munson, P. L., Tashjian, A. H. Jnr. and Levine, L. (1965). 'Evidence for parathyroid hormone in non-parathyroid mass associated with hypercalcemia.' *Cancer Res.* **25,** 1062.

Oates, J. A., Melmon, K., Sjoersdma, A., Gillespie, L. and Mason, D. T. (1964). 'Release of a kinin peptide in the carcinoid syndrome.' *Lancet* **1,** 514.

Odell, W. D., Bates, R. W., Rivlin, R. S., Lipsett, M. B. and Hertz, R. (1963). 'Increased thyroid function without clinical hyperthyroidism in patients with choriocarcinoma.' *J. clin. Endocr. Metab.* **23,** 658.

Pfohl, R. A. and Doe, R. P. (1963). 'Adrenal and pituitary studies in a patient with brochogenic carcinoma and Cushing's syndrome.' *Ann. intern. Med.* **58,** 993.

Pisapia, M. (1965). 'Sindrome éndocrine assosciate a neoplasie: segnalazione di due casi di tumori broncogeno con ipercorticismo e ipertiroidismo.' *Nunt. radiol.* **31,** 887.

Rees, J. R., Rosalki, S. B. and Maclean, A. D. W. (1960). 'Hyponatraemia and impaired renal tubular function with carcinoma of bronchus.' *Lancet* **2,** 1005.

Rosen, S. W., Becker, C. E., Schlaff, S., Easton, J. and Gluck, M. C. (1968). 'Ectopic gonadotropin production before clinical recognition of bronchogenic carcinoma.' *New Engl. J. Med.* **279,** 640.

Ross, E. J. (1963). 'Hyponatraemic syndromes associated with carcinoma of the bronchus.' *Q. Jl Med.* **32,** 297.

Schwartz, W. B., Tassel, D. and Bartter, F. C. (1960). 'Observations of hyponatremia and renal sodium loss resulting from inappropriate secretions of antidiuretic hormone.' *New Engl. J. Med.* **262,** 743.

— Bennett, W., Curelop, S. and Bartter, F. C. (1957). 'A syndrome of renal sodium loss and hyponatremia probably resulting from inappropriate secretion of antidiuretic hormone.' *Am. J. Med.* **23,** 529.

Steiner, H., Dahlback, O. and Waldenstrom, J. (1968). 'Ectopic growth hormone production and osteoarthropathy in carcinoma of the bronchus.' *Lancet* **1,** 783.

Thalassinos, N. and Joplin, J. F. (1968). 'Phosphate treatment of hypercalcaemia due to carcinoma.' *Br. med. J.* **2,** 14.

Thorn, N. A. and Transbøl, I. (1964). 'Hyponatremia and bronchogenic carcinoma associated with renal excretion of large amounts of antidiuretic material.' *Am. J. Med.* **35,** 257.

Tisné, L., Barzalatto, J. and Stevenson, C. (1955). 'Estudio de la functión tiroidea durante el estado grávido-puerperal con el yodo radioactivo.' *Boln Soc. chil. Obstet. Ginec.* **20,** 246 (English abstract in *J. Obstet. Gynaec. Br. Emp.* 1957, **2,** 11).

Turkington, R. W., Goldman, J. K., Ruffner, B. W. and Dobson, J. L. (1966). 'Bronchogenic carcinoma simulating hyperparathyroidism.' *Cancer, N.Y.*, **19,** 406.

Uttiger, R. D. (1966). 'Inappropriate antidiuresis and carcinoma of the lung: detection of arginine vasopressin in tumour extracts by immunoassay.' *J. Clin. Endocr. Metab.* **26,** 970.

Weisenfeld, S., Hecht, N. and Goldner, M. G. (1962). 'Tests of carbohydrate metabolism in carcinomatosis.' *Cancer, N.Y.* **15,** 18.

Winkler, A. W. and Crankshaw, O. F. (1938). 'Chloride depletion in conditions other than Addison's disease.' *J. clin. Invest.* **17,** 1.

Williams, E. D. and Azzopardi, J. G. (1960). 'Tumours of the lung and the carcinoid syndrome.' *Thorax* **15,** 30.

II—Neuromuscular Syndromes

J. R. Heron

'Disease often tells its secrets in a casual parenthesis.'

The remote effects of cancer on the nervous system have received increasing attention over the past two decades since an early description by Denny-Brown (1948) of a sensory neuropathy occurring in association with bronchial carcinoma. A well-defined group of syndromes has become recognized clinically and pathologically. The nervous system may be affected at all levels from its most peripheral nerve endings to the cerebral cortex, and often different levels of the nervous system are simultaneously affected so that clinical groupings of symptoms and signs overlap. Brain and Adams (1965) produced a comprehensive guide to classification, grouping the disorders according to the level at which the nervous system was involved, their main groups being encephalopathy, myelopathy, neuropathy and muscular disorders.

The prime cause of these syndromes is as obscure as the cause of cancer itself. They are considered by some to be a direct result of the cancer, and by others to be caused by the same intrinsic mechanism which is responsible for the development of the neoplasm. Recognition of these manifestations of central nervous system involvement in an individual with cancer is useful in so far as early recognition may lead in some instances to appropriate treatment before the malignancy becomes untreatable.

Academic interest in the epiphenomena of cancer rests on the premise that they are a possible viaduct into cancer research. It is possible, for example, that these multicentric non-infiltrative lesions in the nervous system represent a different stage of cancer development in an individual, or a different host response to the disease process, which could have implications in research into the alteration of the immune status of the affected patient.

INCIDENCE OF NEUROMYOPATHY

The highest incidence of neuromyopathy is found in carcinoma of the lung and of the ovary. Of 250 patients with carcinoma of the lung

(Croft and Wilkinson, 1965), 16 per cent showed neurological abnormalities indicating neuromyopathy. The incidence in women was 13 per cent. Neuromuscular disorders were the commonest presentation, occurring in 80 per cent of the affected males. The next most common syndrome was the polyneuritic disorder, and other forms of disorder were seen in combination in the remainder of cases.

The incidence of neuromyopathy increases slightly with age and is higher in treated than in untreated patients. It bears no relation to the method of treatment of the carcinoma and is not dependent on the duration of the tumour. Histologically undifferentiated or anaplastic carcinoma is less liable to be associated with signs of neuromyopathy than squamous carcinoma or adenocarcinoma (4 per cent compared with 15 per cent). The incidence of neuromyopathy is also higher in patients who have evidence of metastases than in those who do not.

Although these figures in general represent the overall incidence in a population, Wilner and Brody (1968) compared 106 patients with histologically diagnosed lung cancer and 44 control patients with non-cancerous chronic lung disease, assessing each group for the presence of unexplained neurological signs. Their findings were at variance with previously published reports in that neurological signs were at least as frequent among the controls as among the cancer patients. Their control population consisted of patients suffering from chronic disease, in poor general health, and with similar smoking and drinking habits to the cancer patients. Unexplained neurological signs were much commoner in their controls than in previous control studies, and in their cancer patients the frequency of such signs was lower than in most other series and the signs were modified by successful treatment.

Accurate incidence figures will only become available when larger series of unselected patients with lung cancer are carefully documented.

CLASSIFICATION

Multifocal Leuco-encephalopathy

This is a rare association with carcinoma more commonly seen in Hodgkin's disease, leukaemia and reticulo-endothelial malignancy. Widely disseminated lesions occur in the central nervous system. There is demyelination in the cerebral hemispheres, the brain stem and the cerebellum. Occasionally the spinal cord may be similarly affected, and lesions can also occur in the grey matter. This rare syndrome (Richardson, 1965) is a rapidly evolving rostral neurological disorder, with evidence of progressive neurological signs developing often over a period of a few months. Death usually occurs within a year of the first development of neurological signs.

Diffuse Polio-encephalopathy

This includes the groups of psychiatric disorders, subacute cerebellar degeneration and lesions of the brain stem. The psychiatric syndrome presents as a disorder of thought, memory or mood, or with the symptoms of a progressive organic dementia. The clinical picture may be suggestive of a frontal lobe lesion and, in the context of bronchial carcinoma, may lead to the suspicion of secondary deposits in this area. Focal neurological signs are often absent in the early stages, and the syndrome needs to be differentiated from other primary psychiatric disorders and progressive dementing processes such as cerebrovascular disease, presenile dementia, vitamin B_{12} deficiency, portal systemic encephalopathy and encephalitis. However, where a systemic carcinoma is known to be present, the commonest form of the clinical presentation of dementia is metastasis from the primary tumour. The syndrome rarely occurs in complete isolation, and other signs of nervous system involvement such as cerebellar degeneration or peripheral neuropathy are frequently seen.

The association of a limbic encephalitis with carcinoma of the bronchus, where damage centres on the limbic grey matter and the medial temporal areas, has been described (Corsellis, Goldberg and Norton, 1968). The clinical presentation is with severe anxiety or depression and profound disturbance of affect. Hallucinations occur and occasionally epilepsy. The most characteristic feature is disturbance of recent memory, progressing to a global dementia. Cerebrospinal fluid examination often shows lymphocytes, elevation of protein and a paretic Lange curve. Electroencephalographic changes are not specific but can show a generalized background abnormality, sometimes with localizing temporal lobe features. The dementia of diffuse polio-encephalopathy is usually subacute. However, even where it is the presenting feature of the carcinoma of the bronchus, it may present as an acute fulminating dementing illness.

Subacute Cerebellar Degeneration

Brouwer and Biemond (1938) suggested a causal link between carcinoma and this now well-established syndrome. Brain and

Wilkinson (1965) reviewed the syndrome, adding 19 personal cases whose average age was 56·4 years. The site of the neoplasm was in the lung in ten of these patients, four being of the oat cell variety, three squamous cell, one adenocarcinoma and one undifferentiated carcinoma.

The cerebellar lesion, as in other central and neuromuscular syndromes, may complicate an already disclosed cancer developing after a period of months or, more rarely, years. In such instances the possibility of secondary invasion of the cerebellum with metastatic deposits should be considered as the first probability. A cerebellar disorder may precede the detection of the carcinoma by a similar latent period and, where other causes for a progressive cerebellar syndrome have been excluded, this clinical picture should initiate full investigation and frequent review to detect a possible occult neoplasm at its earliest detectable stage. Serial chest x-rays should be supplemented by bronchoscopy.

The clinical presentation consists of a progressive cerebellar ataxia of the limbs, truncal ataxia, dysarthria of speech, dysphagia and signs of progressive bulbar involvement. Varying degrees of dementia, muscular weakness and peripheral neuropathy are seen within the spectrum of the disorder. Nystagmus is infrequent. The plantar responses are extensor in about a third of patients with subacute cerebellar degeneration.

Lumbar puncture will reveal a normal pressure and may show cellular reaction, elevation of the protein content and a mid-zone rise in the Lange curve. Pathologically the changes consist of loss of Purkinje cells, a thin molecular layer and loss of granular cells (Greenfield, 1954) (*Figure 1*). There is, in addition, degeneration in the spino-cerebellar and pyramidal tracts and the dorsal columns, perivascular infiltration and lymphocytic infiltration of the meninges.

The differential diagnosis in this progressive cerebellar syndrome is between metastatic deposits from primary carcinoma; an intrinsic tumour of the cerebellum, posterior fossa or brain stem; multiple sclerosis; chronic alcoholism; drug intoxication; myxoedema; late onset of spino-cerebellar degeneration or sporadic cerebellar degeneration; and progressive ischaemic damage to the brain stem and cerebellar connections in cerebrovascular disease affecting the vertebro-basilar system.

Encephalomyelitis

Malignancy may be associated with damage to brain stem structures and the spinal cord (Henson, Russell and Wilkinson, 1954; Henson,

Figure 1. Cerebellar degeneration with carcinoma of the breast. (a) Loss of Purkinje cells. Proliferation of Bergmann's astrocytes. Thinning of granular layer. Haematoxylin and Van Giesen (HVG) stain. (b) Loss of Purkinje cell and 'empty' baskets. Roger's impregnation. (c) Normal control. Purkinje cells surrounded by basket fibres. Glees' impregnation

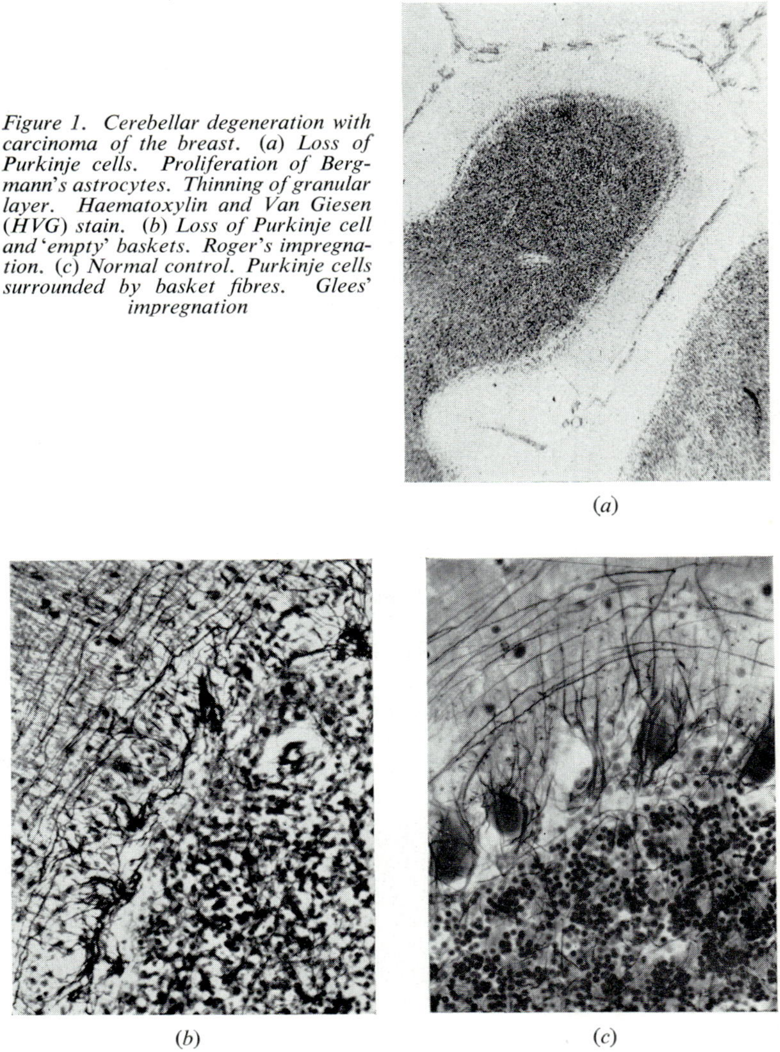

(*a*) (*b*) (*c*)

Lovell, Hoffman and Urich, 1965). The pathological findings consist of brain stem encephalitis, anterior horn cell damage and ganglio-radiculitis. Occasionally associated changes of limbic encephalitis are seen.

A spectrum of physical signs of varying severity results and can include ophthalmoplegia, gaze palsies, pupillary changes, bulbar palsy, cerebellar signs, and motor and sensory deficit in the limbs. An associated sensory neuropathy is not uncommon. A high incidence (80 per cent) of oat cell carcinoma of the bronchus is found in this group. The neurological disorder is steadily progressive over the course of 6–18 months, although spontaneous arrest may occur, particularly in those cases where there is an associated sensory neuropathy.

In the more rapidly progressive disease with severe brain stem damage, differentiation from secondary deposits and carcinomatous meningitis may be difficult. Alternative diagnoses which may require exclusion include multiple sclerosis, intrinsic neoplasms of the brain stem, brain stem infarction, encephalitis and progressive supranuclear palsy.

Necrotizing Myelopathy

Mancall and Rosales (1964) described two patients with bronchial carcinoma who developed flaccid paraplegia with sphincter paralysis and segmental loss of all modalities of sensation, and reviewed nine other cases from the literature. The destruction is acute in onset and rapid in evolution. Death usually occurs in a few days or weeks. Pathologically there is tissue necrosis of the grey and white matter of the cord, the thoracic cord being particularly vulnerable. The usual cause, however, of such an acute transverse cord lesion in the presence of carcinoma is spinal or extradural secondary deposits.

Motor Neurone Disease

A clinical picture of selective muscle weakness, atrophy and fasciculation with cortico-spinal signs, bulbar palsy and preservation of sensory pathways, often indistinguishable from classical motor neurone disease, may coexist with visceral carcinoma. Norris and Engel (1965) studied 130 consecutive hospitalized cases of amyotrophic lateral sclerosis and compared the incidence of cancer in these patients with a near-concurrent selected series of 200 adult stroke patients. Of those patients with motor neurone disease, 13 (10 per cent) had malignant disease, and in three the lesion was a bronchial carcinoma. Only two instances of malignancy were found in the stroke series (1 per cent).

Brain, Croft and Wilkinson (1965) studied 11 patients in whom a combined diagnosis of carcinoma and motor neurone disease had been made. The mean age at onset was 58 years for the neurological disorder. In five patients the site of malignancy was in the lung. The physical signs included in varying combination bulbar palsy, fasciculation in the tongue and upper limbs, weakness and wasting of the upper more commonly than the lower limbs, spasticity, increase or absence of reflexes, and extensor plantar responses. The pathological changes in two patients resembled those seen in motor neurone disease but were less marked than those commonly seen in the classical disease (*Figure 2*). In addition, changes were shown in the dorsal root ganglia and posterior columns. These authors concluded that motor neurone disease may on occasion be a manifestation of carcinomatous neuromyopathy and that, when it is, it may be atypical and more slowly progressive than classical motor neurone disease.

Where atypical features are found in the clinical presentation or natural history of motor neurone disease, a search for malignant disease is mandatory. Other disorders which may clinically mimic atypical motor neurone disease are cervical spondylosis, diabetic amyotrophy, and the neuroglycopenic signs of an insulin-secreting tumour of the pancreas. Cerebrospinal fluid examination is usually normal. Electrodiagnostic tests show the changes of chronic partial denervation; motor and sensory conduction velocities are within the normal range.

Sensory Neuropathy

A pure sensory neuropathy of the type described by Denny-Brown (1948) in association with malignancy is uncommon. It is more usual for evidence of neuromyopathy to coexist. Clinically, the neuropathy presents as a tingling in the extremities, or as a feeling of deadness of the toes and feet and later of the hands. This progresses to painful dysaesthesia in the limbs, with loss of tendon reflexes and with impairment and later loss of any or all modalities of sensation. Difficulty in walking and in using the hands and arms results, together with ataxia. Spontaneous remissions may occur, but the course of the disease is usually subacute and progressive or chronic. In addition to signs of peripheral neuropathy, muscle weakness and wasting, pyramidal signs and evidence of dementia

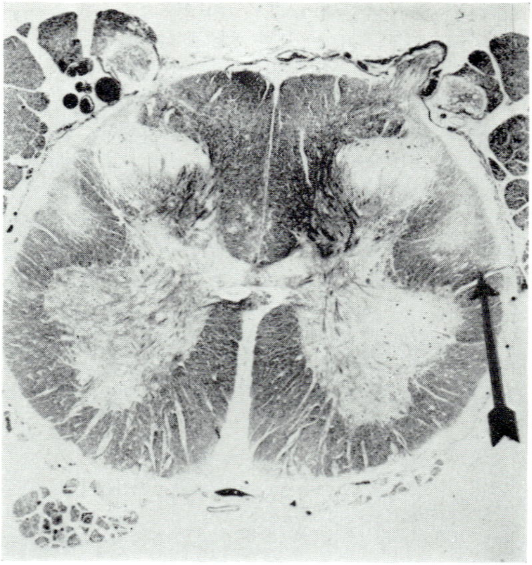

(*a*)

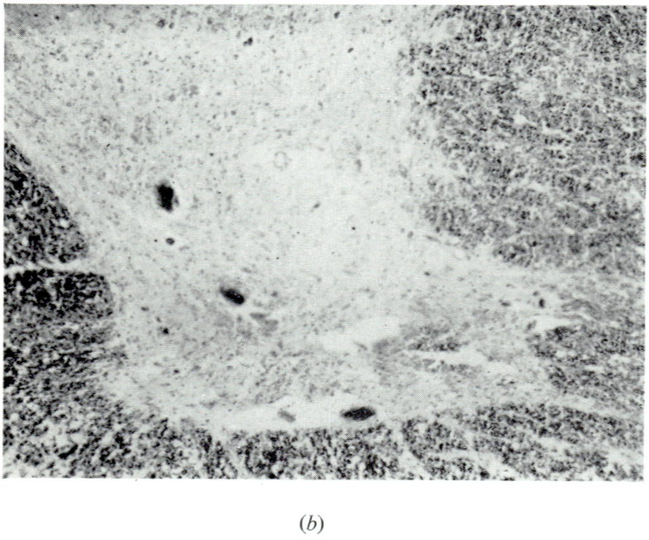

(*b*)

Figure 2. Motor neurone disease and carcinoma of the bronchus. (*a*) *Lumbar cord. Demyelination of pyramidal tracts (arrowed). Luxol fast blue (LFB) stain.* (*b*) *Thoracic cord. Complete loss of nervous in anterior horn. LFB stain*

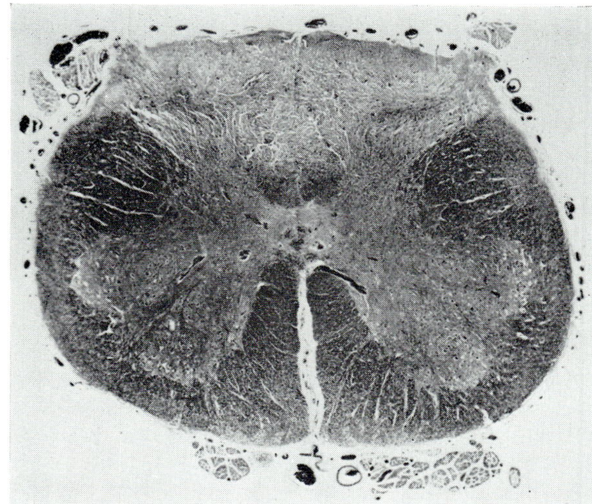

(*a*)

(*b*)

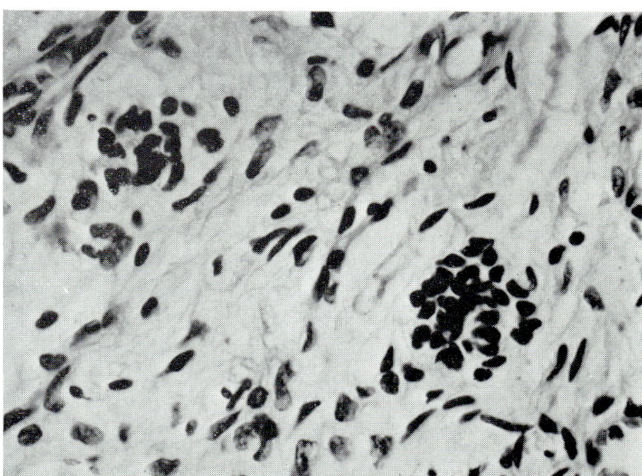

Figure 3. Sensory neuropathy and bronchogenic carcinoma. (a) Lumbar cord. Demyelination of dorsal columns. LFB stain. (b) Sensory ganglion. Loss of nervous. Neuronophagic nodules (residual nodules of Nageotte). Haematoxylin and eosin (HE) stain

are common. The lung is the site of the primary growth in 75 per cent of such cases.

The CSF protein is frequently raised, and circulating organ-specific antibodies reacting against whole human brain in complement fixation tests have been demonstrated (Wilkinson, 1964; Croft and colleagues, 1965). It has been suggested that the antibodies may arise in response to damage to the nervous system by a primary immunological mechanism. The pathological findings in the nervous system consist of Wallerian degeneration and neuronal loss in posterior root ganglia and degeneration in the peripheral nerves and dorsal columns (*Figure 3*). Scattered inflammatory lesions are also present in the brain and spinal cord.

When a sensory neuropathy is the presenting symptom, although other causes of sensory neuropathy such as diabetes mellitus, vitamin B_{12} deficiency, drugs, alcohol, uraemia, porphyria and connective tissue disorders must be excluded, the possibility of a coexisting or occult malignancy must be fully investigated. Where no cause is found, careful follow-up is essential.

NEUROMUSCULAR DISORDERS

In addition to generalized tissue and muscle wasting in chronic debilitating disease due to disuse of the limbs and cachexia, there exists in carcinoma, particularly carcinoma of the lung, a clearly defined syndrome of progressive symmetrical proximal muscle weakness and wasting. The muscles may also be tender, and those most prominently affected are the limb girdle and trunk muscles. The patient in the early stages complains of difficulty in rising from a low chair, and sometimes of difficulty in standing or climbing stairs and weakness on exertion. In the upper limbs there may be cramps and weakness on lifting, reaching or combing the hair. The muscle weakness may fluctuate, with clinical features suggestive of myasthenia in the absence of true myasthenia. Associated signs of neural involvement at other levels are often seen, such as ptosis, bulbar weakness, loss of reflexes and peripheral neuropathy. However, a pure muscular syndrome is seen in which there is primary muscle involvement without neural involvement, and it is then indistinguishable from polymyositis.

It has been known for many years that patients with polymyositis and dermatomyositis may harbour a carcinoma (Walton and Adams, 1958; Williams, 1959), and the incidence of carcinoma in dermatomyositis has been estimated as varying between 5 and

20 per cent. There have also been reports of the association of pulmonary neoplasms, particularly alveolar cell carcinoma, with progressive systemic sclerosis (Holt, 1961; Montgomery, Sterling and Hamer, 1964).

In addition to the primary muscle weakness and wasting of 'carcinomatous myopathy', patients who have a carcinoma secreting ACTH with Cushing's syndrome may present with myopathy similar to that seen in classical Cushing's disease. Muscle biopsy shows changes which are not specific but indicate a primary muscle disorder. There is loss of cross-striation with floccular, cloudy and granular changes and an increase in connective tissue. Inflammatory changes with muscle degeneration and regeneration are seen. Electromyography of affected muscles will confirm primary muscle involvement.

When proximal muscle disease is the presenting clinical problem, polymyositis in connective tissue disorders, thyrotoxic myopathy, diabetic amyotrophy and late onset myopathy may require elimination, but in older age groups carcinoma should be suspected. Shy and Silverstein (1965) estimated that 60 per cent of male patients over the age of 50 years with symptoms and signs of symmetrical proximal muscle weakness and wasting will be shown at investigation to have a systemic cancer.

Myasthenia

The occurrence of myasthenia with tumours of the lung was first observed by Anderson, Churchill-Davidson and Richardson in 1953. This led to speculation, subsequently not confirmed, that myasthenia gravis might have a higher incidence in association with carcinoma than in the general population. Henson, Russell and Wilkinson (1954) and Heathfield and Williams (1954), in studying this problem, showed that the clinical findings in these patients were not typical of myasthenia gravis. The clinical and electrophysiological characteristics of myasthenia in association with cancer were later studied in more detail by Lambert and co-workers (Lambert, Eaton and Rooke, 1956; Lambert and colleagues, 1961; Lambert, Okihiro and Rooke, 1965). Clear abnormality of neuromuscular transmission was shown in these patients, the majority of whom had an associated small cell carcinoma of the lung, usually unsuspected prior to the diagnosis of the neuromuscular syndrome.

The classical feature of this syndrome is increased fatigability of muscles, particularly the proximal and limb girdle muscles and those of the trunk. Additional symptoms of dryness of the mouth, blurring of vision, ptosis, diplopia, depressed or absent tendon reflexes, dysarthria, pains in the muscles and impotence are also described in association with the myasthenia. It is a rare syndrome, probably occurring in fewer than 1 per cent of patients with primary lung cancer and in about 6 per cent of those with small cell carcinoma.

The electrodiagnostic tests in this syndrome are diagnostic. These are a low-voltage muscle action potential elicited by a single supermaximal stimulation of the motor nerve with a progressive decline in amplitude of the muscle action potential at slow rates of repetitive stimulation of the motor nerves (2 per second), while at rapid rates of stimulation (50 per second) there is facilitation of the response leading to an increase in the voltage of muscle action potential. There is a paradoxical build-up in strength during the first phases of voluntary contraction.

These patients are unusually sensitive to neuromuscular blocking agents which can give rise to complications during anaesthesia, with prolonged muscle paralysis and respiratory paralysis. In patients with the myasthenic syndrome as opposed to myasthenia gravis, the response to anticholinergic drugs such as neostigmine and edrophonium is usually poor, although some benefit may be obtained. Some patients show a useful response to guanidine hydrochloride. It is suggested that defect in neuromuscular transmission is caused by interference in the release of acetylcholine at the presynaptic terminal.

CONCLUSION

Involvement of the central nervous system in patients with cancer of the bronchus usually implies secondary invasion of the nervous system. The presence of neurological signs may, however, represent damage to the nervous system which is not due to infiltration with malignant cells, but does indicate the simultaneous presence of a carcinoma.

The neurological signs can precede by months or years the clinical detection of the cancer, and this latent period should lead to intensive search for a primary tumour so that early effective treatment can be instituted. The commonest neurological signs which suggest an undisclosed cancer are loss of tendon reflexes, proximal muscle weakness and wasting, and intellectual deterioration with dementia, cerebellar ataxia or peripheral neuropathy.

When features suggestive of these syndromes are detected in a patient, careful and repeated examination and investigation are obligatory. Screening tests for malignancy should include chest x-rays, haematological investigations, serum proteins and electrophoresis, barium studies and bronchoscopy.

The aetiology of these syndromes is not yet known. Hypotheses which have received attention are that they are due to toxins released by the tumour, to secondary endocrine or metabolic effects on the nervous system, to nutritional deficiency or folate deprivation, to susceptibility to viral or fungal infections in affected patients, to virus infection or to a combination of virus infection and auto-immune disease.

At the present time there is no concrete or comprehensive explanation of the aetiology of the remote effects of cancer on the nervous system, nor of why the nervous system is selectively vulnerable in some patients with cancer and not in others.

ACKNOWLEDGEMENT

I wish to thank Professor W. Thomas Smith of the University of Birmingham for permission to publish his pathological photographs.

REFERENCES

Anderson, R. J., Churchill-Davidson, H. C. and Richardson, A. T. (1953). *Lancet* **2,** 1291.

Brain, W. R. and Adams, R. D. (1965). In *The Remote Effects of Cancer on the Nervous System*, Chapter XI, p. 216. Ed. by W. R. Brain and F. H. Norris. New York: Grune & Stratton.

— and Wilkinson, M. (1965). *Brain* **88,** 465.

— Croft, P. B. and Wilkinson, M. (1965). *Brain* **88,** 479.

Brouwer, B. and Biemond, A. (1938). *J. belge Neurol. Psychiat.* **38,** 691.

Corsellis, J. A. N., Goldberg, G. J. and Norton, A. R. (1968). *Brain* **91,** 481.

Croft, P. B. and Wilkinson, M. (1965). In *The Remote Effects of Cancer on the Nervous System*, Chapter VI, p. 44. Ed. by W. R. Brain and F. H. Norris. New York: Grune & Stratton.

— Henson, R. A., Urich, H. and Wilkinson, P. C. (1965). *Brain* **88,** 501.

Dayan, A. D., Croft, P. B. and Wilkinson, M. (1965). *Brain* **88,** 435.

Denny-Brown, D. (1948). *J. Neurol Neurosurg. Psychiat.* **11,** 73.

Greenfield, J. G. (1954). *The Spino-cerebellar Degenerations.* Oxford: Blackwell.

Heathfield, K. W. G. and Williams, J. R. B. (1954). *Brain* **77,** 122.

Henson, R. A., Lovell Hoffman, H. and Urich H. (1965). *Brain* **88,** 449.

— Russell, D. S. and Wilkinson, M. I. P. (1954). *Brain* **77,** 82.

Holt, G. W. (1961). *Am. J. med. Sci.* **242,** 93.

Lambert, E. H., Eaton, L. M. and Rooke, E. D. (1956). *Am. J. Physiol.* **187,** 612.

— Okihiro, M. and Rooke, E. D. (1965). In *Muscle*, ed. by W. M. Paul, E. E. Daniel, C. M. Kay and G. Monckton. Oxford and New York: Pergamon.

— Rooke, E. D., Eaton, L. M. and Hodgson, C. H. (1961). In *Myasthenia Gravis*, ed. by H. R. Viets. Springfield, Ill.: Thomas.

Mancall, E. L. and Rosales, R. K. (1964). *Brain* **87,** 639.

Montgomery, R. D., Sterling, G. A. and Hamer, N. A. J. (1964). *Lancet* **1,** 586.

Norris, F. H. and Engel, W. K. (1965). In *The Remote Effects of Cancer on the Nervous System*, Chapter IV, p. 25. Ed. by W. R. Brain and F. H. Norris. New York: Grune & Stratton.

Richardson, E. P. (1965). In *The Remote Effects of Cancer on the Nervous System*, Chapter II, p. 6. Ed. by W. R. Brain and F. H. Norris. New York: Grune & Stratton.

Shy, G. M. and Silverstein, I. (1965). *Brain* **88,** 515.

Walton, J. N. and Adams, R. D. (1958). *Polymyositis.* Baltimore: Williams & Wilkins.

Wilkinson, P. C. (1964). *Lancet* **1,** 1301.

Williams, R. C. (1959). *Ann. intern. Med.* **50,** 1174.

Wilner, E. C. and Brody, J. A. (1968). *Neurology, Minneap.* **18,** 11, 1120.

8—*The Place of Surgery in the Treatment of Carcinoma of the Bronchus*

W. P. Cleland

The surgical extirpation of a primary lung cancer with the associated lymph nodes remains the treatment of choice when elimination of the disease and long-term survival are contemplated. The requisite operation can be performed at the present time in suitable centres with an operative mortality of less than 10 per cent. Follow-up statistics from many centres indicate a five-year survival rate of 25–30 per cent. Such figures can be obtained only by careful selection of the patients being accepted for surgery and by meticulous attention to the many details of management. Regrettably, suitability for surgical exploration is limited to a minority of sufferers from the disease, and probably fewer than 20 per cent of all sufferers are deemed suitable after assessment.

HISTORICAL SURVEY

Early surgical endeavour involved the use of pneumonectomy even for peripheral circumscribed lesions in one lobe. At this time survival of the patient was of paramount importance and every endeavour was being made to reduce operative mortality, without too much concern for the quality of survival.

With the evolution of thoracic surgery following the introduction of antibiotics, the development of safe anaesthesia for thoracic surgery, improvements in blood transfusion techniques and a better understanding of post-operative care, operative mortality gradually fell to acceptable levels and attention was focused more and more on the disease and its local manifestations.

Extensive anatomical and histological studies by Nohl (1956) and others mapped out the expected extensions of the disease originating in different portions of the lung. They demonstrated the spread of infection in mediastinal nodes from one side to the other in a significant number of patients, and also showed that in upper lobe disease the lower lobes were often completely unaffected.

Safe surgery brought with it a realization that total lung removal was not always necessary, and that often it was possible to perform a good radical operation and yet preserve part of the lung on the operated side. Such physiological conservation widened the indications appreciably. A further step forward was introduced by Price Thomas (1956) with the operation of sleeve resection, a procedure again aimed at conserving useful lung tissue.

At the present time, radical surgery aims at removing the primary lung lesion and the associated lymph nodes in the lung hilum and the mediastinum, while at the same time conserving as much functioning lung tissue as possible on the affected side.

Various attempts have been made to improve the results of surgery by combining it with other forms of therapy. Pre-operative irradiation and chemotherapy have both been employed, but results have not been materially affected (Bromley and Szur, 1955).

Recently considerable attention has been paid to the histological type of the lesion in assessing suitability for surgical treatment. The best long-term results have been obtained in squamous carcinomas, and the worst in the 'oat-celled' type and in undifferentiated tumours generally. A comprehensive survey and comparison between patients treated by surgery or radiotherapy with oat-celled carcinomas was recently carried out by the Medical Research Council (Miller, Fox and Tall, 1969). The results in terms of survival at two years were extremely poor in both series, with the radiotherapy patients slightly the better overall, these having avoided the consequences of a major surgical adventure. Clearly account must be taken in future of the histological type in assessing suitability for surgical treatment. It should be emphasized, however, that bronchial biopsies are notoriously difficult to assess histologically and do not always reflect the character of the greater part of the tumour, and reports must therefore be interpreted with caution.

Perhaps more important even than histological type is the general behaviour of the tumour, particularly its rate of growth. Generally the more slowly growing tumours give better survival rates whatever form of therapy is employed. Unfortunately it is rarely possible to keep a lesion under observation long enough to make this assessment.

THE SURGICAL PROCEDURES

Radical Operations

In radical operations, the aim is to remove the whole of the primary tumour in the lung and the lymph nodes liable to be involved and at the same time to preserve as much uninvolved lung as possible.

When patients are accepted for surgery, it is assumed that they are accepted for radical resection, and only if the latter should prove impossible at thoracotomy will a palliative resection be performed. Only rarely are patients deliberately accepted for a palliative resection, a classical example being a patient with a breaking-down lesion with much infected sputum or persistent bleeding.

On opening the chest at thoracotomy, a careful assessment of the lesion is made with the minimum of disturbance to the lung. The size, site and distribution of the primary are noted and extensions into the mediastinum, pericardium or chest wall are excluded. The paratracheal and subcarinal lymph nodes are palpated to exclude involvement. If total removal seems practicable, the first step is to secure and occlude the relevant pulmonary vein in order to reduce the chances of dislodging tumour emboli during mobilization of the lung. If radical removal is not practicable, a decision will have to be made between palliative resection and abandonment of the operation.

Ideally the primary tumour and the lymph nodes in the mediastinum should be removed in one piece (Brock and Whytehead, 1955). However, this is often difficult to achieve, and most surgeons remove the lung lesion initially and then do a block dissection of the mediastinum. Radical resection can be carried out with removal of the whole lung or of a lobe with or without sleeve resection of the stem bronchus. Lesser (segmental) resections are unlikely to result in extirpation of the lesion, although in exceptional circumstances they may be indicated.

Palliative Resections

These are rarely embarked on as deliberate policy, although they are occasionally indicated for the removal of a grossly infected lung or a lesion producing severe or repeated bleeding.

They are usually performed on patients thought to have a removable tumour when it is found at thoracotomy that the whole lesion cannot be removed. The usual cause is infiltration of some vital structure (for example, the aorta, vena cava or oesophagus), sometimes by mediastinal lymph node involvement. Opinion is divided about the wisest course to be adopted in such instances. Abbey Smith (1957) has for long advocated an aggressive policy and attempts a resection in the vast majority of patients. He maintains that a worthwhile result—that is, a reasonable span of life and relief of disabling symptoms—is obtained in most of such cases. Other surgeons will not attempt resection unless the way seems clear to doing a radical excision. This is largely a matter for individual surgical decision. The removal rate in any series will vary from 80 to nearly 100 per cent, depending on the attitude of the surgeon.

Palliative resections can be supplemented by radiotherapy postoperatively, or radioactive gold grains can be inserted into residual tumour at the time of thoracotomy.

A special indication for palliative surgery exists where there is limited invasion of the chest wall, especially in the region of the apex of the chest—the so-called Pancoast syndrome. Here experience has shown that the patient may suffer considerable pain over many months, and there seems to be every justification for a radical excision of the invaded chest wall. Although long-term survival figures are not an encouraging feature, the relief of pain resulting from nerve excision has often been very gratifying.

ASSESSMENT OF SUITABILITY FOR SURGERY

It has already been emphasized that the aim of surgical treatment should be the removal of the primary lesion and the associated lymph node bed without leaving the patient crippled. The object of preoperative investigation is to determine whether such a course is likely to be possible. Investigations are designed to indicate (1) whether the primary tumour has involved important adjacent organs or tissues; (2) whether the primary tumour has spread to distant sites; (3) the condition of the patient's cardio-respiratory reserve.

To elucidate these matters, some or all of the following inquiries, tests or investigations will be employed.

The History

Apart from the routine account of the patient's symptoms, answers should be sought to the following direct questions:

(1) Have there been any headaches or abnormalities of behaviour, suggesting cerebral secondaries?

(2) Has there been fixed or constant chest wall pain, suggesting invasion of the chest wall?

(3) Has there been any constant skeletal pain, suggesting bone secondaries?

(4) Has there been any difficulty in swallowing, suggesting oesophageal involvement?

Direct questioning should also provide valuable information about the patient's respiratory reserve, and a careful assessment should be made of his reactions to the efforts of everyday life such as going upstairs, walking on the flat or up inclines, and running.

Clinical Examination

This should pay special attention to the neck for enlarged nodes, to the abdomen for liver enlargement, and to the skin and the skeleton for signs of secondaries. Special attention should also be paid to chest wall movements on respiration and to signs suggesting chronic bronchitis or emphysema.

Radiological Examinations

These play a very important part in the assessment of the extent of the lesion and possible extensions. The importance of special views, and the value of both antero-posterior and lateral tomography of the hilar region and the mediastinum, are fully discussed in Chapter 5.

Bronchography usually has little part to play in assessment of a proven lesion, but is often invaluable in providing information about doubtful conditions.

Bronchoscopy

This examination not only provides evidence of diagnostic value and enables biopsies to be taken for histology, but will show the precise location of the tumour and indicate the type of resection which will be necessary. Paralysis of the vocal cord, widening of the carina, and generalized rigidity of the trachea and main bronchi are features suggesting inoperability.

Lung Function Tests

Overall function can usually be fairly accurately assessed by talking to the patient about his capabilities and watching his performance in the ward and on the stairs. A poorly mobile chest and bronchitic signs in the opposite or good lung call for a careful appraisal. When in doubt, lung function studies can be carried out. The chief value of routine studies lies in their provision of evidence of airway obstruction and its potential relief by isoprenaline. The vital capacity and forced expiratory volumes in one second before and after the inhalation of isoprenaline supply the evidence. Beyond this, highly sophisticated differential studies are required, and these are rarely justified.

When there is doubt, a period of treatment with physiotherapy, bronchodilators and possibly antibiotics, followed by reassessment, may be of value.

Scalene Node Biopsy and Mediastinoscopy

The presence of a palpable supraclavicular node or of paratracheal swelling demands these investigations to determine whether there are involved nodes. Should a positive node be found, then clearly complete excision of all the tumour at thoracotomy will be unlikely and other forms of treatment are advisable.

Routine scalene node biopsy and mediastinoscopy are advised by some surgeons on the grounds that if involved nodes are found, thoracotomy will be avoided (Pearson and Kergin, 1965). Others believe that only clinically or radiologically enlarged nodes should be so investigated, on the basis that minor involvement of paratracheal nodes can be dealt with by mediastinal block dissection and does not necessarily render the condition inoperable. This is the view taken by the author, a view supported by well-documented long-term (five-year) survival after the resection of involved paratracheal nodes. The histology of the tumour will influence decisions significantly, the less favourable prospects being in oat cell or undifferentiated lesions.

Liver Scanning

Secondaries in the liver occur relatively frequently and are difficult to detect. Until recently the only reliable way to exclude involvement of the liver was by laparotomy. However, the introduction of liver scanning or coeliac axis arteriograms now enables the clinician to detect solitary or multiple metastases with reasonable certainty if they are of moderate size. Routine liver scanning may occasionally reveal unsuspected deposits, but regular use of this procedure is hardly justified at present.

CONTRA-INDICATIONS TO OPERATION

The following are generally regarded as contra-indications to an exploratory thoracotomy.

(1) Spread of the primary tumour with involvement of the chest wall, trachea, oesophagus, superior vena cava, or phrenic or recurrent laryngeal nerves.

(2) Proven involvement of mediastinal or supraclavicular lymph nodes.

(3) Distal blood-borne metastases, especially in the brain, bone, liver, suprarenals and skin.

(4) Invasion of the pleura or the chest wall as indicated by persistent blood-stained pleural effusions, fixed chest pain, or erosion of ribs.

(5) Severe limitation of respiratory reserve, suggesting that lung resection would leave the patient a respiratory cripple.

(6) Age is a less important factor than general condition in assessing operability; as a general rule, patients over the age of 65 are poor subjects for pneumonectomy, but many patients over 70 have survived a lobectomy without distress.

THE PANCOAST SYNDROME

This lesion is essentially caused by a carcinoma arising in the apical portion of the lung. The tumour differs in no essential way from a peripheral carcinoma, but owing to the frequent occurrence of adhesions between the apex and the chest wall (the aftermath of old tuberculous disease) the tumour can fairly rapidly invade the adhesions and involve the surrounding structures. Those involved are the brachial plexus (giving rise to pain along the medial side of the arm and forearm and weakness and wasting of the small muscles of the hand), the sympathetic chain and stellate ganglion (causing Horner's syndrome), and erosion of the upper ribs and vertebral bodies.

The tumours are frequently squamous cell in type and only slowly progressive. Invasion of bone and nerve produces intolerable pain. Treatment is difficult and radiotherapy has proved disappointing. Even though the chest wall is already invaded, a radical surgical approach seems justified if only for the relief of pain. At operation the lung lesion is excised together with a block of the upper involved ribs and adjacent vertebral processes. The sheath of the subclavian vessels should be removed, and if the lower root of the brachial plexus is involved, it is wise to excise this since the resulting disability is often surprisingly little. The remaining tissue bed can then be injected with radioactive gold grains, or post-operative irradiation can be given if residual tumour remains (*Figures 1* and *2*).

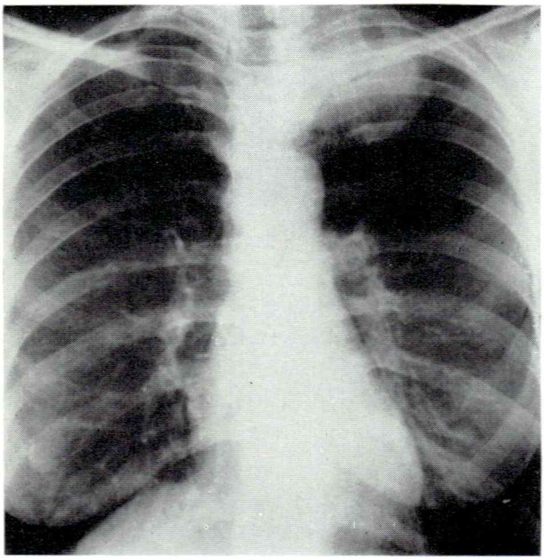

Figure 1. Pancoast tumour at left apex in November 1962. Treated by lobectomy and excision of involved chest wall and vertebral processes

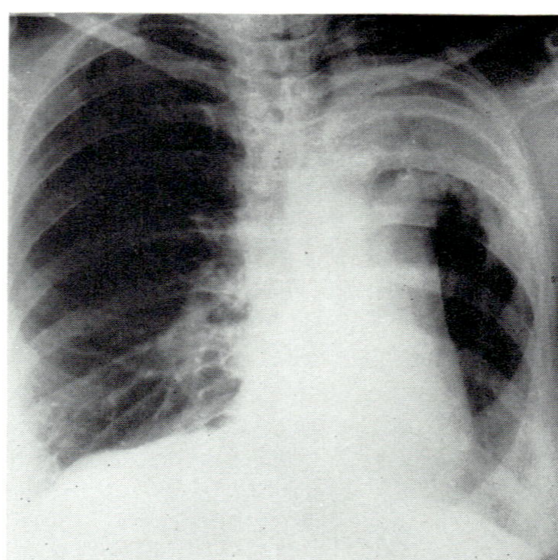

Figure 2. Same patient in May 1969, when she was fit and well and free from pain

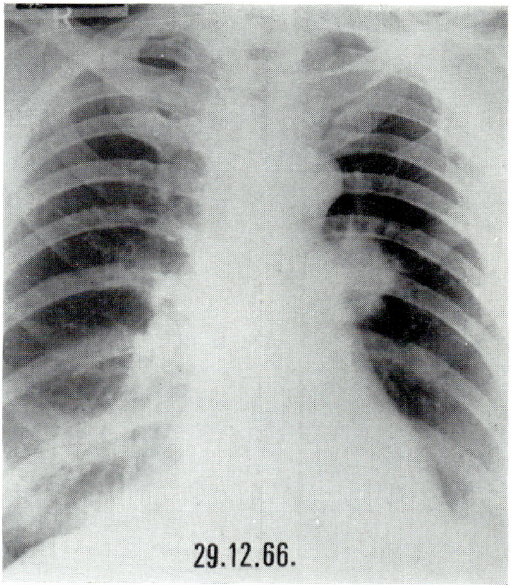

Figure 3. Tumour in hilum of left lung, found inoperable at thoracotomy

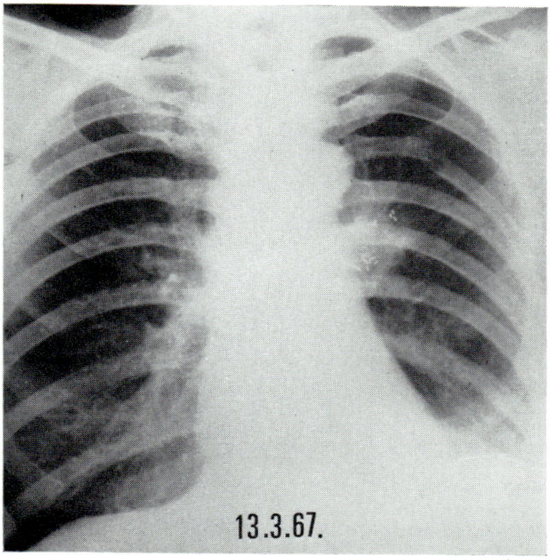

Figure 4. Gold grains distributed throughout tumour at thoracotomy

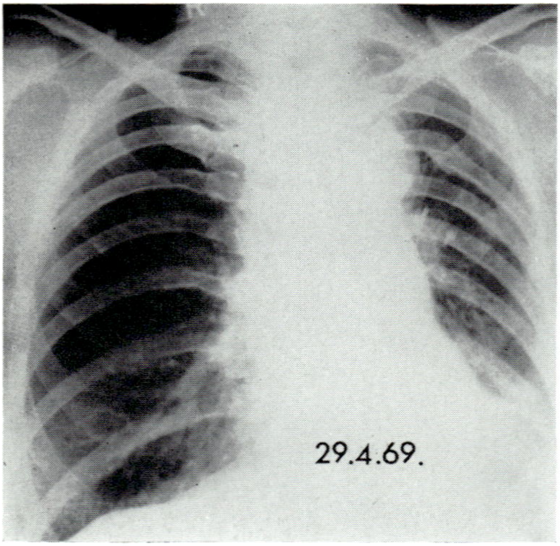

Figure 5. Same patient two years after thoracotomy and interstitial irradiation. There has been some contraction of the left lung; the patient is clinically well and free from tumour

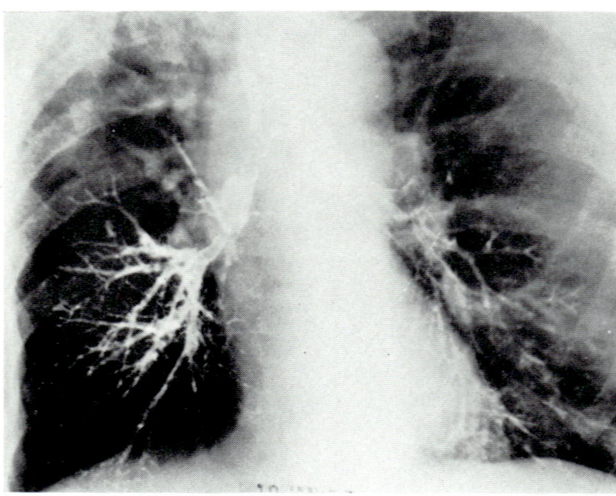

Figure 6. Carcinoma of right main bronchus involving lower end of trachea. Treated by bronchoscopic insertion of gold grains supplemented by external irradiation (January 1957)

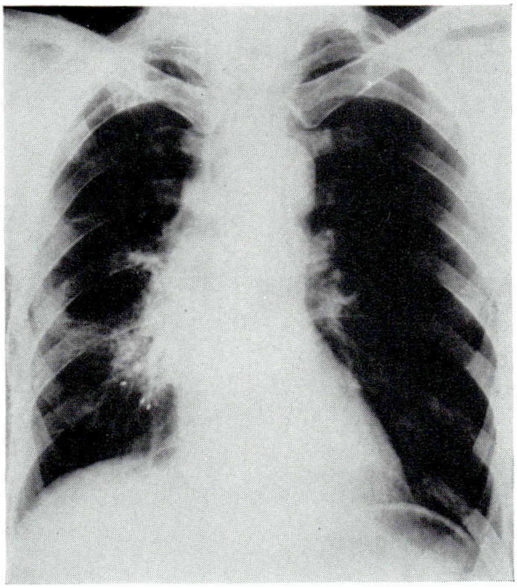

(*a*)

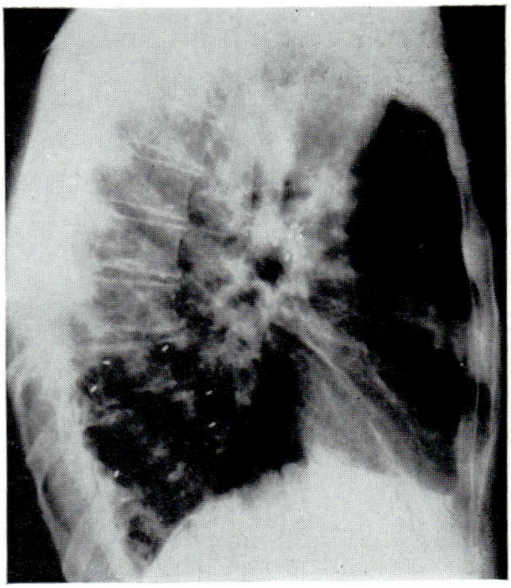

(*b*)

Figure 7a and b. Postero-anterior and right lateral radiographs of same patient 15 months after irradiation (May 1958). The tumour recurred, however, and the patient died two years after treatment

Although survival after this heroic procedure is often not prolonged, relief of the severe pain is often gratifying and alone justifies the procedure.

INTERSTITIAL IRRADIATION

Patients found to be inoperable at thoracotomy or in whom only incomplete removal of tumour is possible can often be helped by insertion of the isotope of gold ^{198}Au. This is delivered in the form of small gold rods (grains), covered with platinum, which have been activated by exposure in an atomic pile. The half-life of the activated gold is about 2·7 days. Grains placed at 1 cm intervals in a tumour will give a tumour dose of about 5,000 r units. The grains are provided in cartridges containing 14 units and are injected into the tumour with a special gun and needle. Tumours up to 5–6 cm in diameter (*Figures 3*, *4* and *5*) or the equivalent size in plaques can be successfully treated by this means, but larger tumours are less effectively managed. Special long needles are available for injecting grains into intrabronchial tumours at bronchoscopy (*Figures 6* and *7*).

Worthwhile palliation has been achieved in a significant number of patients (Johnston, Cleland and Howard, 1961), and experience subsequent to this report is still favourable (Gibbons and Baker, 1969). The technique has the advantage of applying a full tumour dose just where it is needed at one time and with few of the systemic side effects usually associated with radical radiotherapy. Inadequate interstitial irradiation can be supplemented by external irradiation if necessary.

REFERENCES

Abbey Smith, R. (1957). 'The results of raising the resectability rate in operations for lung carcinoma.' *Thorax* **12,** 79.

Brock, Sir Russell and Whytehead, L. L. (1955). 'Radical pneumonectomy for bronchial carcinoma.' *Br. J. Surg.* **43,** 8.

Bromley, L. L. and Szur, L. (1955). 'Combined radiotherapy and resection for carcinoma of the bronchus: experience with 66 patients.' *Lancet* **2,** 937.

Gibbons, J. R. P. and Baker, R. (1969). 'Treatment of carcinoma of the bronchus by interstitial irradiation.' *Thorax* **24,** 451.

Johnston, J. B., Cleland, W. P. and Howard, N. (1961). 'Treatment of carcinoma of the bronchus by interstitial irradiation.' *J. thorac. cardiovasc. Surg.* **42,** 527.

REFERENCES

Miller, A. B., Fox, W. and Tall, R. (1969). 'Five-year follow-up of the Medical Research Council comparative trial of surgery and radiotherapy for the primary treatment of small-celled or oat-celled carcinoma of the bronchus.' *Lancet* **2,** 501.

Nohl, H. C. (1956). 'An investigation into the lymphatic and vascular spread of carcinoma of the bronchus.' *Thorax* **11,** 172.

Pearson, F. G. and Kergin, F. G. (1965). 'Mediastinoscopy: a method of biopsy in the superior mediastinum.' *J. thorac. cardiovasc. Surg.* **49,** 527.

Price Thomas, Sir Clement (1956). 'Conservative resection of the bronchial tree.' *Jl R. Coll. Surg. Edinb.* **1,** 169.

9—Surgery and Radiotherapy

I—Pre-operative Radiotherpay

A. H. W. Nias

The three methods of treating lung cancer have been surgery, radiotherapy and chemotherapy. Until recently each of these has been used independently with no particular plan. Combinations of two or all three of these methods may be advantageous if a rationale can be shown to exist. Pre-operative radiotherapy is one such planned combination—radiotherapy, then surgery. The rationale for this combination is discussed below, together with experimental evidence which suggests that there is a basis for clinical trials in the right circumstances. Under laboratory conditions it is comparatively easy to design experiments which avoid confusion by factors, such as heterogeneity of populations and ethical considerations, which are inherent in clinical trials. It is therefore important to consider the clinical aspects of pre-operative radiotherapy first. The circumstances must be defined in which a clinical trial may both be useful to the patient and provide a meaningful result. Having defined these circumstances, one can then consider those radiobiological aspects which are relevant.

CLINICAL ASPECTS

The clinical evidence was reviewed by Glicksman (1965), who concluded that there were good arguments for 'properly designed prospective clinical trials' of pre-operative irradiation when certain circumstances applied. He stated: 'Combined radiation and surgery should not be considered if the patient has distant metastases or has a very small primary lesion with no regional nodes. The situation optimal for combined treatment is that in which the patient has neither a very high nor a very low probability of survival. In the former instance it is not necessary. In the latter it is not sufficient.'

There are four basic assumptions that will be made. The first follows from Glicksman's conclusion: we have to assume, when considering pre-operative irradiation of a particular tumour, that neither radical surgery nor radical radiotherapy is curative on its own, although the tumour is operable.

Secondly, we have to assume that a significant clinical problem arises from cells disseminated at the time of operation. From this it follows that local recurrence at the operation site and/or metastases occurring at the time of operation must present an important problem in the long-term management of the patient.

The third assumption is that cancer cells disseminated both locally and distantly at the time of operation are oxygenated and fully radiosensitive. This assumption follows from the knowledge that anoxic cells occur in the tumour *substance* rather than at the periphery (Thomlinson and Gray, 1955). Unless the surgeon cuts through the tumour, he can only disseminate cells *locally* by spill from the peripheral region and *distantly* by vascular spread from the substance of the tumour. Vascular spread will concern cells lying close to vessels, and such cells will be oxygenated.

The fourth assumption concerns the growth rate of tumours. Although we have all too little information about the kinetics of tumour cell populations, we must assume the most pessimistic value, that is, that cells may divide daily. At this rate single cells could grow into macroscopic tumours within one month (10^9 cells, weighing 1 g and measuring 1 cm in diameter). Such tumours may already contain anoxic cells; if a tumour is large enough to be palpable, it contains these. Suit and Maeda (1966) have demonstrated anoxic cells in tumours as small as 1 mm in diameter.

HIGH VERSUS LOW DOSAGE

The biological basis of pre-operative radiotherapy has been demonstrated by W. E. Powers and his collaborators, using both laboratory and clinical studies. In a recent review (Powers and Palmer, 1968), the two alternatives of high and low radiation dosage were contrasted. High dosage may be indicated in situations where an extensive tumour involves vital structures. With such high dosage (approaching the maximum tolerance dose) there is a greater incidence of operative complications (even when operation is delayed), but this was thought to be acceptable in those cases where there was a low chance of cure.

The first alternative, high dosage pre-operative radiotherapy, was chosen by Bloedorn and colleagues (1961). They reviewed the natural history of bronchogenic carcinoma and estimated that of the patients first seen in any clinic, 30 per cent will already have distant metastases (although these are not always clinically evident when the patient is first examined). Another 30 per cent will have mediastinal lymph node metastases, and a further 15 per cent will develop metastases in the scalene, supraclavicular or neck lymph nodes. In another 15 per cent the disease is locally so advanced as to preclude surgery. The authors deducted 5 per cent for the patients who die due to operative and post-operative complications. This left only 5 per cent of the patients as being potentially curable, a figure which equalled the cure rate obtained by surgery in any large series at that time.

Bloedorn and his co-workers assumed that high dosage pre-operative radiotherapy would sterilize half of the local extensions of the primary tumour together with half the mediastinal, scalene and supraclavicular lymph node metastases. On this assumption the potential cure rate would rise by 30 per cent, but they deducted 15 per cent from this because some patients develop metastases while under treatment. Even so, the net effect of their assumptions was a potential cure rate of 20 per cent, and they presented some preliminary results to support this optimistic approach. These were selected patients, however, and not part of a controlled trial.

The hypothesis has since been tested in a random trial (Collaborative Study, 1969) organized by the Committee for Radiation Therapy Studies established by the National Cancer Institute, United States Public Health Service. This trial included a series of 568 patients with lesions considered operable at the time of diagnosis. These were randomized, half receiving immediate surgery and the other half receiving a full course of radiotherapy followed by surgery up to eight weeks later. There was no significant difference between the survival rates of the two groups at three years. Surgical complications were more frequent in the group given pre-operative radiotherapy. It was concluded that, although differences in survival might still appear when the patients had been followed up for a longer period, this random trial indicated that a substantial part of the favourable results reported in non-randomized studies must be accounted for by the selection of patients.

If high dosage pre-operative radiotherapy is not effective in the treatment of carcinoma of the bronchus, it might be reasonable to doubt whether there is any place for the second alternative using low dosage, but here the rationale is different. The irradiation is not intended to be curative on its own, but only to reduce the proportion of cancer cells which may survive dissemination at the time of operation. Because of the smaller dosage, operative complications are negligible and there need be no delay before surgery. This regimen is suitable for those potentially curable patients in whom local recurrence and/or freshly disseminated metastases lead to a significant degree of morbidity and mortality.

Malignant cells are undoubtedly disseminated at the time of operation (Cole and colleagues, 1961), and contamination of the operative site has been shown to be associated with an increase in local recurrence and distant metastases, together with a higher death rate (Smith, Thomas and Hilberg, 1958). It may be that an unfavourable biochemical environment and/or an active immunological response prevents the growth of many disseminated cancer cells. Until there is more evidence for such rejection mechanisms, however, the most pessimistic assumption is required: namely, that every single cancer cell is capable of growth into a lethal tumour. The problem is how to destroy those cells disseminated at operation.

Dose–Response Curves

Recent radiobiological studies have shown a phenomenon that is common to cells from all types of tissue. This is the exponential dose–response relationship whereby a linear increase in radiation dosage is associated with a logarithmic increase in the probability of cell sterilization. This relationship is illustrated in *Figure 1*, where HeLa cells (derived from human carcinoma of the cervix) were irradiated either in air or in nitrogen (Nias and colleagues, 1967). After an initial shoulder, both the cell survival curves follow an exponential slope, but the slope for cells irradiated in nitrogen is less steep. These curves illustrate the importance of assuming that cells disseminated at the time of operation are oxygenated. A single dose of 500 rads reduces the surviving fraction to 10 per cent with oxygenated cells, but only to 50 per cent with anoxic cells.

While this phenomenon has most often been demonstrated with tissue cultures *in vitro*, the same sort of dose–response curves are obtainable *in vivo*. *Figure 2* is an example where L1210 leukaemia cells irradiated in the bone marrow of $DBA/_2$ mice have been assayed for the survival of their ability to form colonies in the spleens of recipient mice. A single dose of gamma rays as low as 500 rads reduces the surviving fraction to 2 per cent in this case. The various cell types from bronchogenic carcinoma have not been studied in this way, but there is no reason to suppose that their radiation

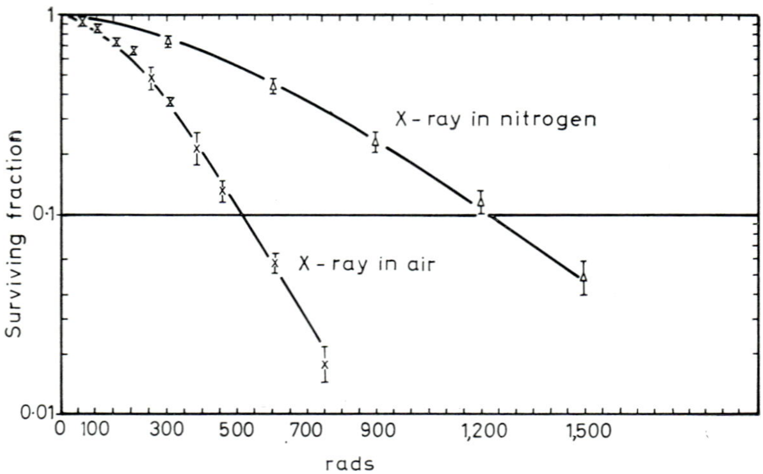

Figure 1 (above). Survival curves of HeLa cells irradiated in vitro. ×, *x-rays in air;* △, *x-rays in nitrogen. (Reproduced from Nias and colleagues, 1967, by courtesy of the Editor of* International Journal of Radiation Biology)

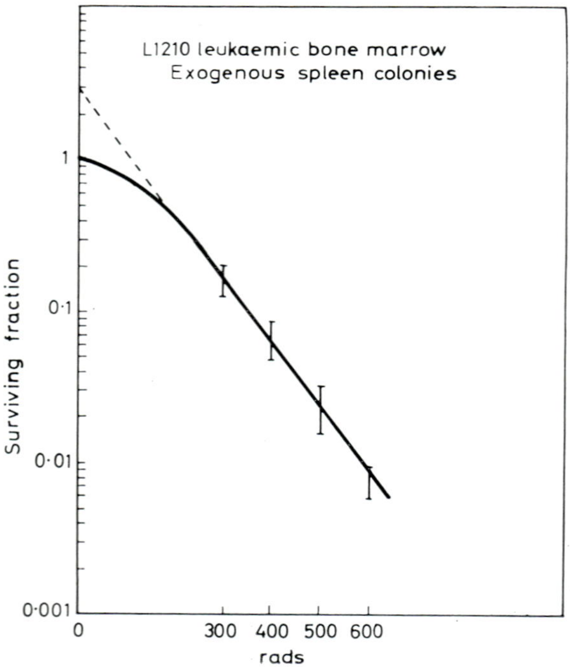

Figure 2. Survival curve of L1210 leukaemic bone marrow cells gamma-irradiated in vivo *and assayed in recipient mice*

dose–response curves would lie outside the general range, which shows a relatively narrow spread of radiosensitivity as far as single cell survival is concerned, both *in vitro* and *in vivo* (Whitmore and Till, 1964).

The implication of such exponential dose–response curves is that a large single dose of radiation would be required to sterilize *all* the cells in a small bronchogenic carcinoma (for example, more than 3,000 rads for a 4 cm diameter tumour containing 10^{10} cells). On the other hand, a much smaller single dose in the range 500–1,000 rads will still reduce the probability of survival of the majority of the cancer cells. The question of dose level is completely different when the irradiation is not intended to be curative on its own but is only the first step in a plan of treatment of the carcinoma by radiotherapy followed by surgery.

LOW DOSE PRE-OPERATIVE RADIOTHERAPY

With this plan, the dose level will now represent a compromise between the lowest that will sterilize a useful proportion of the cells that may be disseminated at the time of operation and the highest that will allow immediate surgery without operative complications. Three questions must be posed, therefore, when deciding whether this plan of low dose pre-operative radiotherapy merits clinical trial:

(1) What is the lowest 'useful' dose?

(2) What is the highest 'safe' dose?

(3) Is there any evidence that such a dose will influence the survival of patients who undergo surgery?

Clinical data should ideally be used to answer these questions but, in general, laboratory investigations provide the only reliable data. The relevant data are reviewed below.

Lowest 'Useful' Dose

The lowest 'useful' dose is one that reduces the surviving fraction of the tumour cell population by a significant amount. If the sort of survival curve shown in *Figure 1* is relevant to this situation, then 500 rads will be the minimum dose, assuming that the cells are oxygenated. Such a single dose of 500 rads will reduce the surviving fraction of disseminated cells by at least 90 per cent, while with a dose of 1,000 rads the fraction will be reduced by at least 99 per cent. If a corresponding reduction were to be obtained in mortality from local recurrence and/or from those metastases which are freshly disseminated at operation, then this dose range of 500–1,000 rads would be said to be 'useful'.

In some clinical trials of pre-operative radiotherapy, the dose has been delivered in several fractions spaced over several days. This was the method used by Strong and colleagues (1966) in their controlled clinical trial of pre-operative radiotherapy before block dissection of cervical lymph nodes (which showed a significant reduction in the incidence of cervical recurrence). They delivered five daily doses of 400 rads—that is, a total dose of 2,000 rads. This dosage is neither high nor low in the present context; with high dosage, fractionation is known to be essential if the radiation is to be tolerated by the normal tissues and surgical complications are to be avoided.

With the low dosage plan these problems may be negligible. Feder, Blair and Close (1965) have used a mouse tumour system to show that there is no advantage to be gained by fractionation. Indeed, there is a positive advantage in delivering a low dose of pre-operative radiation in one session followed immediately by surgery. If the most is to be made of the moderate degree of cell sterilization, surgery is desirable before there has been time for the small proportion of surviving cells to repopulate the tumour. Furthermore, cells disseminated immediately after irradiation will possess the minimum chance of viability, and this is another reason why it may be important to allow a minimum of delay between irradiation and operation.

Highest 'Safe' Dose

If the smallest 'useful' dose is 500–1,000 rads delivered in one session, what is the highest 'safe' dose? This will be a dose which can immediately be followed by surgery without complications. The main complication to be considered is delay in wound healing, and this has been studied by Powers, Ogura and Palmer (1967). They reported a clinical series of 214 patients, but as these were not randomized among the various pre-operative dose levels and as there was no control group, no conclusion can be reached. They also reported an experimental series of mice, however, and although it may be misleading to extrapolate from such animal data, the results are statistically valid.

They studied groups of C_3H mice which received various single doses of irradiation (0, 1,000, 2,000, 3,000 or 4,000 rads) to the flank. An elliptical piece of skin was then excised from the irradiated area and the wound was sutured. All the animals were checked daily for completion of wound healing as manifested by complete closure of the defect. There was no delay in wound healing after a single pre-operative dose of 1,000 rads. With increasing doses of radiation, however, there was increasing delay, although this could be reduced if surgery was performed either the same day or 15 days after irradiation. Although these are mouse data, it can be concluded that a single pre-operative dose as high as 1,000 rads is 'safe'.

Experimental Evidence

If a pre-operative dose of 500–1,000 rads is both 'useful' and 'safe', the important question is whether there is any evidence that such a dose will influence the survival of patients who undergo surgery. Clinical data should ideally be used to answer this question, but none is available where the low dose plan was used. A dose of 3,000 rads was the lowest pre-operative dose quoted by Deeley (1967) in his review of the treatment of carcinoma of the bronchus. Once again, laboratory investigations provide the only reliable data and very few of these are strictly relevant to the question.

In the absence of a controlled clinical trial, a large series of spontaneous animal tumours might permit a scientific assessment of the plan. That is not practicable either and transplanted tumours must be used instead, although with the advantage of a uniform series of experimental animals and a uniform tumour size at the time of operation. Agostino and Nickson (1960) implanted Walker tumour into the caecal appendix of 200 female Wistar rats in order to simulate carcinoma of the colon. After two weeks half the animals were given pre-operative irradiation, equivalent to 500 rads, and all the animals were then submitted to operation. Nine weeks later the non-irradiated group contained 33 survivors, 21 of whom had no disease, while the irradiated group had 49 survivors, 40 of whom had no disease. These differences are all significant ($P = <0{\cdot}01$).

Perhaps the most conclusive experiment is that of Powers and Tolmach (1964), who used the Gardner lymphosarcoma in C_3H mice. By performing serial dilutions of a suspension of the tumour cells, they had earlier determined (Powers and Tolmach, 1963) the number of cells required to produce a tumour when injected into an animal. Their *in vivo* assay showed that 99 per cent of the cells were sterilized by a single dose of 500 rads although, of course, no tumours containing more than 100 cells would be cured by such a dose.

For their test of the efficacy of small dose pre-operative radiation, they used four groups of mice bearing transplanted tumours in the flank. Group 1 was left untreated. Group 2 was given a single dose of 500 rads to the tumour site and surrounding skin. Group 3 had surgery in which the tumour and a wide flap of skin were excised with minimum manipulation of the tumour bed. Group 4 had the combination of 500 rads followed immediately by surgery. The results in Table 1 show a highly significant difference (P = <0·001) in survival rates between Groups 3 and 4 when these were assessed at the end of six months. Perez and Olson (1970) used this system to compare pre-operative and post-operative radiotherapy and found the pre-operative regimen to be more effective.

TABLE 1

Survival after Excision of Gardner Lymphosarcoma (reproduced from Powers and Tolmach, 1964, by courtesy of the Editor of *Nature*)

Group	*Treatment*	*Number of mice*	*Percentage of survivors*
1	Nil	50	0
2	500 rads	50	0
3	Surgery	106	53
4	500 rads + surgery	116	85

The Case for Clinical Trials

These experimental data suggest that a good case exists for mounting clinical trials of low dose pre-operative radiotherapy. In a previous review of this subject (Nias, 1967), it was emphasized that care must be taken to choose only those clinical situations where local recurrence and/or freshly disseminated metastases lead to a significant degree of morbidity and mortality. Furthermore, there is no purpose in mounting a clinical trial unless a large enough sample of patients is available to provide two well-matched groups. This was clearly the problem in the comparative trial of the Medical Research Council Working Party (1966), where even a number of centres could provide a total of only 166 patients, and the ultimate comparison was blurred because of the different frequencies of implementation of the two treatment policies (radiotherapy or surgery for oat cell carcinoma of the bronchus).

By contrast, Evans and Todd (1969) were able to report a trial involving 504 patients with bronchial carcinoma from one centre. This was a good example of a random trial devoted to a simple question (is Synkavit a radiosensitizer in the treatment of bronchial carcinoma?). The patients in the two groups were matched for age, stage and duration of treatment, and this confirmed the random nature of the selection of the groups. The differences in survival rates up to three years were no greater than those which could be expected in a random trial based on 504 patients; that is, there was no significant difference. Although this trial was not concerned with the question of pre-operative radiotherapy, it illustrates the sort of design necessary for a random trial to examine the efficacy of this regimen.

In conclusion, the evidence suggests that low dose pre-operative radiotherapy may reduce mortality and morbidity in those cases of carcinoma of the bronchus where local recurrence and newly disseminated metastases are significant problems. There are thus good ethical reasons for mounting a controlled clinical trial to investigate this possibility. Such a trial would ordinarily be limited to the small percentage of patients who present with an operable tumour. However, the regimen might usefully be extended to include the preliminary biopsy procedure (which itself may be associated with the dissemination of tumour cells). Although benign histology may be shown in some cases, only a small radiation dosage is involved and this may be acceptable. Whether pre-operative or pre-biopsy, the small dose of radiation is best delivered on the day of operation, ideally on the way to the theatre.

SUMMARY

Pre-operative radiotherapy has a limited place in the treatment of carcinoma of the bronchus. It may reduce mortality and morbidity from local recurrence and from metastases freshly disseminated at the time of operation. This may be achieved by the administration of a single low dose (500–1,000 rads) just before surgery. Such a dose is sufficient to reduce to a low level the proportion of viable cells disseminated at operation, while operative complications remain negligible. Experimental evidence is quoted and clinical trials are suggested in carefully chosen circumstances.

REFERENCES

Agostino, D. and Nickson, J. J. (1960). *Radiology* **74,** 816.

Bloedorn, F. G., Cowley, R. A., Cuccia, C. A. and Mercado, R. (1961). *Am. J. Roentg.* **85,** 875.

Cole, W. H., MacDonald, G. O., Roberts, S. S. and Southwick, H. W. (1961). *Dissemination of Cancer: Prevention and Therapy.* New York: Appleton-Century-Crofts.

Collaborative Study (1969). *Cancer, N.Y.* **23,** 419.

Deeley, T. J. (1967). *Br. J. Radiol.* **40,** 801.

Evans, C. M. and Todd, I. D. H. (1969). *Clin. Radiol.* **20,** 228.

Feder, B. H., Blair, P. B. and Close, P. (1965). *Radiology* **84,** 447.
Glicksman, A. S. (1965). *Rhode Isl. med. J.* **48,** 538.
Medical Research Council Working Party (1966). *Lancet* **2,** 979.
Nias, A. H. W. (1967). *Br. J. Radiol.* **40,** 166.
— Greene, D., Fox, M. and Thomas, R. L. (1967). *Int. J. Radiat. Biol.* **13,** 449.
Perez, C. A. and Olson, J. (1970). *Am. J. Roentg.* **108,** 396.
Powers, W. E. and Palmer, L. A. (1968). *Am. J. Roentg.* **102,** 176.
— and Tolmach, L. J. (1963). *Nature, Lond.* **197,** 710.
— — (1964). *Nature, Lond.* **201,** 272.
— Ogura, J. H. and Palmer, L. A. (1967). *Radiology* **89,** 112.
Smith, R. R., Thomas, L. B. and Hilberg, A. W. (1958). *Cancer, N.Y.* **11,** 53.
Strong, E. W., Henschke, U. K., Nickson, J. J., Frazell, E. L., Tollefsen, H. R. and Hilaris, B. S. (1966). *Cancer, N.Y.* **19,** 1509.
Suit, H. and Maeda, M. (1966). *Am. J. Roentg.* **96,** 177.
Tomlinson, R. H. and Gray, L. H. (1955). *Br. J. Cancer* **9,** 539.
Whitmore, G. F. and Till, J. E. (1964). *A. Rev. nucl. Sci.* **14,** 374.

II—Post-operative Radiotherapy

P. J. Bangma

INTRODUCTION

The results obtained in the treatment of bronchial carcinoma were studied in a material of 1,613 patients, from various Dutch clinics, in whom a diagnosis of primary bronchial carcinoma was verified during the period 1947–59 and in whom a cytological or histological classification according to Kreyberg was possible (Bangma, 1963). In 785 of these patients a resection of curative design was performed: 103 of them died from post-operative complications within a month of the intervention. Of the remaining 682 patients, 275 (40·3 per cent) were still alive three years after resection. In 389 of the 682 patients, operation and examination of resected specimens had failed to reveal regional metastases or extrapulmonary tumour growth: the tumour appeared to be confined to the original bronchus. Of these 389 patients, 219 (56·3 per cent) were still alive three years after operation. In the other 293 of the 682 patients, examination of resected specimens, including suspected lymph nodes, showed extensions or metastases in the hilus and/or the mediastinum. Of these 293 patients, only 56 (19·1 per cent) survived three years after operation.

These figures show that after a resection of curative design in the most favourable stage of dissemination, the mortality within three years of the operation still exceeds 40 per cent. The question is, what factors are responsible for the fatal course in patients treated by what was meant to be curative surgery?

To begin with, unresected lymph nodes of the hilus and/or the mediastinum may contain micrometastases, A second possibility is the pre-operative presence of distant metastases which are not clinically manifest. Many investigators (for example, Aylwin, 1951; Ballantyne, Clagett and McDonald, 1957; Collier and colleagues, 1957; Nohl, 1962; Vossenaar, 1963) point out the significance of haematogenous dissemination of tumour embolisms which originate from carcinomatous tissue that has invaded the wall of a pulmonary vein. The third possibility is that detachment and dissemination of tumour embolisms and formation of telemetastases are promoted by surgical manipulations in the tumour area.

The question arises whether x-irradiation following extirpation of the primary tumour can so arrest the growth of micrometastases remaining in the hilus and/or mediastinum that the prognosis is substantially improved.

Endrei and Fridrich (1963) compared the four-year survival rate in 24 patients treated for bronchial carcinoma by pneumonectomy with that in 17 patients treated by operation and subsequent radiotherapy. No significant difference was found. The dosage of irradiation is not specified.

Burr, Mackay and Sellers (1963) compared 135 patients treated by resection and radiotherapy with 50 who had surgery only. In terms of one-year survival, no significant difference was demonstrable.

Ennuyer (1963) compared 61 patients given post-operative radiotherapy with 60 treated by operation only. The irradiation (telecobalt) was aimed at the full length of the mediastinum; the dosage was 6,000–6,500 rads. After two years, 29 of the irradiated and 22 of the non-irradiated patients were still alive; this difference was not significant.

METHOD OF INVESTIGATION

In the Department of Lung Diseases, Utrecht University Clinic, a study was started in 1958 in an effort to establish whether, after curative resection for bronchial carcinoma, radiotherapy to the hilar area and the homolateral side of the mediastinum could improve the prognosis (Bangma and Tonkes, 1965). The operations were performed in the Surgical Clinic and the subsequent treatment was given in the Department of Medical Radiology. All patients reported to have undergone resection of curative design for bronchial carcinoma were given consecutive numbers. Those with odd numbers received post-operative radiotherapy, while those with even numbers served as controls. The following patients were given numbers but not included in the study:

(1) Patients who died due to post-operative complications.

(2) Patients with odd numbers whose irradiation had to be discontinued prematurely for any reason.

(3) Patients of both categories for whom radiotherapy was contra-indicated on clinical grounds.

(4) Patients on whose resected specimens the pathologist reported that microscopic examination revealed carcinomatous tissue in the plane of resection. These cases were not regarded as having had operations of curative design.

In the evaluation of results, only those patients were considered whose operation was performed one year or longer before conclusion of the study.

Of the total of 73 patients (all men) covered by the study, 36 received post-operative radiotherapy; the remaining 37 did not. The former group comprised 26 cases of lobectomy and 10 of pneumonectomy, while the latter group consisted of 20 cases of lobectomy and 17 of pneumonectomy.

Radiotherapy was given by the rotation method in 14 cases and consisted of field irradiation in 22 (2 fields in 1 case, 3 fields in 3 cases, 4 fields in 18 cases). With the rotation method, the calculated mean dose on the hilus and mediastinum was 4,643 r (standard deviation $s_{\bar{x}} = 525$); the mean dose attained in field irradiation was 4,369 r (standard deviation $s_{\bar{x}} = 474$). The mean time required to attain these doses was 5 weeks ($s_{\bar{x}} = 1{\cdot}2$) for rotation irradiation and 5·6 weeks ($s^{-} = 1{\cdot}4$) for field irradiation.

RESULTS

The figures in Table 1 show that, of the 17 deaths among the 36 irradiated patients, 12 occurred within a year after the operation;

TABLE 1

Survival, Mortality and Causes of Death in 73 Patients with Lung Cancer Treated by Operation With or Without Post-operative Radiotherapy

	Number of patients	*Alive > 1 year after operation*	*Deceased **					
			< 1 year			*> 1 year*		
			T	*O*	*U*	*T*	*O*	*U*
Irradiation	36	19†	7	3	2	4	1	—
No irradiation	37	25‡	4	1	—	5	1	1

*T = death from tumour metastases.
O = other known causes of death.
U = cause of death unknown.
† Including none with signs of tumour relapse.
‡ Including two with signs of tumour relapse.

in 7 of these the verified cause of death was tumour metastases. The autopsy on one patient who died showing symptoms of pneumonia (three months after pneumonectomy and a few weeks after the last irradiation) disclosed extensive irradiation fibrosis with interstitial pneumonitis of the remaining lung. In 2 patients who died three months after pneumonectomy, the chest x-ray shortly before death showed infiltrative changes in the remaining lung. Of the 5 irradiated patients who died after the first post-operative year, 4 died due to tumour metastases. The fifth died more than two years after operation, possibly from pneumonia. Radiological examination disclosed marked irradiation fibrosis.

Of the 37 controls, 12 were dead when the study was concluded. Of these, 5 died within the first post-operative year, tumour metastases being verified cause of death in 4. Tumour metastases were likewise the cause of death in 5 of the 7 patients who died after the first post-operative year. The two groups, therefore, did not significantly differ in their mortality from tumour metastases, either within a year or later ($0{\cdot}50 < P < 0{\cdot}70$)*.

For further substantiation of the conclusions reached, efforts were made to establish whether the groups compared were indeed of the same composition as to (1) average age of patients; (2) regional tumour spread at time of operation; (3) type of carcinoma; and (4) lobectomy: pneumonectomy ratio.

(1) The average age of the irradiated patients was 58·7 years (standard deviation 5·7); the corresponding values in the control group were 57·9 and 6·0, the difference being of no significance.

(2) The stage of tumour spread according to surgeon and pathologist is of great prognostic importance. The regional tumour spread was recorded using the classification proposed for bronchial carcinoma by Thomas (1963):

Stage I: tumour of peripheral localization without metastases†.

Stage II: tumour of central localization without metastases.

Stage III: tumour with metastases in hilar glands or invasive growth.

Stage IV: tumour with metastases in mediastinal glands or invasive growth.

Table 2 shows that the two groups did not significantly differ in the ratio between stage I and stage II cases and the prognostically less favourable cases (stages III and IV). Nor was the difference in incidence of stage III or stage IV significant ($0{\cdot}10 > P > 0{\cdot}05$). Of the 7 patients classified as stage IV, 6 died from tumour metastases

* χ^2 test on mxn tables.

† A bronchial tumour distal to the orifice of a segmental bronchus was regarded as peripheral.

within 2 years; the seventh (not irradiated) was still alive 16 months after operation but had developed telemetastases.

(3) The type of carcinoma is likewise of prognostic significance. It was established that even when, after resection of curative design, examination of the resected specimen showed that the tumour was apparently confined to the original bronchus, patients with anaplastic small cell carcinomas had poor survival chances compared with cases of other types of carcinoma.

The figures of Table 3 show that the distribution of the four types of carcinoma was virtually the same in the two groups of patients.

TABLE 2

The 73 Patients Divided According to Stage of Tumour Spread

Stage	*Irradiation*	*No irradiation*
I	13	11
II	14	17
III	4	7
IV	5	2
Total	36	37

TABLE 3

The 73 Patients Divided According to Type of Carcinoma

Type	*Irradiation*	*No irradiation*
Squamous cell carcinoma	27	29
Anaplastic small cell carcinoma	4	3
Anaplastic large cell carcinoma	4	5
Adenocarcinoma	1	—
Total	36	37

Table 4 reviews only those patients in both groups who suffered from tumours of the squamous cell type in stages I and II. The possible influence of a difference in the composition of the two groups as to type and stage of tumour spread is thus eliminated. The figures show a higher mortality within the first post-operative year among the irradiated patients (6 of 8 deaths) than among the controls (1 of 6 deaths) ($0{\cdot}05 < P < 0{\cdot}02$). No significant difference was found between the two groups in mortality from tumour metastases.

(4) Table 5 summarizes the data on pneumonectomies and lobectomies of curative design for squamous cell carcinoma without regional spread. Neither in the lobectomy nor in the pneumonectomy group did post-operative irradiation influence the results. Even if the deaths of the two patients who died of unknown causes within a year of pneumonectomy with irradiation are ascribed to tumour metastases, this does not significantly influence the statistics ($0{\cdot}10 < P < 0{\cdot}20$).

TABLE 4

Survival, Mortality and Causes of Death in 43 Patients with Squamous Cell Carcinoma in Stages I and II, Treated by Operations of Curative Design

	Number of patients	*Alive > 1 year after operation*	*Deceased** < 1 year T			*Deceased** > 1 year T		
			T	*O*	*U*	*T*	*O*	*U*
Irradiation	21	13†	2	2	2	1	1	—
No irradiation	23	17‡	—	1	—	3	1	1

*T = death from tumour metastases.
O = other known causes of death.
U = cause of death unknown.
† Including none with signs of tumour relapse.
‡ Including one with signs of tumour relapse.

TABLE 5

Survival, Mortality and Causes of Death in Patients with Squamous Cell Carcinoma Without Regional Spread, Treated by Operations of Curative Design

	Number of patients	*Alive > 1 year after operation*	*Deceased** < 1 year			*Deceased** > 1 year		
			T	*O*	*U*	*T*	*O*	*U*
Pneumonectomy:								
Irradiation	6	1†	—	2	2	1	—	—
No irradiation	11	9‡	—	1	—	—	1	—
Lobectomy:								
Irradiation	15	12†	2	—	—	—	1	—
No irradiation	12	8‡	—	—	—	3	—	1

*T = death from tumour metastases.
O = other known cause of death.
U = cause of death unknown.
† Including none with signs of tumour relapse.
‡ Including one with signs of tumour relapse.

Post-operative radiotherapy can be expected only to inhibit the growth of micrometastases remaining in glands of the hilus and the mediastinum. It cannot be expected to have any effect on overlooked pre-operative telemetastases or on dissemination of tumour cells during the operation.

In 14 patients who died from tumour metastases within the period of observation, the first signs of relapse were identified as distant metastases or intrathoracic glandular metastases. Of these 14 patients, 8 had received post-operative irradiation (Table 6).

TABLE 6

Deaths from Tumour Metastases After Lobectomy (14 Patients)

First signs of relapse	*Irradiation*	*No irradiation*
Extrathoracic metastasis	6	1
Intrathoracic metastasis	2	5
Total	8	6

There are indications that radiotherapy prevents intrathoracic metastases from becoming manifest.

COMMENT

Radiotherapy following resection for bronchial carcinoma could not be demonstrated to improve the prognosis.

A disadvantage of radiotherapy is the occurrence of pulmonary fibrosis. This complication was observed chiefly after lobectomy and occurred on the homolateral side. In 12 of 26 patients treated by lobectomy and post-operative irradiation, the degree of fibrosis which developed in the course of a few months was such that the tissue-saving effect of the lobectomy was entirely lost.

Recent investigations (Brady, Germon and Cander, 1965; Germon and Brady, 1968) have shown that radiotherapy reduces the perfusing and diffusing capacity of the lung.

In a few cases, an irradiation reaction occurred in the remaining lung following pneumonectomy; in one case this was the verified cause of death.

REFERENCES

Aylwin, J. A. (1951). 'Avoidable vascular spread in resection for bronchial carcinoma.' *Thorax* **6,** 250.

Ballantyne, A. J., Clagett, O. T. and McDonald, J. R. (1957). 'Vascular invasion in bronchogenic carcinoma.' *Thorax* **12,** 294.

Bangma, P. J. (1963). *De resultaten van de behandeling van het bronchus-carcinoom.* Thesis, Utrecht.

— and Tonkes, E. (1965). 'De waarde van postoperatieve röntgen-bestraling bij bronchuscarcinoom.' *Ned. Tijdschr. Geneesk.* **109,** 653.

Brady, L. W., Germon, P. A. and Cander, L. (1965). 'Effects of radiation therapy on pulmonary function in carcinoma of the lung.' *Radiology* **85,** 130.

Burr, R. C., Mackay, E. N. and Sellers, A. H. (1963). 'Radiation therapy in the treatment of carcinoma of the lung.' *Can med. Ass. J.* **88,** 1181.

Collier, F. C., Blakemore, W. S., Kyle, R. H., Enterline, H. T., Kirby, C. K. and Johnson, J. (1957). 'Carcinoma of the lung. Factors with influence on five-year survival with special reference to blood vessel invasion.' *Ann. Surg.* **146,** 417.

Endrei, E. and Fridrich, R. (1963). 'Zur Frage der chirurgisch-radiologischen Behandlung des Lungenkarzinoms.' *Radiologia clin., Basel* **32,** 353.

Ennuyer, A. (1963). 'L'irradation du médiastin après pneumonectomie pour cancer bronchique.' *Poumon Coeur* **19,** 1093.

Germon, P. A. and Brady, L. W. (1968). 'Physiologic changes before and after radiation treatment for carcinoma of the lung.' *J. Am. med. Ass.* **206,** 809.

Nohl, H. C. (1962). *The Spread of Carcinoma of the Bronchus.* London: Lloyd-Luke.

Thomas, P. 1963. *Bronchuscarcinoom.* Thesis, Leiden.

Vossenaar, T. (1963). 'Pathologisch-anatomisch onderzoek van bronchus-carcinomen'. *Ned. Tijdschr. Geneesk.* **107,** 673.

10—The Organization of Co-operative Controlled Clinical Trials

Wallace Fox and A. B. Miller

There is a large literature dealing with the general principles involved in the organization of controlled clinical trials (Hill, 1951, 1962; Royal Society of Medicine, 1958; Council for International Organizations of Medical Sciences, 1960; Witts, 1964; Hayward, 1965; Paterson, 1965; Atkins, 1966). A particularly valuable recent publication is the report by a W.H.O. scientific group (World Health Organization, 1968). In this chapter it is therefore intended only to consider certain specific issues and problems which are of special importance in co-operative controlled clinical trials in carcinoma of the bronchus.

ROLE OF LARGE-SCALE CO-OPERATIVE TRIALS

Controlled clinical trials of bronchial carcinoma require substantial numbers of patients. This is particularly so if it is proposed to study patients with all histological types of tumour, since the analysis will need to take account of the histology, not only in order to confirm equality in the distribution of tumour types between the treatments under study but also to evaluate the results of therapy in the different types. Although the disease is common, it is likely to take a single centre several years to achieve an intake adequate to yield clear-cut answers on almost any aspect of therapy. It is thus much more efficient to undertake large-scale multi-centre co-operative trials and substantially reduce the period of intake. This is especially desirable since (advanced inoperable disease apart) a five-year follow-up of every patient under study must be the aim, so that even with a rapid intake a study is likely to take up to seven years or more from the start of the intake to the publication of the five-year results. Although interim reports may be published, the minimum period of observation for these is likely to be two or three years. A further advantage of a multi-centre trial is that it is more illuminating to know that a method of treatment—whether this be a drug, a form of radiotherapy or a surgical technique—has proved beneficial in the hands of a number of different workers than in a single centre.

CENTRAL CO-ORDINATION

In any co-operative investigation, it is essential that all the investigators adhere strictly to the experimental design. All the observations, measurements and interpretations need to be as standardized as possible, and this is only likely to be achieved through a central co-ordinating organization with adequate medical, statistical and clerical facilities. The role of the central co-ordinating group is not only to supervise the centres but to keep them informed, at regular intervals, of the progress of the intake and of any important problems or issues which have arisen and might be of general interest. Good central co-ordination stimulates flagging enthusiasm. The long time-scale of studies of carcinoma of the bronchus makes highly organized central co-ordination particularly important.

ETHICAL CONSIDERATIONS

There are now a number of statements and guide-lines referring to the ethical considerations involved in experimentation on man (World Medical Association, 1964; Medical Research Council, 1964; World Health Organization, 1968). All who work in the field of the controlled clinical trial should be fully acquainted with the general problems which inevitably arise. Needless to say, research workers must also consider the ethical issues specific to each trial in which they engage.

Ethical problems in studies of cancer therapy can best be considered by stages. The first stage is usually undertaken at a committee level, whether this is formally or informally constituted. In the studies of bronchial carcinoma undertaken by the Medical Research Council, the Working Party on the Treatment of Carcinoma of the Bronchus discusses in detail, at a very early stage in planning, the ethical issues involved in any study under consideration, in order to satisfy itself that in the experimental design the best interests of the patients do not suffer. The second stage arises when the co-ordinators discuss the proposed investigation with clinicians who are being approached with a view to obtaining their co-operation in it. This will establish whether or not they are prepared to submit their own patients to the study. Only if it meets with enthusiastic support at this stage will the study commence and the third stage arise. This stage continues throughout the period of intake, for each time a clinician proposes to admit an individual patient to the investigation he must satisfy himself, after considering both the medical and the social circumstances, that it is not against that particular patient's interests to be admitted.

In studies of the treatment of malignant disease, it is not practicable in most countries to obtain *fully informed* consent from the patients in the full meaning of the phrase. It is not normally considered good medical practice to discuss the diagnosis and prognosis with the patient in full detail because it is seldom regarded as being in his best interests to do so. Hence it is particularly important to safeguard the patient's interests in the three ways referred to above.

The co-ordinators of controlled clinical trials have a further responsibility falling within the realm of ethics. They must carefully scrutinize progress reports as they are received and review from time to time the results as they accumulate in order to be fully aware of any problems that may be arising and to look for evidence of the superiority of one regimen over another. They must see that no group of patients under study is running unnecessary risks, and if a regimen is toxic or clearly inferior therapeutically, the whole plan of the study must be reviewed. The co-ordinators must be ready to refer back problems to the study's steering committee (or, if it has been disbanded, consider reconvening it) and report to it interim analyses which suggest important differences between regimens. However, with a fixed sample the investigator periodically analysing his results must realize that such analyses invalidate ordinary tests of significance, and great care must be taken in deciding during the course of the study that one regimen is, in fact, inferior to another (Paterson and Russell, 1962). The committee's chairman should be kept closely in touch with important developments even in individual cases, such as an unexpected severe toxic manifestation.

SELECTION OF PATIENTS FOR STUDY

The objects of the investigation may well predetermine a degree of selection of patients. For example, studies of pre-operative radiotherapy will normally involve patients who have been assessed and regarded as having an operable lesion, and the surgeon should, indeed, have agreed to perform a thoracotomy before a patient is allocated. Even here, however, two types of patient can be differentiated. Thus in the Collaborative Study (1969) undertaken in the

U.S.A., patients were classified as initially operable if they had no evidence of extension of the tumour beyond the lung and as potentially operable if they had only regional involvement. In this study the potentially operable group actually included patients with chest wall invasion, with confirmed metastasis in ipsilateral or contralateral supraclavicular, scalene or mediastinal lymph nodes, and with nerve involvement as shown by Horner's syndrome, vocal cord paralysis or phrenic nerve paralysis. It is evident that further selection or subdivision of patients would have been readily possible within this group. For studies of post-operative radiotherapy, a decision will also have to be taken whether to restrict this treatment to patients who have had a complete resection of the primary growth and have no evidence of metastases, even including involvement of the regional lymph nodes; whether, on the contrary, involvement of the nodes leaves the patient eligible or is indeed a condition of eligibility; and also whether further extension of the growth, discovered at operation, leaves the patient eligible. The decision will clearly depend on the defined objects of the particular investigation.

In studies in which one of the forms of treatment under investigation is cytotoxic chemotherapy, it may be considered necessary, as in a current Medical Research Council study, to exclude women aged under 45 years in order to avoid hazard to the foetus from the cytotoxic drug should pregnancy occur.

The failure to appreciate the element of patient selection which unavoidably exists in all controlled clinical trials can lead to confusion. Thus the Medical Research Council (1966) trial, comparing surgery with radical radiotherapy in the primary treatment of small-celled or oat-celled carcinoma of the bronchus, was restricted to patients who were diagnosed pre-operatively on bronchial biopsy. Because of this special selection, the findings relate to a quite different patient population from those with oat cell carcinoma reported in surgical series, most of which contain a high but all too often unstated proportion of patients who had an undiagnosed intrapulmonary tumour which was resected in order to make a diagnosis. Patients in the latter group present a completely different clinical problem from that investigated in the Medical Research Council trial (Scadding, 1968; Miller, Fox and Tall, 1969).

HISTOLOGY

If patients are to be selected for study on the basis of the histological type of their growth, it is important to ensure uniformity of histological diagnosis. For example, in the Medical Research Council

(1966) trial of surgery and radical radiotherapy it was decided to investigate only one histological type, namely small-celled or oat-celled growths in a bronchial biopsy specimen. As this trial involved over 40 centres and the histological diagnosis was being made by the local pathologists, it was possible that the interpretation of what constituted small-celled or oat-celled carcinoma would vary from centre to centre. This problem was overcome in two ways. First, before the start of the study, all the local pathologists were sent slides which the reference pathologist regarded as showing the typical appearances of small-celled or oat-celled carcinoma. Secondly, slides from every patient were collected by the co-ordinators for independent assessment by the reference pathologist. It was on his assessment that the eligibility of the patients for the final analysis, in terms of the histological type of their growth, was based. In the event, of the total of 166 patients submitted to the study, in only 7 cases did the reference pathologist disagree with the histological classification made by the local pathologist.

Even if all histological types are to be included in a study, it is still desirable for a systematic classification of the growths to be made by one observer, since this will improve the grouping of patients in attempts to find prognostic associations.

THE ROLE OF DOUBLE-BLIND STUDIES

An essential aim of any controlled clinical trial is to ensure that in all respects, apart from the differences in the regimens under study, all the patients are treated equally. This can usually best be achieved by conducting (if possible) the study double-blind—that is, the nature of the treatment received by a subject at any time being unknown to both the subject and the observer—since this will remove the risk of bias which might otherwise arise. For example, Wolf and colleagues (1966) have reported the results of a controlled clinical trial of radiotherapy, with a control group receiving a placebo tablet, in which there was an advantage to the radiotherapy series. However, the interpretation of this finding was uncertain, because patients in the radiotherapy series received more chemotherapy for intercurrent infections and this might well have been the explanation of the differences observed. Had all the patients in the study received a placebo tablet, and had all been put under the radiotherapy apparatus whether or not they were due to receive radiotherapy, it would have been possible to conduct the study double-blind, although this would have necessitated considerable organizational elaboration.

If the roles of radiotherapy and of different dosage schedules and techniques are to be investigated accurately and systematically in controlled clinical trials, the need to ensure that the studies are really conducted double-blind cannot be overstressed. The mere act of putting the patient under a radiotherapy apparatus may result in the quality of patient care being improved and thereby prolong survival, as appears to have happened in the study of Wolf and colleagues (1966). If a study settles conclusively one way or another the place of radiotherapy or of a particular dosage schedule in treatment, the valuable time of the radiotherapy apparatus will indeed have been well used.

ASSESSMENT OF RESULTS

Survival

Survival is the main assessment in carcinoma of the bronchus. In the Medical Research Council (1966) trial, when the proportion of survivors in the two series was compared, the difference was not statistically significant except at two months, when the early post-operative mortality in the surgery series made itself felt. A more sensitive method is to take into account the actual survival time of each patient and to calculate the mean of the individual survival times. However, the prolonged survival of a few individuals, which often occurs in malignant disease, can have a disturbing effect on an ordinary arithmetic mean survival time, and this must be allowed for appropriately in the analysis. One method, used in the Medical Research Council trial, is to calculate the mean of the square roots of the individual survival times. With this measure, it was shown that the difference in mean survival time between the two series was unlikely to be a chance effect because it attained statistical significance at the 5 per cent level (Miller, Fox and Tall, 1969).

Cause of Death

Comparisons of survival times are most meaningful when they are supported by a full post-mortem examination for every fatality to confirm the cause of death, the extent of recurrence of the primary growth, and the absence or presence of metastases and their distribution. Unfortunately it may be difficult to obtain autopsies, and valuable information is often lost. However, the importance of making every effort to obtain a full post-mortem examination cannot be overstressed, for without such examinations there is, in all probability, over-certification of cancer as the cause of death. This is because of the natural tendency of the patient's general practitioner and other medical attendants to attribute subsequent illnesses to the malignancy or to complications associated with its spread. The co-ordinators of controlled trials have an important role in reminding all co-operating clinicians to try to ensure that relatives are at least asked for permission to perform an autopsy.

It is not always appreciated that within the framework of a controlled clinical trial, the case for performing autopsies in malignant disease is much stronger than in normal clinical practice. This is because in such a trial, post-mortem findings may result in a decisive evaluation of the relative merits of the different methods of therapy under study in preventing or minimizing recurrence or metastases. Outside a controlled clinical trial, it is only by excluding or confirming drug toxicity that post-mortem examination is likely to yield decisive information about an individual patient's treatment. The physician co-operating in a controlled trial can therefore truthfully explain to relatives of a deceased patient that an autopsy might well help other patients suffering from the same disease, and many relatives find this a positive source of consolation.

Presence of Metastases

A record should be made, on all progress report forms, of the presence of definite or suspected metastases. Such data provide supporting evidence on the course of the disease. However, scrutiny of individual patient records in controlled trials will readily demonstrate that reports of suspected and of definite metastases are both to some extent unreliable and that a clinician may, in a subsequent report, withdraw such earlier reports. It is for this reason that clinical reports are no substitute for a detailed post-mortem examination, which may also reveal unexpected recurrence of metastases in patients who have died of other conditions. Even so, the length of the period from allocation of treatment to recurrence of the disease is an important measure of the influence of the primary therapy. This is especially so in view of the fact that further treatment cannot be withheld once a definite recurrence has been diagnosed. Once the growth has recurred, it is therefore likely that an increasing proportion of patients will have subsidiary treatments which may very well complicate the interpretation of subsequent results.

Assessment of Quality of Survival

A very important aspect of survival in malignant disease is not merely its duration but its quality. A form of therapy which prolongs survival by a month or two may not be in the best interests of the

M.R.C.B.—14

patient if it results in an increase in or a prolongation of the distress of the terminal illness. Unfortunately, there are still no satisfactory methods of measuring the quality of survival. Standard assessments which are commonly obtained, such as a classification of the patient's general state of wellbeing, the degree of dyspnoea or the degree of physical activity, are not very informative. They also give no information on the patient's psychological state, which is often disturbed (Hinton, 1963). In any case, if the standard assessments are recorded by the clinician in charge of the patient's treatment they may, unless it has been possible to conduct the study double-blind, contain a systematic bias and so be unreliable for making comparisons between groups of patients treated by different methods. For example, in the Medical Research Council's (1966) trial of surgery and radical radiotherapy, the radiotherapists reported on the progress and clinical condition of the patients in the radiotherapy series and the surgeons on the patients in the surgery series. Because of this, it is possible that the assessments obtained reflected not the true clinical state of the patients in the two series but the views of the radiotherapists on the one hand and the surgeons on the other. Even had an attempt been made at each centre to obtain the assessments of a third party, say a physician, it would still have been possible for this assessment also to be unconsciously yet systematically influenced by a knowledge of the treatment each individual patient had received.

A way of overcoming this difficulty in obtaining an unbiased assessment might be to get the patient himself to complete at intervals questionnaires providing information on his own sense of well-being, activity and mood. Such questionnaires can be undertaken when the patient attends for follow-up. They need, however, to be completed before he sees the clinician in charge of his case—that is, before he is submitted to the possibility of suggestion from his medical supervisor. Such an approach is currently being explored in the Medical Research Council's study of cytotoxic chemotherapy.

SPECIAL OPPORTUNITIES FOR RESEARCH

The opportunity may well arise within a large-scale co-operative controlled clinical trial to explore side-issues of special interest. For example, the M.R.C. study of cytotoxic chemotherapy (*see above*) has provided an opportunity to study whether these drugs produce *specific* and characteristic changes in the lung, as has been reported for both cyclophosphamide and busulphan (Oliner and colleagues, 1961; Leake, Smith and Woodliff, 1963; André and colleagues,

1967; Heard and Cooke, 1968; Annotation, 1968), with the special advantage that lungs from patients who received a placebo will serve as controls. Provided that specimens from a sufficient number of patients can be collected for examination 'blind' by the reference pathologist, valuable information should be obtained.

The same study also offers an opportunity to test the W.H.O. classification of histological typing of lung tumours (World Health Organization, 1967) and to compare, in a series of 'blind' readings, the tumour type of the lung lesion, of the affected regional nodes and of the bronchial biopsy specimen. The prognostic value of the W.H.O. classification can also be tested.

One of the functions of a co-ordinating group is to remain alert to such research opportunities and for co-operating clinicians to suggest further research projects so that the maximum yield of information can be obtained from the trial.

CONCLUSION

The methodology of the controlled clinical trial in the treatment of cancer of the bronchus is in a relatively early stage of development, and very few studies have yet been undertaken in this disease. In particular, the methods of assessment are not satisfactorily established. The field is a difficult one, partly for methodological reasons and partly because large numbers of patients and a long period of observation are necessary. However, it is only by means of well-conducted controlled clinical trials that the present empiricism in the therapy of the disease will be replaced by scientifically established facts.

REFERENCES

André, R., Rochant, H., Dreyfus, B., Duhamel, G. and Péchère, J. C. (1967). 'Diffuse interstitial fibrosis of the lung in a case of Hodgkin's disease treated with high doses of Endoxan.' *Bull. Soc. méd. Hôp. Paris* **118,** 1133.

Annotation (1968). 'Toxic Effects of Busulphan.' *Lancet* **1,** 854.

Atkins, H. (1966). 'Conduct of a controlled clinical trial.' *Br. med. J.* **2,** 377.

Collaborative Study (1969). 'Preoperative irradiation of cancer of the lung.' *Cancer, N.Y.* **2,** 419.

Council for International Organizations of Medical Sciences (1960). *Controlled Clinical Trials* (Papers delivered at the Conference convened by the Council). Oxford: Blackwell.

Hayward, J. L. (1965). 'Planning and conducting cancer clinical trials.' *Proc. R. Soc. Med.* **58,** 626.

Heard, B. E. and Cooke, R. A. (1968). 'Busulphan lung.' *Thorax* **23,** 187.

Hill, A. B. (1951). 'The clinical trial.' *Br. med. Bull.* **4,** 278.

— (1962). *Statistical Methods of Clinical and Preventive Medicine*. Edinburgh: Livingstone.

Hinton, J. M. (1963). 'The physical and mental distress of the dying.' *Q. Jl Med.* **32,** 1.

Leake, E., Smith, W. G. and Woodliff, H. J. (1963). 'Diffuse interstitial pulmonary fibrosis after busulphan therapy.' *Lancet* **2,** 432.

Medical Research Council (1964). 'Responsibility in investigations on human subjects.' *Br. med. J.* **2,** 178.

— (1966). 'Comparative trial of surgery and radiotherapy for the primary treatment of small-celled or oat-celled carcinoma of the bronchus.' *Lancet* **2,** 979.

Miller, A. B., Fox, W. and Tall, R. (1969). 'Five-year follow-up of the Medical Research Council comparative trial of surgery and radiotherapy for the primary treatment of small-celled or oat-celled carcinoma of the bronchus.' *Lancet* **2,** 501.

Oliner, H., Schwartz, R., Rubio, F. and Dameshek, W. (1961). 'Interstitial pulmonary fibrosis following busulfan therapy.' *Am. J. Med.* **31,** 134.

Paterson, R. (1965). 'Clinical trials in malignant disease. Part IV: general principles.' *Proc. R. Soc. Med.* **58,** 625.

— and Russell, M. H. (1962). 'Clinical trials in malignant disease: lung cancer.' *Clin. Radiol.* **2,** 141.

Royal Society of Medicine (1958). *A Symposium on Clinical Trials.* Pfizer Ltd.

Scadding, J. G. (1968). 'Treatment of oat-cell carcinoma of lung.' *Lancet* **2,** 1145.

Witts, L. J. (1964). 'Medical surveys and clinical trials.' In *Methods and Applications of Group Research in Medicine.* London and New York: Oxford University Press.

Wolf, J., Patno, M. E., Roswit, B. and D'Esopo, N. (1966). 'Controlled study of survival of patients with clinically inoperable lung cancer treated with radiation therapy.' *Am. J. Med.* **40,** 360.

World Health Organization (1967). *Histological Typing of Lung Tumours.* Geneva: W.H.O.

— (1968). *Principles for the Clinical Evaluation of Drugs.* Technical Report Series No. 403. Geneva: W.H.O.

World Medical Association (1964). 'Human experimentation: code of ethics of the World Medical Association.' *Br. med. J.* **2,** 177.

11—Radical Supervoltage Therapy in Inoperable Carcinoma of the Lung

Ruth Guttmann

INTRODUCTION

This chapter will deal with the role of supervoltage irradiation in the treatment of inoperable carcinoma of the lung and will cover selection of patient material, approach and technique with 2 million volt irradiation, tolerance and side effects, subjective response, influence of microscopic diagnosis and of dosage on response, and results.

The steadily increasing number of patients with advanced inoperable cancer of the lung has during the past years become a challenge and a problem for the radiotherapist. Because of the known poor prognosis of this disease, many have refused to accept these patients for radiotherapy as they question the value of any type of therapeutic interference in such a hopeless situation. They feel that no treatment whatever is indicated unless the patients are threatened by serious complications—for instance, by compression of vital organs. Others have thought that aggressive therapy was imperative and worthwhile. I have always felt that there was an indication for treating these patients, especially those in good general condition, and have been of the opinion that supervoltage irradiation might offer some advantages. This clinical impression was borne out by some of the findings which were reported by the late Alfred Hocker and myself in a preliminary report on our experience with the 1,000 kV unit at the Memorial Hospital in New York (Hocker and Guttmann, 1944).

The literature did not offer much information to support either of the conflicting opinions mentioned above. For this reason, I started 15 years ago to outline a systematic radiation treatment for all patients with inoperable carcinoma of the lung (Guttmann, 1955). This I hoped would give me the opportunity to accumulate a large series of patients whose cases could be evaluated critically and documented in order to establish the success or failure of the therapeutic method.

REPORT ON 150 UNSELECTED CASES MICROSCOPICALLY PROVED INOPERABLE

A group of 150 unselected patients with microscopically proved inoperable lung cancer has been treated and followed in the Department of Radiotherapy of the Francis Delafield Hospital in New York since 1955 (Guttmann, 1958). It was our policy to accept every patient, no matter how far the disease had advanced, as we were interested in providing symptomatic relief and in accumulating and studying a large series in a short time. The most pertinent facts and observations which were collected by studying this group can be outlined as follows.

Method of Treatment

The patients were treated with a daily tumour dose of 200 rads for a total of 5,000–6,000 rads delivered over 5–6 weeks with a 2 MV roentgen ray unit. The therapeutic approach with a machine which operates at a target skin distance of 100 cm and is connected with a half-value layer of 7 mm of lead was chosen as an example, as we have used this unit for the treatment of patients with lung lesions. When other supervoltage machines are used, minor adjustments have to be made as certain differences between the machines do exist, but the basic approach and the underlying thoughts remain the same. Two large opposing fields, including the mediastinum on the involved side, were utilized as shown in *Figure 1*, but no rotation or scanning was applied as it is essential to maintain the normal function of the opposite lung. We have calculated that even with a partial scan the opposing hilar area would receive a dose of 1,250 rads when 5,000 rads were given to the diseased hilar area, while the dose with full rotation would amount to 2,500 rads (*Figures 2* and *3*).

Advantages of Supervoltage Radiotherapy

It is the goal of any radiotherapeutic programme to deliver a high dose of radiation to the neoplasm with minimal effects upon the normal contiguous structures. Irradiation in the higher energy

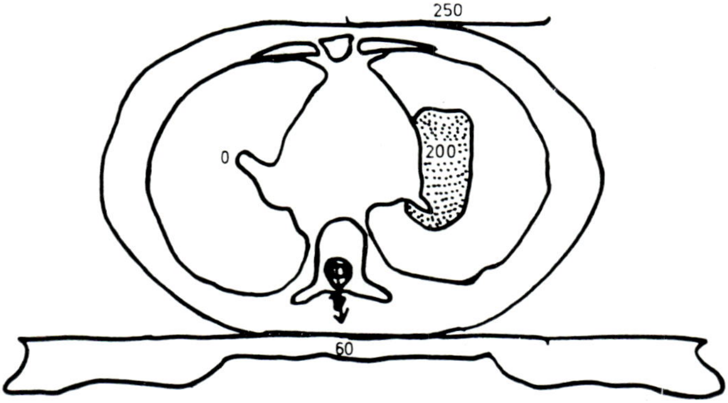

Figure 1. Treatment with 2,000 kV; opposing 15 × 15 cm fields

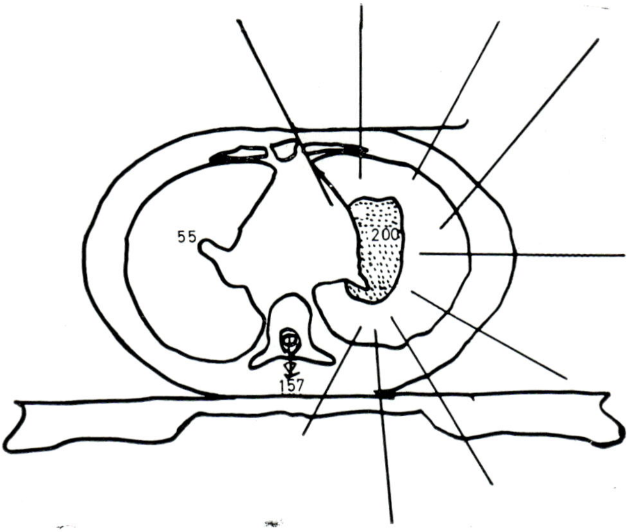

Figure 2. Cobalt-60; scanning from 330 to 210 degrees; 15 × 15 cm field

range, which includes any radiation of and above 1,000 kV, can accomplish this better than any radiation in the orthovoltage range. This gain is due to the superior physical qualities of the hard beam of radiation of supervoltage units, which are different from the

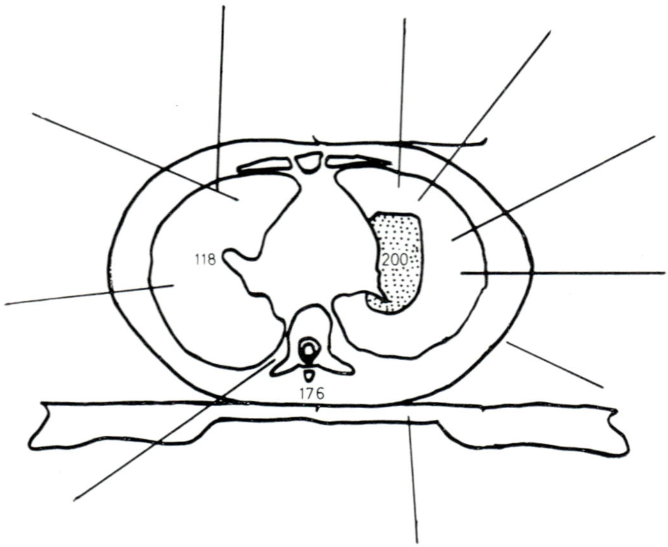

Figure 3. Cobalt-60; full rotation; 15 × 15 cm field

previously used conventional deep x-ray therapy units. There is no advantageous biological difference between supervoltage and conventional irradiation. However, the following physical qualities are responsible for the greater effectiveness of the former:

(1) Better penetration, resulting in better depth dosages.

(2) Maximum ionization of the beam of radiation below the surface, resulting in a skin-sparing effect.

(3) Diminished side-scatter, resulting in better general tolerance.

(4) Decreased absorption of this hard beam of radiation in bone and cartilage, resulting in (*a*) fewer complications in bone and cartilage, and (*b*) less depression of the bone marrow.

Methods of Accurate Localization

In planning and actually carrying out the therapy, accuracy is of the utmost importance. For this reason we make use of every diagnostic method that will enable us to determine the size and location of the lesion, for even a near miss would impair the result.

Contours are taken with narrow strips of wet plaster of Paris over the centre of the area to be treated, and these contours are traced on paper as soon as the plaster has hardened. With the help of roentgenograms, normal organs and the tumour area are drawn into anatomical cross-sections which bear the actual measurements of the patient. The next steps are the determination of the field size for the treatment and the calculation of the tumour dose. When arranging the fields we try to avoid the adjacent normal, healthy structures as far as possible, as has been demonstrated above in *Figures 1*, *2* and *3*.

Before starting the actual therapy, localization films are taken on the treatment unit with the patient in the proper treatment position, because only these films will assure us that the size and position of the outlined field correspond with the area intended for irradiation.

Results

The immediate tolerance to this amount of radiation given in the specified time has been excellent, and no late serious complications have been observed in our series. Subjective improvement of symptoms was experienced in 75 per cent of the cases, with relief from cough, haemoptysis, pain and dyspnoea. It has been interesting to note that malignant lesions of the epithelium have responded better than those of glandular tissues.

There has been microscopic evidence that with this amount of radiation, squamous cell carcinomas of the lung have been completely destroyed in some cases. Twenty autopsies were performed in this patient group, and in four of these the pathologists failed to find evidence of disease in the treated areas. Drs. A. P. Stout and E. Sproul, who were the pathologists at that time at the Francis Delafield Hospital, sectioned these irradiated lungs most carefully before they were willing to describe their findings as 'extensive fibrosis in the form of complete replacement and an advanced healed interstitial pneumonia'.

Of the total group of 150 patients, 40 per cent were alive for more than one year after the completion of radiotherapy, 13 per cent were alive for two years, and 7 per cent for three years.

It is evident that the bare statistical figures cannot give a true picture of the achievements of a method when the survival rates of an unselected material like this were burdened by the inclusion of patients with such a grave initial prognosis that some of them died during or immediately following the completion of therapy. Nevertheless, there was the subjective improvement in 75 per cent of the patients; there was the microscopic evidence that a number of squamous cell carcinomas had been completely destroyed; and there was the fact that 40 per cent of the patients were alive more than a year after completion of treatment. The question has been asked whether such beneficial results could not have been achieved with smaller dosages of radiation, and the following rather interesting comparative data will help to provide an answer.

Comparative Data

After the publication of my treatment results (Guttmann, 1958), Rubenfeld and Kaplan (1959) published their experience in the treatment of 43 patients with inoperable carcinoma of the lung who received a tumour dose of 3,000 r delivered over two weeks. This dosage was chosen in an attempt to shorten the overall treatment time for this type of therapy, and was given with a conventional 250 kV machine through two opposing fields. The authors were impressed by the subjective improvement in 72 per cent of their patients, a figure which is almost identical with ours of 75 per cent. However, there is a drastic difference in the survival rates of the two groups. Only 2 of the 43 patients treated with a tumour dose of 3,000 r have survived 12 months—that is, 4·5 per cent. This is in sharp contrast to our group of patients who were given a tumour dose of 5,000–6,000 rads over 5–6 weeks. Sixty of our 150 patients (that is, 40 per cent) have survived for 12 months.

The opinion that there is a definite correlation between the increase in the tumour dose and the survival rate of patients who have been treated for inoperable carcinoma of the lung is further supported by the findings reported by Hocker and Guttmann (1944). Ninety-three patients with inoperable lung cancer who were included in this report were treated with a tumour dose of 4,000 r over 3–4 weeks on a 1,000 kV roentgen ray unit. We were impressed by the subjective improvement in most cases, and even more by the fact that 20 of these 93 patients with advanced inoperable disease (that is, 21·5 per cent) survived longer than one year. These figures do not reach the results in our series of unselected patients (Guttmann, 1958), but they are definitely better than those obtained with the smaller dosages (Rubenfeld and Kaplan, 1959). It is interesting to note that the treatment results in the three groups can be expressed in an ascending curve in which the improved survival rates correspond to the higher tumour dose (*Figure 4*).

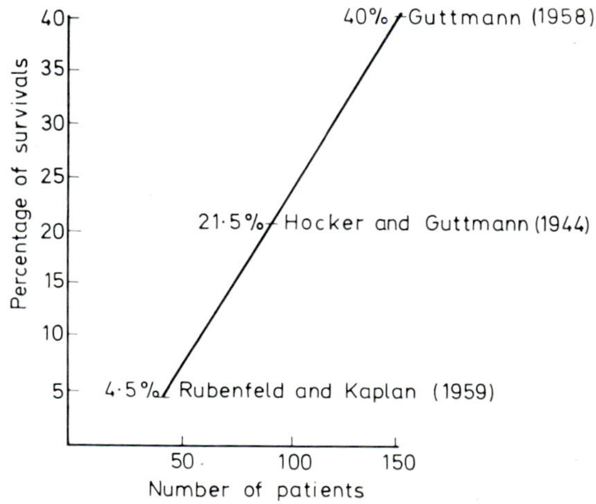

Figure 4. Comparison of percentage of survivals in the three series, showing that the higher the tumour dose, the better the results

While it is conceivable that any one of the groups treated may have been made up of more favourable patient material than the others, the details obtainable from the original publications as to the extent of the disease reveal a striking similarity which makes the statistical results as comparable as statistics ever can be.

REPORT ON 103 CASES FOUND AT OPERATION TO BE UNRESECTABLE

The cases discussed above include all patients with inoperable carcinoma of the lung—those who were inoperable because of clinical evidence of distant metastases as well as those who were found to be unresectable at the time of an exploratory thoracotomy. The next phase of this investigation has concentrated on patients who did lend themselves to an exploratory thoracotomy but were found to be inoperable at the time of surgery. This project seemed to be of special importance, as many surgeons and radiotherapists do not even offer such patients any therapy after an unsuccessful thoracotomy as long as they are asymptomatic. I hope the following review will prove that it is worth while to revise this attitude.

This report will centre on 103 patients with malignant tumours of the lung who were found to be unresectable at the time of an exploratory thoracotomy and who were treated with irradiation between July 1955 and July 1962. This is a selected group consisting of only those patients who underwent an exploratory thoracotomy, who had their diagnosis verified by a microscopic examination of the tumour, and who were treated with a full course of supervoltage therapy. Patients who were not referred for radiotherapy immediately after the exploratory thoracotomy, but some months later for symptomatic relief or for the treatment of metastases, are not included.

The microscopic classification of the 103 patients is shown in Table 1.

TABLE 1

Microscopic Classification of 103 Patients with Unresectable Malignant Disease of the Lung at Thoracotomy

Classification	*Number of patients*	
Squamous cell carcinoma	56	
Anaplastic carcinoma	12	73
Oat cell carcinoma	5	
Carcinoma		17
Alveolar carcinoma		1
Adenocarcinoma		10
Thymoma		1
Mesothelioma		1
Total		103

Technique and Results

The treatment approach has been a rather uniform one. A total tumour dose of 5,000 rads was delivered over five weeks. Included in the field of radiation were the entire involved lung and the involved side of the mediastinum. A 2 MV roentgen ray unit operating at a target skin distance of 100 cm with a half-value layer of 7 mm of lead was utilized. Large opposing fields were used as described above, but no rotation or scanning was applied as either of these methods contributes some radiation to the healthy opposing side.

Figures 5 and *6* bear out clearly that this additional radiation is undesirable, that the preservation of unimpaired function of the healthy opposite lung is essential for survival since the treatment results in complete fibrosis of the diseased side. *Figure 5* represents the chest film of a patient with unresectable carcinoma of the right lung after an exploratory thoracotomy. *Figure 6* shows the same

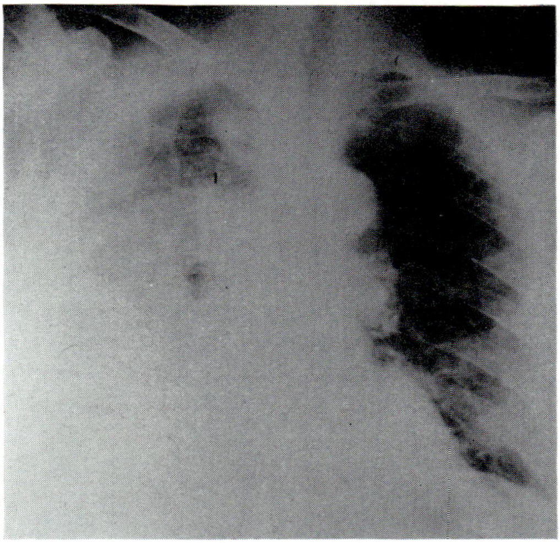

Figure 5. Chest film after exploratory thoracotomy. The tumour was inoperable because of extensive involvement of the mediastinum

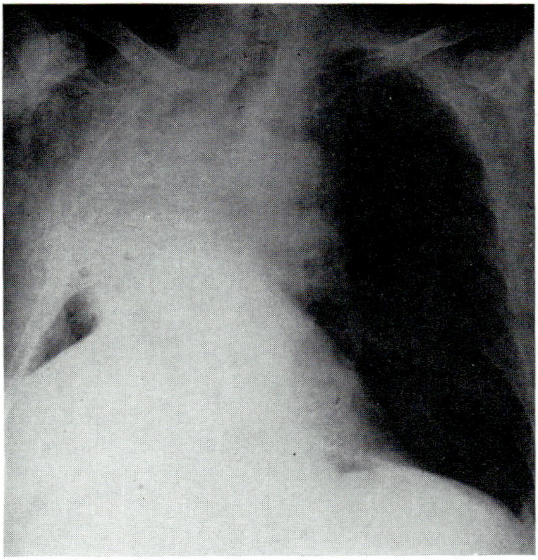

Figure 6. Chest film 2½ years after radiotherapy. The treated lung shows complete fibrosis

patient $2\frac{1}{2}$ years after therapy and demonstrates the complete fibrosis of the treated side. The patient was alive and asymptomatic three years after radiotherapy. Had the other lung received some irradiation by scan or rotation, it would have shown unavoidable fibrotic changes which would make the patient a respiratory cripple to say the least. This film (*Figure 6*) is rather typical of the roentgenological appearance of a heavily radiated lung, showing the expected—and, in this situation, even desired—complete fibrosis.

Again it should be pointed out that a similar approach can be used with other supervoltage units—for instance, with a cobalt-60 unit operating at a STD of 75 cm, with a linear accelerator or with a betatron.

The immediate tolerance to this amount of radiation is excellent, and we have not encountered any serious side effects. In none of our patients have we seen damage to the spinal cord or to any of the vital healthy surrounding organs.

Roentgenographically, the majority of these patients show relatively slight changes, while only in a minority is there complete disappearance of the lesion after therapy. One such case is shown in *Figures 7* and *8*.

The patient presented with a two months' history of cough, fever and right chest pain. A large mass, histologically diagnosed as adenocarcinoma, was found to be filling the right upper lobe and extending into the hilar and mediastinal nodes, and was deemed to be inoperable because of the extensive mediastinal involvement. The patient was referred for radiotherapy. He was treated in the way described above, receiving a tumour dose of 5,400 rads over $5\frac{1}{2}$ weeks. He tolerated the treatments extremely well; his complaints disappeared, and so did the lesion roentgenographically.

It must be emphasized that the lack of dramatic changes in the roentgenograms is not necessarily a poor prognostic sign. Obviously, large tumours which have often caused changes in surrounding tissues do not melt away under radiotherapy. Radiation pneumonitis, pleurisy and later fibrosis appear and frequently persist for the duration of the patient's life. How much, therefore, of the original tumour shadow remains is impossible to determine by follow-up roentgenological studies.

Survival Rates

The results of applying this treatment method in the total group of 103 patients who were explored, found to be unresectable and

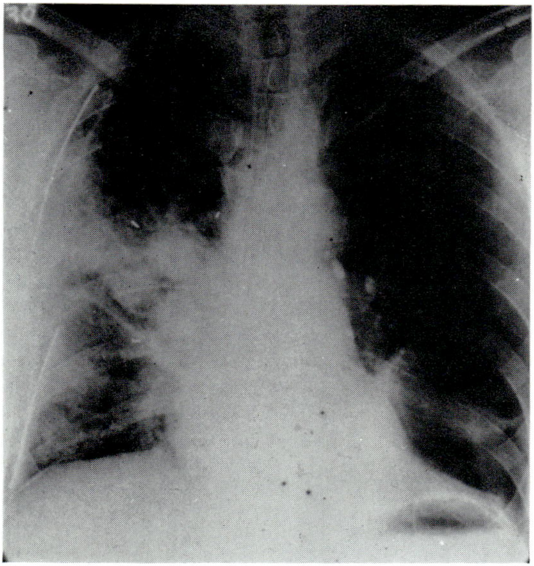

(*a*)

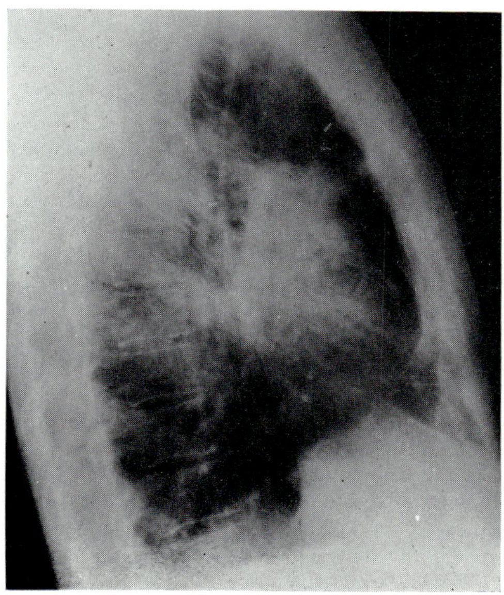

(*b*)

Figure 7. (a) Antero-posterior and (b) lateral chest film after exploratory thoracotomy. The tumour was inoperable because of extensive mediastinal involvement

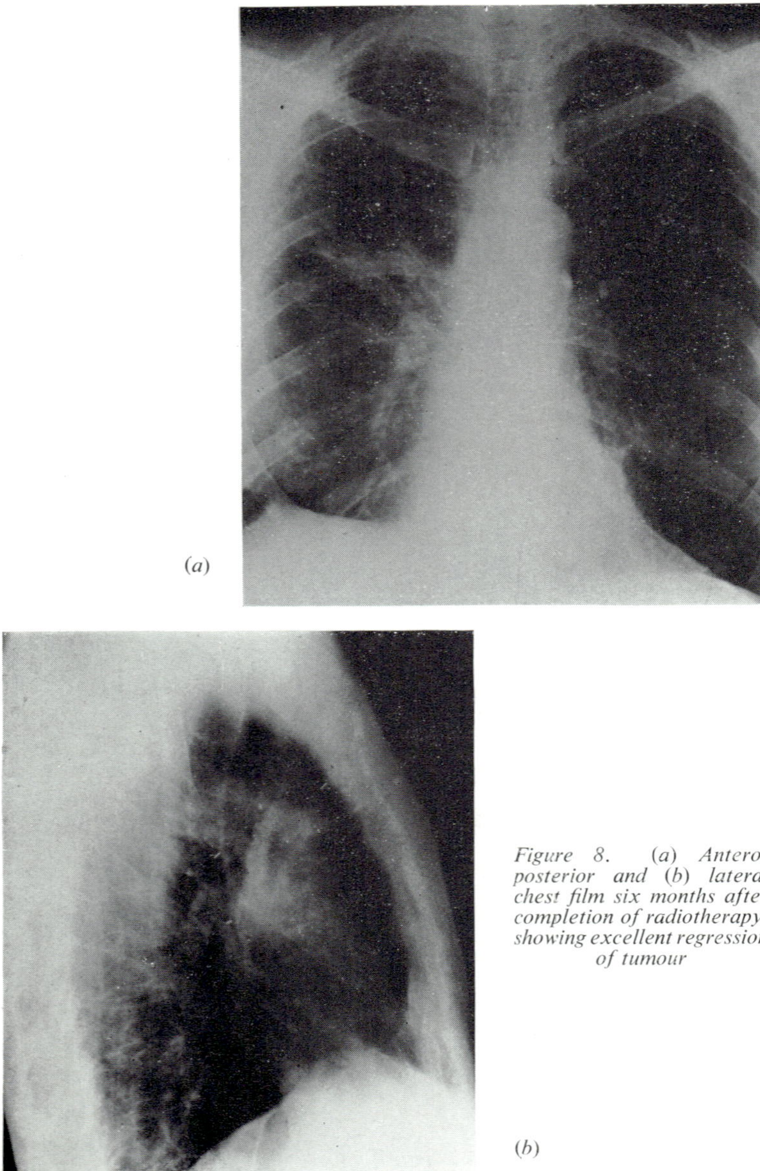

(*a*)

(*b*)

Figure 8. (*a*) *Antero-posterior and* (*b*) *lateral chest film six months after completion of radiotherapy, showing excellent regression of tumour*

given a full course of irradiation are shown in Table 2. Fifty-nine have been alive for one year or more; of these, 29 patients have lived longer than two years; of these 29 patients, 18 have lived more than three years; of these, 11 have lived more than four years, 9 have lived five years, and 7 have lived ten years and are still alive. The average survival time is 27 months, compared with 10 weeks to 9 months in untreated cases as reported in the literature.

TABLE 2

Survival Rates in 103 Patients with Unresectable Malignant Disease of the Lung at Thoracotomy

Duration of survival	*Number of patients*	
More than 1 year	59	(57·2%)
More than 2 years	29	(28·1%)
More than 3 years	18	(17·4%)
More than 4 years	11	(10·6%)
More than 5 years	9	(8·7%)
More than 10 years	7	(6·8%)

TABLE 3

Resectability and Survival Rates in Pulmonary Carcinoma: Data Collected from Six Clinics in the United States

Total number of patients	4,814
Explored	2,792
Resected	1,637
Five-year survival	412
Five-year survival of explored patients	14·75%

These figures take on an even greater significance when some of the overall figures in pulmonary cancer are recalled. Pack and Ariel (1960) have recently published data on resectability and survival rates which were collected from six large clinics in the United States for a total of 4,814 patients (Table 3). Although it was not especially mentioned in this report, it can be assumed that the patients who survived five years came from the group in which resection of the tumour was possible. This would leave, in other words, 1,155 patients in the group undergoing exploratory operations with no five-year survivors, compared with a five-year survival of 8·7 per cent in our patients who had unresectable tumours. In looking at these figures, one has to keep in mind not only the importance of the five-year survival but also that the number of patients who benefited from radiotherapy for one, two, three and four years, and who lived useful lives, must be taken into consideration.

SUMMARY

The treatment of inoperable carcinoma of the lung with irradiation exclusively has been discussed and two patient groups have been evaluated. All patients received a minimal tumour dose of 5,000 rads delivered over five weeks by a 2 MV roentgen ray unit through large opposing fields, including the involved lung and the mediastinum on the involved side. The tolerance to this amount of radiation has been excellent; there has been symptomatic relief in 75 per cent of the cases, and a definite increase in life expectancy from 1 to 14 years. It has been observed that tumours of the epithelium respond better than those of glandular tissue.

The survival rates in the group of 103 patients who were treated with irradiation after an exploratory thoracotomy had revealed an unresectable lung cancer is as follows: the one-year survival has been 57·2 per cent, the two-year survival 28·1 per cent, the three-year survival 17·4 per cent, the four-year survival 10·6 per cent, the five-year survival 8·7 per cent, and the ten-year survival 6·8 per cent. The average survival time of these patients has been raised to 27 months, compared with 10 weeks to 9 months in the untreated patients as reported in the literature.

We therefore believe that the question which we set out to investigate, namely whether definitive treatment with supervoltage irradiation is indicated and can be tolerated in patients suffering from unresectable carcinoma of the lung, can be answered in the affirmative. It is urged that well-planned irradiation, as outlined in this chapter, should be offered immediately after the exploratory thoracotomy, since it cannot be conceived that such beneficial results as we have reported can be achieved when the tumour is permitted to grow and spread after an unsuccessful exploration.

BIBLIOGRAPHY AND REFERENCES

Bauer, R. and Hartweg, H. (1952). 'Erfahrungen und Ergebnisse der Röntgenstrahlenbehandlung des Bronchial-bzw. Lungenkrebses.' *Strahlentherapie* **88,** 8.

Blomfield, G. W. (1953). 'Experience with two million volt x-ray therapy and preliminary assessment of clinical results.' *Proc. R. Soc. Med.* **46,** 219.

Deeley, T. J. (1967). 'Treatment of inoperable carcinoma of the bronchus by megavoltage x-rays.' *Thorax* **22,** 562.

Garland, L. H. and Sisson, M. A. (1956). 'Results of radiotherapy of bronchial cancer.' *Radiology* **67,** 48.

Guttmann, R. J. (1955). 'Two million volt irradiation therapy for inoperable carcinoma of lung.' *Cancer, N.Y.* **8,** 1254.

— (1958). 'Experiences in treatment of inoperable carcinoma of lung with 2 MV and cobalt-60 irradiation.' *Am. J. Roentg.* **79,** 505.

Haas, L. L., Harvey, R. A. and Langer, S. S. (1954). 'Radiation management of otherwise hopeless thoracic neoplasms.' *J. Am. med. Ass.* **154,** 323.

— — and Melchor, C. F. (1957). 'Radiotherapeutic experiences with inoperable lung carcinoma.' *Cancer, N.Y.* **10,** 280.

Hocker, A. F. and Guttmann, R. J. (1944). 'Three and one-half years' experience with 1,000 kilovolt roentgentherapy unit at Memorial Hospital.' *Am. J. Roentg.* **51,** 83.

Hustu, H. O. and Nickson, J. J. (1964). 'Carcinoma of lung: results of radiological treatment.' *Am. J. Roentg.* **91,** 95.

Kutz, E. R. (1958). 'Intensive cobalt-60 teletherapy of lung cancer.' *Radiology* **71,** 327.

Medical Research Council (1966). 'Comparative trial of surgery and radiotherapy for the primary treatment of small-cell or oat-cell carcinoma of the bronchus.' *Lancet* **2,** 979.

Pack, G. T. and Ariel, I. M. (1960). *Tumors of the Breast, Chest and Esophagus,* Vol. 4, p. 323. New York: Hoeber.

Rubenfeld, S. and Kaplan, G. (1959). 'Treatment of bronchogenic cancer with conventional x-rays according to specific time–dose pattern.' *Radiology* **73,** 761.

Rubin, P. (1966). 'Current cancer concepts: bronchogenic carcinoma.' *J. Am. med. Ass.* **195,** 662; **195,** 1036; **196,** 348; **196,** 853.

12—Methods of Improving Results of Radiation

I—Fractionation Technique

D. K. Sambrook

The question to be considered in this chapter is whether any advantages can be gained in the radiation treatment of lung cancer by modifications of fractionation.

The advantages which are sought are of two main kinds:

(1) A *simplification* of treatment so that it is less exhausting and burdensome to the patient, yet without sacrificing any benefits which he may obtain.

(2) An *increase in the efficiency* of treatment in terms of better tumour control, yet without an increase or with an actual reduction in local radiation reactions and damage to adjacent normal tissues.

RESULTS OF RADIOTHERAPY IN LUNG CANCER

It must reluctantly be admitted that despite the great technical advances in radiotherapy during recent years, there has been very little improvement in the prognosis of inoperable lung cancer. Bruce and Ash (1963), reviewing nearly 1,000 cases treated in Toronto between 1930 and 1957, concluded that the survival rates of patients treated for this disease had changed little since 1930 despite the introduction of supervoltage and cobalt therapy.

Roswit and colleagues (1968) have recently reported the results of a large-scale prospective randomized study of over 500 inoperable male patients, in which radiation was compared with a placebo. This was carried out in 17 hospitals in the U.S.A. under the aegis of the Veterans' Administration. Radiotherapy was given to 308 patients, the agreed factors being a tumour dose between 4,000 rads (minimum) and 5,000 rads (maximum), given in five fractions per week over 4–6 weeks; 246 patients were given an inert substance and served as untreated controls. (Patients requiring definitive treatment for palliation were exempted.) The survival rate at one year was 18 per cent in the treated group and 14 per cent in the control group, and the median survival time was 142 days in the treated group as against 112 days in the controls. When patients receiving less than the intended dose were excluded, it made no difference to the survival pattern. The only significant factors influencing survival were a long history and a well-differentiated tumour, these being associated with longer survival in both treated and untreated patients.

This discouraging report spells out only too clearly the failure of radiotherapy to improve significantly the survival of patients with advanced lung cancer. However, the authors emphasize that they were not investigating symptomatic effects, and their experience confirmed that radiation can often give important symptomatic relief. This investigation emphasizes the importance of not aggravating the patient's suffering in advanced cases by giving unnecessarily long and distressing courses of radiotherapy which will not significantly prolong life.

Palliative Treatment

Deeley (1966) compared the effects of two different dose levels in patients with inoperable anaplastic carcinoma of the bronchus. Patients were paired as closely as possible according to factors known to affect the prognosis. The dose level for the first member of each pair was decided from random numbers, and the second member then received the other dose. The two levels compared were 3,000 rads in four weeks and 4,000 rads in four weeks, both given by 8 MV linear accelerator. The average field size was closely similar in each series. There were 51 pairs of patients, and the survival rates are shown in Table 1. These differences are significant at the 5 per cent level. There was no significant difference in the incidence of distant metastases or of residual carcinoma within the chest.

The main difference in effect between the two dose levels was seen in the incidence of radiation fibrosis of the lung. In patients surviving long enough for serial radiographs to be taken, this was shown to occur earlier and to have a higher incidence in those given 4,000 rads. The longer survival and lower morbidity in patients given 3,000 rads was probably attributable to the smaller amount of lung fibrosis following this dose. (Deeley remarks that unit density of tissue was assumed in calculating tumour doses. Owing to the presence of aerated lung in part of the fields, actual doses may have been up to 30 per cent higher.)

TABLE 1

Percentage Survival Rates Compared in 51 Pairs of Patients

Duration of survival after treatment	*Tumour dose in 4 weeks* *3,000 rads*	*4,000 rads*
6 months	56	52
12 months	20	16
18 months	14	—
24 months	6	—

Radical Treatment

From the above reports, it is clear that little or no advantage is to be expected from long courses or high dosage in the palliative treatment of advanced cases. What about radical radiotherapy, with the object of cure of the disease?

In lung cancer, dissemination by the blood stream occurs so commonly and so early that even if the primary tumour could be destroyed in every case, most patients would still die from distant metastases. Nevertheless, if a patient is fortunate enough to be diagnosed when the disease is at an early stage, a chance of cure exists, as can be seen from the results of lobectomy or pneumonectomy in such cases.

Hilton and Smart (1956) and Smart (1966) reported the results of medium-voltage x-ray therapy in 40 carefully selected early cases. Dose–time factors were 5,000–5,500 r given in daily fractions over 7–8 weeks for squamous carcinoma, and 4,000–4,500 r for anaplastic tumours; 22 per cent of the patients survived for more than five years, a result comparable with those of surgical series at that time.

Comparison with Surgery

Since most early cases are still treated surgically, could radiotherapy do as well or better, now that modern apparatus and more accurate dosimetry make radical treatment simpler?

Morrison, Deeley and Cleland (1963) carried out a careful prospective trial in 58 patients with disease confined to the thorax, without evidence of gross mediastinal metastases, who were randomly allocated to surgery or supervoltage radiotherapy (by 8 MV linear accelerator). Twenty patients with squamous cell tumours allocated to surgery showed a four-year survival rate of 30 per cent, whereas of 17 patients allocated to radiotherapy, only one (6 per cent) survived—a significant difference at the 5 per cent level. Patients with anaplastic lesions showed no significant difference in survival after rdiotherapy or surgery. In fact, nine patients allocated to the surgical group were found to be inoperable at thoracotomy, and three others developed extrathoracic metastases and were therefore not operated on. The four-year survival rate of those who did undergo radical surgery (17 patients) was 41 per cent; of these, 82 per cent had squamous carcinoma. The inference must be that for early squamous carcinoma, surgery is much more effective than radiotherapy. Yet an objection may be raised against this conclusion on the grounds that the tumour dose received by the irradiated patients was only 4,500 rads given over four weeks by daily fractions (equivalent to 4,100 r in medium-voltage roentgens)—a dose on the low side for cure of squamous carcinoma.

Curative Dose Level

What evidence is available concerning the dose needed to sterilize carcinoma of the lung?

Bloedorn and colleagues (1961) at the University Hospital, Baltimore, carried out a programme of pre-operative irradiation followed two months later by pneumonectomy or lobectomy. In all patients the diagnosis was proved by biopsy before irradiation. The tumour dose to the primary site and adjacent mediastinum was 6,000 r in six weeks by telecobalt therapy. In 26 patients who completed the programme, careful study of multiple sections of the operation specimens showed no recognizable tumour cells at the primary site in 54 per cent, or in mediastinal lymph nodes in 92 per cent.

A more recent study of autopsy findings in patients who had received megavoltage radiotherapy was reported by Rissanen, Tikka and Holsti (1968). There were 67 patients with histologically verified inoperable lung cancer. In 18 cases where no carcinoma could be detected macroscopically or microscopically in the treated area, tumour doses varied between 4,800 and 6,250 rads over 5–10 weeks. (Eight of these patients died from distant metastases, and ten from other causes.) In 26 cases showing clearly viable carcinoma in the treatment area, therapy had been discontinued at 2,000–3,000 rads in 4 cases, and had been interrupted for long periods due to fever or anaemia in 13 others. In 23 other patients who showed islets of carcinoma cells with fibrosis or necrosis, treatment had been suspended or interrupted in 11. All patients receiving less than 3,000 rads tumour dose showed persistence of malignant tissue in the treated area.

In another study of pre-operatively irradiated lung cancer (Hellman and colleagues, 1964), 24 patients were operated on 4–8 weeks after receiving a tumour dose of 5,500–6,000 r in $5\frac{1}{2}$ to 6 weeks by 2 MV x-rays. Seven patients showed no evidence of any residual primary tumour. Of 15 patients with pre-operative radiographic evidence of hilar or mediastinal lymph node enlargement, only three showed residual tumour on microscopy. These authors also investigated early and late reactions in 132 patients undergoing radical radiotherapy at or approaching the same dose level. Transient oesophagitis during or soon after treatment was common and was dose-related, occurring in 12 per cent of patients having less than 4,000 r but in 46 per cent of those receiving over 5,500 r. It settled in all cases within three weeks, and no case of later stricture was noted.

The other common sequel to irradiation was pulmonary fibrosis. The incidence of this condition increased with the passage of time after radiation; it was seen in 50 per cent of cases at nine months and in nearly 90 per cent at two years, but it caused clinical symptoms in fewer than 5 per cent of patients.

These investigations indicate that a tumour dose of 6,000 rads given in daily fractions over six weeks may be expected to sterilize the primary tumour in up to 50 per cent of cases, and hilar and/or mediastinal lymph node metastases in a rather higher proportion. Furthermore, this is a dose which can be tolerated by most patients without serious immediate or late complications.

The size of the tumour is probably an important factor in determining radio-curability. The successfully sterilized tumours in the Helsinki investigation averaged 4–7 cm, whereas in failed cases the average size was 6–9 cm.

Higher doses might sterilize the primary tumour in a larger percentage of cases, but at the cost of an increase in morbidity.

FRACTIONATION TECHNIQUE

Most patients have in the past been treated by the conventional daily fractionation, with 200–250 rads (TD) given on five days per week. Various departures from this conventional method are now under consideration in the hope of (1) reducing the physical and economic burdens of treatment, and (2) improving the therapeutic ratio, defined as the ratio:

$$\frac{\text{tolerance dose of normal tissues}}{\text{lethal dose to tumour cells}}$$

The first objective, to reduce the burden of treatment, is most important in palliative therapy. This may be achieved by increasing the size of fractional doses and spacing them further apart—for example, instead of giving 250 rad fractions five days per week, giving 400 rad fractions three times per week or 600 rad fractions twice weekly.

The second objective, a gain in therapeutic ratio which would result in more effective sterilization of the tumour without a corresponding increase in morbidity from early or late sequelae, would be of value principally in radical therapy. This has been sought mainly by prolonging the overall treatment time, either by giving the treatment in many small fractions or by introducing gaps or rest periods during treatment so that a higher tumour dose can be given without severe reactions.

The number of possible variations of technique based on different combinations and permutations of fraction size, interval and overall time is almost limitless. Clearly, we need some guide as to the effect of such variations on the biological action of the radiation on both tumour and normal tissue. Fortunately such a guide is now available, even if still incomplete.

RADIOBIOLOGICAL RESEARCH IN RELATION TO FRACTIONATION

Some valuable data are available concerning the effects of both fraction size and time. This is perhaps the most notable instance in which radiobiology has made a practical contribution to radiotherapeutic technique. Cell survival curves for mammalian cells, relating loss of reproductive capacity to dose, show a relatively inefficient 'shoulder' in the curve at the beginning of radiation. This is interpreted as being caused by relatively inefficient sterilization due to 'single-hit' ionizing events at small doses, superseded by much more efficient 'multi-hit' events at larger doses. Due to short-term repair of intracellular damage, when radiation is given in fractions at intervals of 24 hours (or longer) the inefficient 'quasi-threshold' recurs at the beginning of each fraction (Elkind and Sutton, 1960). Consequently, if radiation is given in a few large fractions the effect will be greater than that of the same total dose given in many small fractions.

Fowler (1965) has worked out the relationship between total dose and number and size of fractions with respect to skin reactions, based on clinical and experimental data. His tables and nomogram provide a useful guide in estimating the equivalent total dose for different fractionation regimens, but do not take full account of the time factor. This becomes increasingly important when the overall treatment time extends over several weeks. For example, Fowler and colleagues (1963), in experiments on skin reactions in pigs, using fields comparable in size to those in clinical use, found that the single dose (of x-rays) required to produce desquamation was 2,000 rads. When the radiation was given in five fractions over four days, an increase of 80 per cent to 3,600 rads (that is, 5 × 720 rads) was needed to produce the same reaction. If the five fractions were spaced out over 28 days, a further increase to 4,200 rads (that is, 5 × 840 rads) was required. This further increase is due to long-term repair; that is, repopulation by proliferating surviving skin cells. Although this is less important than the effect of fraction size, it is not negligible over longer periods.

Comparison of Two Systems Based on Clinical Data

In recent years, attempts have been made to arrive at a general equation taking account of both short-term and long-term repair so as to provide a formula applicable to fractionation regimens in clinical practice.

Ellis (1967, 1969) has proposed a model based on clinical data. (Cell survival curves obtained by experiments *in vitro* show too great a variation in parameters to be used as a basis for clinical radiotherapy.)

Not only do skin reactions reflect the response of individual squamous epithelial cells, but late reactions are probably largely dependent on the underlying vasculo-connective tissue, and may therefore serve as a valid model for tissue tolerance in most normal tissues (except bone and brain and also kidney, where pressure within the renal capsule may influence acute effects).

Ellis relates total dose, number of fractions and overall treatment time to a concept called nominal standard dose (NSD). This corresponds to the normal tissue tolerance at the tumour site, expressed in rets (rad equivalent therapy given as cobalt-60 radiation) given as a single dose. Fractionation is allowed for by taking the total dose as proportional to the 0·24 power of the number of fractions (N), and the effect of time by taking the total dose as proportional to the 0·11 power of the treatment time in days (T), thus:

$$\text{Total dose} = \text{NSD} \times N^{0\cdot 24} \times T^{0\cdot 11}$$

The fractionation effect $N^{0\cdot 24}$, due to short-term repair, affects normal tissues and tumour cells in similar fashion. The time effect

($T^{0 \cdot 11}$) was derived from the difference in slope of dose–response curves for skin tolerance and cure of squamous carcinoma. It thus represents long-term repair due to regenerative activity in the skin, it being assumed that no such regenerative repair due to homoeostatic mechanisms takes place in tumours, and that repopulation due to inherent proliferation would be relatively unimportant.

Ellis compared the clinical dose schedules for patients treated to tolerance level at various sites in four different radiotherapy centres (Ellis, 1969) and, by application of his equation, derived corresponding values for NSD. These show considerable scatter, as would be expected to occur between different sites and with different field sizes, but there is also some variation in values of NSD for the same site treated at different centres. This is due, no doubt, to the well-known variation in the biological effect of the rad in different centres! Ellis advised, in fact, that each centre should determine its own values for NSD so as to allow for differences in dosimetry and criteria of tolerance. Nevertheless, the values of NSD cluster around a mean of about 1,860 rets. Corresponding values for NSD for tumours were calculated by omitting the regression coefficient for the time factor, that is:

$$\text{NSD tumour} = \frac{\text{total dose}}{N^{0 \cdot 24}}$$

This, in effect, ignores the possibility of a significant degree of tumour cell repopulation during treatment. While this is probably not important over treatment times up to 4–6 weeks (since tumour cells do not have homoeostatic repair mechanisms, and successive doses of radiation should inhibit or delay mitosis), it may not be negligible in treatment schedules extending over longer periods, either with very small fractions or with rest periods of several weeks as in the split course method.

Cohen (1968) in Johannesburg has also proposed a model to describe both skin and tumour response to radiation, based on established radiobiological principles. The optimal parameters for his equation were obtained by fitting the model to published data of clinically observed dose–time relationships—in fact, much the same data as those used by Ellis. A later development (Cohen and Scott, 1968) replaced the simple exponential coefficient for the regeneration of surviving viable cells by a much more sophisticated logistic function.

Hall (1969) has undertaken a comparison of these two systems (which were developed independently in different parts of the world, but were both based on the same clinical data from daily fractionated regimens). Iso-effect curves produced by the two systems agree closely for daily treatments five days per week, as would be expected. However, when the curves are drawn for a regimen in which fractions are given every four days, there is not such close agreement. There is also an increasing divergence between the curves predicting tolerance doses for regimens protracted over longer times than those commonly used, for example 5–6 weeks.

These disparities follow from a difference in the basic premises on which the two models are based. In Cohen and Scott's system, total dose is taken initially to be proportional to the number of fractions (N) in almost the same way as in Ellis's system, that is:

Ellis: Dose $\propto N^{0 \cdot 24}$
Cohen and Scott: Dose $\propto N^{0 \cdot 25}$

This is held to apply, however, over only a limited range of 2–15 fractions. When treatment is given in a large number of fractions, each fraction will be small, and the smaller the fraction the higher its effect will fall on the flat part of the 'Elkind shoulder' region of the cell survival curve. This is simply another way of saying that cell-killing or loss of reproductive capacity with smaller doses of radiation not only becomes disproportionately less than with larger doses, but is increasingly due to single-hit events, and this effect is simply additive and independent of the number of fractions in which the total dose is delivered. Conversely, with time, for short treatments of 4–15 fractions the coefficient is $T^{0 \cdot 14}$ to $T^{0 \cdot 18}$ and is not very different from Ellis's $T^{0 \cdot 11}$. However, for longer treatment times it increases rapidly and continuously, reaching a value of $T^{0 \cdot 6}$ for overall times of 80–100 days. This is due to an assumption that the regeneration of normal cells on which tolerance depends can restore the population to its original level, given sufficient time. This would lead to the prediction that tolerance would be virtually unlimited if time were sufficiently prolonged. This is not in accordance with clinical observation. Once a tissue has had a maximum tolerance dose, it cannot tolerate such a dose again, no matter how long afterwards it is given. There is also a definite top limit of tolerance dose, even with very long protraction of treatment.

Baclesse (1955), reporting the results of treatment of carcinoma of the breast by high doses fractionated over periods of 3–4 months, noted that 'beyond a certain dose the fractionation does not give assurance against immediate or late damage'. At least two patients receiving 9,000 r tumour dose developed radionecrosis.

Andrews (1965), in a clinical study of extremes of dose and time factors in radiotherapy of cancers of the mouth and upper air passages, found that a tumour dose of 10,000 r in 43 fractions over 100 days represented an absolute upper limit of normal tissue tolerance. This regimen, analysed by Ellis's equation, gives a value of NSD of 2,400 ret (for normal tissues). In a group of 43 patients given doses of this order there were 22 instances of serious complications due to radiation damage, so it may well be that the tolerance limit should be lower.

The writer also has met with delayed radionecrosis in rather a high percentage of patients given doses in excess of 7,500 r by the split course technique, although severe immediate reactions were avoided by this method (Sambrook, 1968).

A practical objection to Cohen and Scott's system is the complexity of the mathematics needed to solve the equation for the various parameters; as Hall remarks, access to a digital computer would be necessary. On the other hand, Ellis's system provides a relatively simple and readily applicable method of assessing and comparing the biological effects of different fractionation schedules, and is reliable over a range of 4–30 fractions and for times from 3 to 60 days. Furthermore, it can be employed to calculate 'partial tolerance' values for limited treatments, and can also be used to estimate NSD in split course treatments and when changes have been made in the size of dose per fraction. Ellis's values for NSD show a close correspondence with Fowler's figures based on skin reaction experiments in pigs (Fowler and colleagues, 1963).

An indication of the gain in therapeutic ratio can be obtained from Ellis's system by omitting the time factor in calculating NSD for the tumour. As mentioned above, this must be treated with some reserve, especially where rapidly growing tumours are concerned. In the case of a split course treatment, an increase in total dose of the order of 10 per cent is estimated to compensate for any likely tumour repopulation during a three-week rest interval (Sambrook, 1968).

CLINICAL EXPERIENCE WITH UNORTHODOX FRACTIONATION IN LUNG CANCER

Levitt, Bogardus and Ladd (1967) reported the results of a prospective randomized clinical trial, comparing an intensive split-dose technique with conventional daily fractionated therapy in 29 patients with inoperable histologically confirmed squamous carcinoma of the bronchus.

The split-dose course (in 15 patients) consisted of 3 doses of 600 rads (TD) delivered on 3 consecutive days and repeated 28 days later, thus giving a total dose of 3,600 rads in 6 fractions over 31 days. The daily fractionated course (in 14 patients) consisted of a tumour dose of 6,000 rads given over 6–8 weeks. No significant differences were found in symptomatic relief or survival between the two groups. The incidence of dysphagia due to treatment was similar. Monthly follow-up radiographs showed a somewhat higher incidence of lung fibrosis in the split-dose group, and recurrence in the treated area was seen more often. The authors concluded that the split-dose technique was preferable in symptomatic treatment of advanced lung cancer because of the great advantage of fewer attendances.

A comparison of these techniques using Ellis's formula gives the values for NSD (or partial tolerance) shown in Table 2. The biological effect of the split-dose course is only a little less than with the six weeks' daily fractionated course.

TABLE 2

Comparison of Split Dose with Daily Fractionated Course

Dosage	*NSD (or PT)*	*NSD (tumour)*
6,000 rads in 6 weeks (daily, 5 per week)	1,770 ret	2,650
3 × 600 rads daily; 4 weeks' rest; 3 × 600 rads again	1,740 ret	2,340

Dutreix, Schlienger and le Peigneux (1967) at the Institut Gustave Roussy, near Paris, report satisfactory palliative results from a similar technique in which 2 doses of 650 rads are given in 48 hours, followed by 3 weeks' rest, and then 9 fractions of 300 rads given 3 times per week.

Deeley (1966) has conducted a comparative trial of twice weekly and five times weekly fractionation in carcinoma of the bronchus. Somewhat different dose levels were given to anaplastic and squamous carcinomas (Table 3). The preliminary results for two years have shown no differences in survival rates, morbidity or incidence of metastatic spread between the groups of patients treated in 20 and in 8 treatments. The NSD as calculated by Ellis' equation for each pair of techniques is identical. Clearly the twice weekly technique is greatly preferable from the patients' point of view, especially if they are treated as out-patients.

TABLE 3

Comparison of Twice Weekly and Five Times Weekly Fractionation

	Five times weekly	*Twice weekly*
Anaplastic bronchial carcinoma	3,000 r/28 days, given as 20 × 150 rads	2,400 r/28 days, given as 8 × 300 rads
Squamous bronchial carcinoma	4,000 r/28 days, given as 20 × 200 rads	3,200 r/28 days, given as 8 × 400 rads

Somewhat similar techniques employing a few large fractions are currently employed in several large radiotherapy centres in Britain in palliative treatment of carcinoma of the bronchus, for example:

3 × 600 r in 1 week (Newcastle)
5 × 500 r in 1 week (Liverpool)

A note of caution should perhaps be sounded regarding treatment of patients with partial obstruction of the trachea or the main bronchi. A recent study carried out at Edinburgh (Cameron and colleagues, 1969) showed a significant reduction in forced expiratory volume during the first four days of irradiation in 22 of 28 patients with a carcinoma situated in a main or lobar bronchus, the reduction being greatest in the case of proximally situated tumours. This appeared to be caused by swelling of the tumour as a result of intracellular and extracellular oedema due to early cell damage. Improvement in ventilatory function consequent on tumour shrinkage did not counteract this effect until the fourth to the sixth day after commencing irradiation. The fractions in this series were only 250 or 330 rads, given daily. Larger fractions at the inception of treatment might have an even greater immediate oedema-inducing effect. Where dangerous narrowing of the trachea or of both main bronchi is present, it might be prudent to start treatment with small daily fractions and to administer corticosteroids for the first 3–4 days.

RADICAL TREATMENT: THE VALUE OF SPLIT COURSE TECHNIQUE

Radical therapy may reasonably be decided on as an elective procedure in the following classes of case:

(1) Early operable cases of squamous carcinoma where pneumonectomy is contra-indicated by inadequate pulmonary or cardiac function, or where the patient refuses operation.

(2) Early localized tumours too close to the carina to permit complete removal and safe closure of the bronchial stump.

(3) Early localized cases of anaplastic or oat cell tumours.

There remains a group of cases of more advanced disease in which the wisdom of attempting radical treatment may be in doubt.

Superior Mediastinal Obstruction

This may occur early in the evolution of the disease due to the site of the tumour, and provided there is no sign of distant metastases it does not necessarily contra-indicate radical treatment.

Pleural Effusion

A serous effusion may occur due to local hilar obstructive effects. This does not necessarily indicate wide pleural spread, which generally causes a blood-stained effusion containing clusters of malignant cells.

A Large Radiographic Shadow

This may be largely due to atelectasis of the lung distal to a blocked bronchus or division. Alternatively, pneumonitis resulting from sepsis around a tumour may account for much of the shadow. Both conditions often resolve in the course of treatment.

Supraclavicular Node Metastases

When these are present, distant metastases are generally present or will soon develop, but Deeley and Line (1969) found that in 11 per cent of autopsies of patients with involvement of these nodes there was no evidence of spread elsewhere in the body.

It is suggested that patients in these groups should be selected for what may be called 'provisional radical treatment'. In fact, almost any patient in whom the disease is confined to the thorax and whose general condition is good might be placed in this category. Treatment is planned and commenced as in an elective course of radical therapy. When approximately half the intended dose has been given—for example, 2,500–3,000 rads in 2–3 weeks—treatment is suspended for 3–4 weeks. The patient is then reassessed clinically and radiologically after this rest interval. At this point it will be found that most patients fall naturally into one of two groups. Some will show clear evidence of improvement, or at least no deterioration, in their general condition; in others there will be equally clear evidence of deterioration in general condition in such ways as increasing weakness, wasting, anaemia or signs of distant metastases, with or without some relief of local symptoms. The first group, with local and general improvement, may then resume treatment and continue to the full tumour dose decided on. This now amounts to a 'split course', which has been used as an elective technique in several centres.

Holsti and Vuorinen (1967), in Helsinki, have employed the split course technique in lung cancer since 1963. Treatment was by telecobalt or 33 MV x-rays. Minimum tumour doses were 5,000–6,000 rads in 5–6 weeks in continuous therapy, given 6 days per week, and about 5–10 per cent more in split course therapy, with an additional 2–3 weeks' overall time due to the rest interval interposed as described and averaging 16–17 days. Although selection was not truly random, Holsti treated all his cases by split course, whereas the other therapist treated his by the continuous method. The composition of the two groups was similar except that metastases outside the thorax were present in 20 per cent of the split course group but in only 7 per cent of the continuously treated patients. The results are shown in Table 4. The recurrence-free rate at one year was the same in both groups, namely 28 per cent.

TABLE 4

Survival Rates after Split Course and Continuous Therapy

Technique	*Survival after treatment* 6 months	1 year	2 years
Split course	91/130 (70%)	46/130 (35%)	5/51 (10%)
Continuous	29/54 (54%)	18/54 (33%)	1/27 (4%)

In a later paper from the same centre (Rissanen, Tikka and Holsit, 1968) analysing autopsy findings in cases of lung cancer treated by megavoltage radiotherapy, 14 of 38 cases (37 per cent) treated by split course had complete microscopic destruction of the tumour, whereas of 29 treated by the continuous method, only 4 (14 per cent) showed no tumour in the treated area. The incidence of distant metastases in the split course group was 76 per cent, and in the continuous group 93 per cent. On this evidence, it would appear that patients treated by the split course as described certainly do no worse, at least, than those given conventional continuous treatment.

In one respect, a definite advantage has been demonstrated for the split course method. Holsti and Vuorinen (1967) compared the incidence and severity of radiation pneumonitis in 74 patients treated by a split course with those in 33 patients treated by a continuous regimen. Dose levels were similar, but were a little higher in the split course group—nearly one-third of these having a tumour dose between 6,000 and 7,000 r, while only a quarter of the continuous group had over 6,000 r. The incidence of radiological signs of pneumonitis and later fibrosis was the same after split course as after continuous therapy, but both symptoms and signs of the reaction occurred about two months later in the split course group and were unquestionably milder. It was noted that patients tolerated a split course much better, and dysphagia disappeared during the rest interval.

Cook, West and Kraft (1968) described the results of split course irradiation (with 2 MV x-rays) in 332 cases of inoperable lung cancer (all histologically confirmed), some of whom had undergone incomplete surgery. The first course of treatment consisted of a tumour dose of 2,000–2,400 rads given in 8 daily fractions or 2,500–3,000 rads given in 20 treatment days. (No correction was made for increased transmission through the lung.) A full radiological and clinical assessment was made eight weeks after completing the first course, and a second similar course was then given if feasible. In practice, 50 per cent of their patients did not complete the second course. This fact, as the authors remark, reflects a certain advantage, in that patients with a short life-expectancy are spared the ordeal of a more lengthy course of treatment. They found the short intensive course (8 × 250–300 rads) was well tolerated, and preferred this in the majority of cases to the longer course over $3\frac{1}{2}$ weeks. Of those patients completing irradiation, 37·5 per cent survived one year and 12·7 per cent survived two years. The rest interval was found to be valuable in increasing the patients' tolerance of a long course of treatment.

The writer has for several years been using a split course technique in the occasional elective radical treatment as well as in the more numerous provisional radical cases. Of 88 patients treated from mid-1962 until 1966, 18 per cent were alive over one year and 12 per cent more than two years after treatment. All these patients were treated by 250 kV x-rays. The technique employed at present (with telecobalt therapy) consists of 8 fractions of 400 rads tumour dose, given three times per week, followed by a 3–4 week rest interval and repeated if the patient is fit to undergo the second course. This is well tolerated and, examined by Ellis's formula, gives a value for NSD of 2,120 ret and 3,280 NSD tumour.

OPTIMAL FRACTION SIZE AND SPACING

So far, the size and spacing of fractionated doses have been considered mainly from the point of view of socio-economic convenience, subject only to the condition that the new regimen should not be less effective therapeutically. Is it possible that these factors may be manipulated so as to give a positive therapeutic advantage—that is, an enhanced effect on the tumour without a corresponding increase in damage to normal tissues?

The radiobiological factors particularly relevant to this question are:

(1) The presence of hypoxic tumour cells, and the effect of fraction size and spacing on their subsequent recruitment into a better oxygenated state.

(2) Variation in radiosensitivity of tumour cells at different phases of their mitotic–intermitotic cell cycle.

Evidence of recruitment of anoxic cells to a more radiosensitive aerobic state following a dose of radiation has been obtained by Field, Jones and Thomlinson (1968) and by Hawkes and colleagues (1968) at St. Bartholomew's Hospital, London, in certain animal tumours. In some cases the increase in sensitivity more than offset the effect of short-term repair and continued after 24 hours to 48 or 72 hours. The optimal intervals between fractions may vary in different tumours and at different periods during a course of treatment, and reliable data for human tumours are lacking. Since shrinkage of the tumour is instrumental in improving the blood supply, intervals of several days may be better than 24 hours.

Mitchell (1968) made an interesting observation of the effect of different timing of the weekend two-day break in a course of deep x-ray therapy in carcinoma of the lip. Some patients commenced (daily fractionated) treatment on Monday, the course being represented as 5002. Others commenced on Thursday, so that their course was numbered 2005. The placing of the two-day rest interval near the end of the course instead of near the beginning apparently led to a significant improvement in results. This may be explicable as being due to recruitment of hypoxic cells remaining after the first five fractions into an aerobic state before the last two fractions were given.

Kallman (1967) reviewed the experimental evidence for cyclic fluctuations in radiosensitivity at various times after an initial dose of radiation. In a variety of target tissues, after an initial dose of moderate size, a surprising degree of synchronization of mitosis resulted, following which cyclical fluctuations in sensitivity to a subsequent dose were demonstrable during the next few days. However, in order to exploit this effect in therapy, the time of occurrence of sensitive phases would need to be known fairly accurately not only for the tumour cells but also for normal tissues in the irradiated field, so as to time the administration of further doses to coincide with sensitive tumour cell and resistant normal cell phases.

Hahn (1968) calculated the possible relative gain in killing a strain of cancer cells growing in tissue culture by appropriate cell cycle modulation. A computer was used to calculate the optimal spacing of 300 r fractions so as to cause maximal killing of a strain of malignant (HeLa) cells and minimal damage to another strain (L cells), with a different cell cycle, growing in the same area. The resultant gain from optimizing these intervals was of the order of 10^4. Again, data relating to human tumours and tissues are lacking, and research to elucidate them will probably be difficult and time-consuming. Empirical guide-lines to advantageous techniques may come in time from computer analysis of pooled data for tumour control and normal tissue reactions for different fractionation techniques from many different centres.

Investigations show that changes in the rate of proliferation of epidermoid cells following radiation damage may be very important, as is shown in the work of Devik (1962) and Breur (1968). There was evidence of a dramatic shortening of the cell cycle of irradiated epidermal cells following a dose of radiation which had produced a clinically evident reaction. Van den Brenk (1966—personal communication) found similar evidence of regenerative activity following radiation damage, and also noted that it varied from tissue to tissue and even from region to region in human skin. Since these homoeostatic mechanisms in epidermal tissues become operative only after a fairly large dose has been given, advantage can best be taken of them by some such technique as the split course. In the case of bowel reactions, where a rapidly dividing cell-replenishing mechanism is already present under normal conditions, spacing larger fractional doses at intervals of several days should lead to improved tolerance.

Probably one of the most critically significant factors in tolerance is the response of vasculo-endothelial structures. The parameters for damage and repair of these tissues, which form the supporting stroma of nearly all normal tissues, still remain to be worked out.

REFERENCES

Andrews, J. R. (1965). 'Dose–time relationships in cancer radiotherapy.' *Am. J. Roentg.* **93,** 56.

Baclesse, F. J. (1955). 'Pre-operative x-ray therapy in breast cancer.' *J. Fac. Radiol.* **6,** 145.

Bloedorn, F. G., Cowley, R. A., Cuccia, C. A. and Mercado, R. (1961). 'Combined therapy: irradiation and surgery in the treatment of bronchogenic carcinoma.' *Am. J. Roentg.* **85,** 875.

Breur, K. (1968). *The Growth-rate of Tumours.* Lecture to Faculty of Radiologists, London.

Bruce, W. R. and Ash, C. L. (1963). 'Survival of patients treated for cancer at the Ontario Cancer Institute from 1930–1957.' *Radiology* **81,** 861.

Cameron, S. J., Grant, I. W. B., Lutz, W. and Pearson, J. G. (1969). 'The early effect of irradiation on ventilatory function in bronchial carcinoma.' *Clin. Radiol.* **20,** 12.

Cohen, L. (1968). 'Theoretical "iso-survival" formulae for fractionated radiation therapy.' *Br. J. Radiol.* **41,** 522.

— and Scott, M. J. (1968). 'Fractionated procedures in radiation therapy: a computerised approach to evaluation.' *Br. J. Radiol.* **41,** 529.

Cook, J. C., West, H. J. and Kraft, J. W. (1968). 'The treatment of lung cancer by split-dose irradiation.' *Am. J. Roentg.* **103,** 722.

Deeley, T. J. (1966). 'A clinical trial to compare two different dose-levels in the treatment of advanced carcinoma of the bronchus.' *Clin. Radiol.* **17,** 299.

— and Line, D. H. (1969). 'Solitary metastases in carcinoma of the bronchus.' *Br. J. Dis. Chest* **63,** 150.

Devik, F. (1962). 'Changes in cell cycle time following irradiation.' *Int. J. Radiat. Biol.* **5,** 59.

Dutreix, J., Schlienger, M. and le Peigneux, M. (1967). 'Irradiation en deux séries et irradiation pre-opérative en deux jours.' *J. Radiol. Électrol.* **48,** 167.

Elkind, M. M. and Sutton, H. (1960). 'Radiation response of mammalian cells grown in culture.' *Radiation Res.* **13,** 556.

Ellis, F. (1967). 'Fractionation in radiotherapy.' In *Modern Trends in Radiotherapy—1*, Chapter 2. Ed. by T. J. Deeley and C. A. P. Wood. London: Butterworths.

— (1969). 'Dose, time and fractionation: a clinical hypothesis.' *Clin. Radiol.* **20,** 1.

Field, S. B., Jones, T. and Thomlinson, R. H. (1968). 'Relative effects of fast neutrons and x-rays on tumour and normal tissues.' *Br. J. Radiol.* **41,** 597.

Fowler, J. F. (1965). 'The estimation of total dose for different numbers of fractions in radiotherapy.' *Br. J. Radiol.* **38,** 365.

Fowler, J. F., Morgan, R. L., Silvester, J. A., Bewley, D. K. and Turner, B. A. (1963). 'Experiments with fractionated x-ray treatment on the skin of pigs. 1. Fractions up to 28 days.' *Br. J. Radiol.* **56,** 188.

Hahn, G. M. (1968). 'Possible improvement in differential cell killing by cell cycle modulation.' *Br. J. Radiol.* **41,** 239.

Hall, E. J. (1969). 'Time, dose and fractionation in radiotherapy.' *Br. J. Radiol.* **42,** 427.

Hawkes, M. J., Hill, R. P., Lindop, P. J., Ellis, R. E. and Rotblat, J. (1968). 'The response of C_3H mammary tumours to irradiation in single and fractionated doses.' *Br. J. Radiol.* **41,** 134.

Hellman, S., Kligerman, M. M., von Essen, C. F. and Scibietta, C. (1964). 'Sequelae of radical radiotherapy of carcinoma of the lung.' *Radiology* **82,** 1055.

Holsti, L. and Vuorinen, P. (1967). 'Radiation reaction in the lung after continuous and split-course megavoltage radiotherapy of bronchial carcinoma.' *Br. J. Radiol.* **40,** 280.

Kallman, R. (1967). 'Cyclic fluctuations in radiosensitivity.' In *Proceedings of Conference on Radiobiology and Radiotherapy*, 1965. National Cancer Institute Monograph. Bethesda, Maryland: National Cancer Institute.

Levitt, S. H., Bogardus, C. R. and Ladd, G. (1967). 'Split-dose intensive radiation therapy in the treatment of advanced lung cancer.' *Radiology* **88,** 1159.

Mitchell, J. S. (1968). 'Applied science and the development of radiotherapy—past, present and future.' *Br. J. Radiol.* **41,** 729.

Morrison, R., Deeley, T. J. and Cleland, W. P. (1963). 'The treatment of carcinoma of bronchus: a clinical trial to compare surgery with supervoltage radiotherapy.' *Lancet* **1,** 6834.

Rissanen, P. M., Tikka, U. and Holsti, L. (1968). 'Autopsy findings in lung cancer treated with megavoltage radiotherapy.' *Acta Radiol.* **7,** 433.

Roswit, B., Patno, M. E., Rapp, R., Veinbergs, A., Feder, B., Stuhlbarg, J. and Reid, C. B. (1968). 'Survival of patients with inoperable lung cancer: a large-scale randomized study of radiation therapy versus placebo.' *Radiology* **90,** 688.

Sambrook, D. K. (1968). 'Further experience with split-course radiation therapy.' Proceedings of 3rd Annual San Francisco Cancer Symposium. *Frontiers of Radiation Therapy and Oncology*, Vol. 3, p. 180. Basel and New York: Karger.

Shuttleworth, E. and Fowler, J. F. (1966). 'Nomograms for radio-biologically equivalent fractionated x-ray doses.' *Br. J. Radiol.* **39,** 134.

Smart, J. (1966). 'Can lung cancer be cured by irradiation alone?' *J. Am. med. Ass.* **159,** 1034.

— and Hilton, G. (1956). 'Radiotherapy of cancer of the lung: results in a selected group of cases.' *Lancet* **1,** 880.

II—Radiosensitizers

W. M. Ross

The search for a radiosensitizer may be likened to that for the Philosopher's Stone and the need may be thought to be equally great, particularly when one considers the results of present treatment in patients with extensive bronchogenic carcinoma.

A true radiosensitizer is an agent, whether physical or chemical, which increases the effect of a given dose of radiation on a tumour without having any direct effect on the tumour itself. However, in actual patients this is too abstract an ideal, and the great majority of agents which have been employed in this context may in fact themselves be expected to have an effect which is either harmful to the tumour or protective to the patient or his tissues. When substances which are harmful to the tumour are being considered, they should be classed as radiosensitizers only if the effects of radiation plus the substance are greater than would be expected from a simple addition of the separate effects.

In this chapter, reference will be made to the management of patients with advanced brochogenic carcinoma—a large group of patients in any major centre. Despite the effects of improved diagnostic methods, both radiological and cytological, a continuing increased awareness by doctors of the frequency of lung cancer, and education of the public to seek advice at an early stage of their symptoms, the majority of patients with lung cancer present for treatment at a stage when radical surgery is no longer applicable and their expected length of survival is measured in months only. Of this large number of patients, many are treated by radiotherapy, at least as a palliative measure. The treatment frequently results in symptomatic relief, particularly in patients suffering from mediastinal obstruction, haemoptysis or the effects of inflammation distal to an occluded bronchus; but local tumour recurrence or distant metastasis is very often apparent soon after treatment, leading rapidly to death. Attempts have been made to improve the length and quality of survival following such radiotherapy by varying the length of the course of treatment and the dose of radiation given. There is considerable evidence that a dose of approximately 1,800 rads given in a week is as effective in this sense as a more prolonged course delivering a much higher dosage, while tending to reduce the unwanted side effects and also limiting the period of hospitalization. It is considered important that the patient should spend as much as possible of his remaining life-span in his home surroundings.

For these reasons there is great need to use a radiosensitizer in carcinoma of the lung. In addition, this would appear to be a suitable disease in which to assess the effects of substances which may prove to be radiosensitizers.

OXYGEN EFFECT

It is well recognized that cells which are fully oxygenated are considerably more sensitive to radiation than those which are in a state of anoxia, and also that at least some cells in tumours are less well oxygenated than others because of the tendency of tumours, especially rapidly growing ones, to outstrip their blood supply. In particular, some of these tumour cells are less well oxygenated than the cells of the host, the surrounding healthy tissues. It would be expected, therefore, that a given dose of radiation would have a greater effect on these oxygenated healthy cells than on the relatively anoxic tumour cells. For this reason, repeated attempts have been made to improve the effects of radiation either by achieving a greater oxygenation of all the tumour cells or by making all the cells in the treatment volume anoxic, thus reducing the differential between tumour and healthy cells.

Quantitative assessments of the effects of such attempts are difficult to make because the degree of cell oxygenation in a solid tumour is extremely difficult to measure absolutely. Experimental evidence from tissue cultures indicates the possibility of a very rapid change within a given cell from an anoxic to an oxygenated state in a period of time much shorter than the duration of an individual x-ray treatment, to say nothing of the length of a whole course of such therapy.

Several methods have been employed to improve the oxygenation of tumours, the simplest of these being the use of blood transfusion in patients who are anaemic in order to ensure a maximum quantity of haemoglobin to carry oxygen to the tumour cells. Attempts to improve oxygenation by increasing the oxygen capacity of the blood above physiological limits are rather less certain. There is little evidence that breathing pure oxygen under normal pressure has any significant effect. However, breathing either oxygen or air under increased pressure, usually about three atmospheres, has been shown to increase the tissue oxygen pressure above its normal level after a period of about 15 minutes, and advantage is taken of this fact in the use of hyperbaric oxygen chambers in radiotherapy. Another technique which has been attempted is the injection of hydrogen peroxide into the artery supplying the tumour. As hydrogen peroxide is rapidly broken down in the blood, the point of injection must be as close as possible to the actual tumour, requiring an intra-arterial cannula. This technique is therefore seldom applicable to patients with cancer of the lung.

The subject of hyperbaric oxygen treatment is dealt with in another section of this chapter, and therefore it is sufficient to say here that the initial work of Churchill-Davidson, Sanger and Thomlinson (1957) suggested that it might be possible to improve the results of radiotherapy in advanced bronchogenic carcinoma by this technique. Attempts are now being made, by means of a controlled trial, to substantiate this impression (Cade and McEwen, 1967).

The method of exploiting the oxygen effect by applying a tourniquet to the blood supply to the part bearing the tumour, so as to render all the tissues within the treated volume anoxic and thereby eliminate the differential between oxygenated and anoxic cells, is not applicable to cancer of the lung; while the attempt to overcome the problem of anoxic cells by the use of neutrons has not yet been shown to have any significant place in the management of patients with advanced lung cancer.

SYNKAVIT

For many years, Professor Mitchell has investigated the possibility of using Synkavit to improve the effects of radiation on tumours (Mitchell, 1960). Synkavit is an artificially synthesized substance, related to vitamin K, which has been shown to inhibit mitosis in certain cultures of malignant tumour cells, the effect being proportional to the concentration, although it has been found to have little effect when used alone in the treatment of malignant tumours. However, Professor Mitchell showed that an intravenous injection of Synkavit 30 minutes before irradiation of a tumour appeared to increase the biological effect of that dose of radiation by about 40 per cent, though apparently only in a limited range of about

1,400–2,000 rads—a fact which limits the application of the method to palliative treatment of advanced tumours. Results in quite a number of cases treated by Hendry in Newcastle in 1954 (Hendry, 1970) by the regimen advocated by Mitchell—that is, 100 mg intravenously 30 minutes before each fraction of the x-ray treatment —also suggested that there might be a slight benefit to the patient from Synkavit administration. More recently, Evans and Todd (1969) have reported a clinical trial carried out at the Christie Hospital, using the same technique of Synkavit administration but combining it with several different radiotherapy techniques, some radical and some palliative. Analysis of their results does not reveal any apparent benefit from Synkavit, except possibly in the late cases treated palliatively: within this group there was a slightly higher proportion of survivors at three months.

Mitchell (1960) has also investigated a number of other drugs chemically related to Synkavit, but has not found any of them more effective in this respect. In addition, he has carried out many experiments using tritiated Synkavit as a radioactive cancer drug.

STEROIDS

Following the synthesis of steroid chemicals, many attempts have been made to use them for the benefit of patients suffering from cancer. It has been observed empirically that in patients with advanced lung cancer the administration of corticosteroids may produce a feeling of well-being, though the mechanism for this effect is not understood, and in at least some cases it may be related to the presence of adrenal metastases which had been causing a state of subclinical hypo-adrenalism.

Experiments have shown that some of the effects of irradiation on normal tissues may be reduced by the administration of steroids, possibly by reducing the inflammatory response, and there has been a considerable number of animal experiments investigating the effects of these chemicals on tumours, both treated and untreated. In some of these experiments it appeared that the animal tumours were inhibited at the primary site, although the development of secondary deposits seemed to be accelerated. In others, tumours implanted into the anterior chamber of the eye of mice were treated by x-rays. In those animals in which the radiotherapy was supplemented by cortisone, death was delayed, indicating some protective effect.

It is also recognized that the acute effects of radiation on normal lung tissue may be reduced by the administration of steroids, though the incidence and degree of late post-radiation fibrosis do not appear to be reduced by these drugs. This suggested the possibility of greater symptomatic relief for the patients. A clinical trial was therefore mounted (Hendry, 1970) to see whether the effects of deep x-ray therapy given in palliative dosage to patients with inoperable bronchogenic carcinoma could be improved by simultaneous cortisone administration. The dose of 250 kV x-rays used in this trial was 1,600 rads in five fractions over four days, or 1,800 rads in six fractions over eight days, depending on whether a weekend intervened. The patients who were given cortisone received 75 mg daily during the course of treatment, and this dosage was reduced slowly over the following fortnight. Analysis of the results after approximately 400 patients had been admitted to the trial showed that the average survival time among the controls was 157 days, while for those who were also given cortisone it was 113 days. Further analysis of the patients indicated that the older patients who were given cortisone fared rather better than those of a similar age who were not so treated. Similarly, those who had extra-thoracic metastases, usually in supraclavicular lymph nodes, at the time of treatment derived rather more benefit if they were given cortisone than if it was withheld, although none of these differences was statistically significant at the $P \geqslant 0{\cdot}05$ level.

CYTOTOXIC DRUGS

It is to be expected that the cytotoxic or 'radiomimetic' drugs should be considered as possible radiosensitizers, or that at least consideration should be given to their use in conjunction with radiotherapy, even though the effect may be one of addition rather than of sensitization. Experiments with tumours in animals and in human sites other than the lung have not conclusively shown any true sensitization. Nevertheless, a combination of radiotherapy and chemotherapy may occasionally be found to give a rather more satisfactory result than would be expected from either alone, without any undesirable increase in side effects.

In patients with extensive lung cancer, one of the alkylating agents—usually nitrogen mustard—is considered to be the chemotherapeutic agent of choice, and it is recognized that nitrogen mustard can help a patient, particularly one with an advanced tumour or extensive metastases. Nevertheless, at least one attempt to combine intravenous nitrogen mustard and x-ray therapy in inoperable patients with carcinoma of the bronchus was found to give no greater period of survival than x-ray therapy alone.

Bearing in mind that many patients with inoperable lung cancer, who have been given palliative deep x-ray therapy, die with distal metastases which were not present or at least were undetected at the time of palliative radiotherapy, it was felt that it might be possible to augment the benefit derived from this treatment, both immediate and long-term, by adding a cytotoxic agent which could be taken over a prolonged period during and after the course of irradiation. A random clinical trial on these lines was mounted in Newcastle some years ago (Hendry, 1970), employing cyclophosphamide, which was chosen for a number of reasons. The drug is taken orally in a relatively inert form which is activated by enzymes which have been shown to be rather more plentiful in tumour cells than in normal tissues, producing a selective effect on the tumour cells. It was also felt that cyclophosphamide could be given in effective dosage over a long period without the likelihood of troublesome side effects, though alopecia is encountered, and haemorrhagic cystitis does develop in a small proportion of patients and must be borne in mind.

For this trial the patients were treated by deep x-ray therapy in the palliative manner described above. Half of the patients, chosen at random, were also given 100 mg of cyclophosphamide daily during their treatment and continuously thereafter until death or until a complication necessitated the cessation of treatment. Four hundred patients entered the trial, of whom 200 were given cyclophosphamide, and all have been followed till death. The median survival period for the controls, who were given deep x-ray therapy alone, was 132 days, and that for the patients who were also given cyclophosphamide was 128·5 days. No difference in the proportion of survivors could be detected between the two groups at any time up to 600 days from the start of treatment, nor did any particular sub-group appear to derive benefit from the combined treatment.

GENERAL COMMENTS

Over many years dissatisfaction with the results of x-ray treatment, particularly in tumours with such a poor outlook as carcinoma of the bronchus, has stimulated repeated attempts to improve the results of radiotherapy by combining it with chemical or physical agents. True radiosensitization—that is, the situation where the added agent has no independent biological effect on the tumour, but where the addition of this agent increases the effect of the radiation—should be distinguished from combined tumour-inhibiting action, though in many situations the distinction may be difficult or indeed impossible. From the clinical point of view, any form of treatment which improves the benefit offered to the patient must be exploited.

It will be seen from the examples and experiences quoted that as yet, despite repeated efforts, no really effective or generally applicable method of radiosensitization has been devised for patients with advanced lung cancer. It is, of course, still to be hoped that greater success will be achieved in the future, just as advances in knowledge of atomic structure have, at least in part, eliminated the need for the Philosopher's Stone.

REFERENCES

Cade, I. S. and McEwen, J. B. (1967). 'Megavoltage radiotherapy in hyperbaric oxygen.' *Cancer, N.Y.* **20,** 817.

Churchill-Davidson, I., Sanger, C. and Thomlinson, R. H. (1957). 'Oxygenisation in radiotherapy. II. Clinical application.' *Br. J. Radiol.* **30,** 406.

Evans, C. M. and Todd, I. D. H. (1969). 'Synkavit and radiotherapy in the treatment of bronchial carcinoma—a random trial.' *Clin. Radiol.* **20,** 228.

Hendry, G. A. (1970). M.D. Thesis, University of Aberdeen.

Mitchell, J. S. (1960). *Studies in Radiotherapeutics.* Oxford: Blackwell.

III—Adjuvant Chemotherapy

Lars R. Holsti

INTRODUCTION

It has been clearly shown that a primary bronchial tumour can be destroyed by radiation therapy (Rissanen, Tikka and Holsti, 1968). Nonetheless the prognosis of lung carcinoma is poor, due in part to delayed diagnosis and in part to the rapid metastatic spread typical of this type of tumour. Apart from the volume of treatment, metastases may be present which are not influenced by irradiation. Adjuvant chemotherapy offers a means of destroying small secondary neoplasms. This use of the cystostatic agents is more important in lung cancer than the sensitization of a primary tumour to radiotherapy. Moreover, for the latter purpose oxygen is more effective than the cytotoxic drugs.

The use of combination therapy in general has been the object of many good surveys (Tarnowski and colleagues, 1958; Bagshaw, 1963; Foye, 1963; Kligerman, 1965; Doggett, Bagshaw and Kaplan, 1967). This chapter deals only with the treatment of lung cancer.

MECHANISM OF ACTION

The mechanism of action of x-ray therapy and chemotherapeutic adjuvants has recently been reviewed by Vermund and Gollin (1968). Both ionizing radiation and many of the chemotherapeutic agents affect the nucleic acid metabolism of the proliferating cells. The same factors which determine radio-curability are at least partly involved in determining the effectiveness of chemotherapeutic agents: the type, extent and size of the tumour, the tumour bed and the growth rate.

The use of radiotherapy and chemotherapy in conjunction may result in synergism, sensitization, augmentation, potentiation or additivity, as defined by Bagshaw (1963), or in none of these. In the last case the effect of the treatment is not superior to that of irradiation alone.

Enhancement of the radiation effect has been reported for many chemical agents, but details concerning their mechanism of action are lacking. Since many drugs interfere with nucleic acid metabolism, it may be assumed that they enhance the effect of radiation by interfering with the mechanism of the genetic apparatus. Some agents modify the chemical structure or biosynthesis of DNA, others interfere with RNA, while still others inhibit the activity of certain enzymes which play a critical role in the intermediary metabolism (Vermund and Gollin, 1968).

It seems probable that 5-fluorouracil sensitizes the cells to radiation by interfering with DNA synthesis. Actinomycin D forms complexes with DNA and inhibits the formation of messenger RNA. Similar complexes are formed by alkylating agents. In sufficiently large doses many chemotherapeutic agents, 5-fluorouracil and methotrexate in particular, are capable of destroying large numbers of tumour cells. Thus they may also lethally damage tumour cells outside the field of radiation. Under such conditions, a therapeutic synergism between the local effect of radiation and the systemic effect of the drug is produced which results in prolonged survival (Vermund and Gollin, 1968). Bagshawe (1968), who studied tumour growth and the anti-mitotic effect of cytotoxic agents on the basis of theoretical models, emphasized the role of spontaneous cell loss. The higher the potential growth rate and the lower the actual growth rate, the more favourable the conditions for an anti-mitotic effect of such agents on the tumour.

In clinical studies concerning the effect of combined radiotherapy and chemotherapy on lung cancer, attention has been directed on the one hand to the measurable tumour shrinkage and on the other hand to patient survival. The former reflects the combined effect of the two treatments on the primary tumour, and the latter the effect of the cytotoxic agent on unmanifested metastases.

DOSAGE AND FRACTIONATION

In the treatment of lung cancer, various chemotherapeutic agents have been used in combination with radiotherapy. Both radiation and the cytotoxic drugs have been employed at very varied dosage levels. Frequently these have been lower than in the regimens in which only one kind of therapy is given. In regard to radiotherapy, in what follows a distinction is made between dosage levels above and below 4,000 r; the former are considered low, the latter high. Low and high levels of chemotherapy are less readily distinguished, but in classifying the series an attempt has been made to consider the principles applied to drug administration when used alone.

In this review a distinction is also made between series in which the treatment has been continuous and those in which radiation and chemotherapy have been fractionated in an unconventional fashion.

Most series reported have been uncontrolled or small, therefore confident conclusions cannot be readily drawn.

CONTINUOUS TREATMENT

Low Radiation Dosage

Low Dosage of Chemotherapeutic Agent

In carcinoma of the lung, 5-fluorouracil is the drug perhaps most often used in conjunction with radiotherapy. In three investigations (Hall and colleagues, 1960; Foye and colleagues, 1960; Willett and colleagues, 1961), the level of radiation was kept low and 5-fluorouracil was given in sub-toxic doses to avoid moderate to severe toxicity. The dose of fluorouracil was 15 mg/kg body weight for four days, and 7·5 mg/kg on the fifth day and thereafter twice a week until the course of irradiation had been completed. The agent was administered intravenously over a period of 2–3 hours. X-ray treatment was given five times a week at 250 kV; the daily tumour dose was 100–200 r, and the total dose 2,000 r in two weeks. The total dose of 5-fluorouracil was 90 mg/kg body weight. A dosage level of 2,000 r was chosen because, according to many experienced radiotherapists, this rarely leads to a significant response. The patients had histologically confirmed epidermoid carcinomas, and their disease was in an advanced and widespread stage. Marked and rapid regression of the treated tumour was observed in all the 16 patients in question. The authors concluded that the combination therapy used was highly effective and that there seemed to be true synergism. No survival rates were given, and unfortunately none of the series included a control group treated by irradiation alone.

In a partly controlled study of 19 inoperable cases from their private practice described by Helsper and Sharp (1962), a group of five patients received 3,500 r cobalt in four weeks. Another group (eight patients) received 3,500 r in four weeks plus 5-fluorouracil, 10–15 mg/kg intravenously, every second day concomitantly with radiotherapy until toxic symptoms appeared. The total initial dose was 1·5 to 5 g, the mean being 3·5 g. Thereafter a maintenance dose of 15 mg 5-fluorouracil was administered once a week. The dose was reduced if toxic symptoms developed. The total amount supplied was 12–25g. All patients had histologically verified inoperable tumours. A good response and toxic symptoms were noted in all the eight patients given combined treatment. The tumour disappeared entirely in three. In the five patients treated by cobalt radiation alone the response was good, but the tumour did not disappear completely in any of these cases. Data concerning survival are lacking. The authors concluded that the combined treatment had a definite synergistic effect.

Fingerhut and Barnett (1966) were unable to confirm these favourable results. Eleven patients were treated by x-ray alone, consisting of 2,000–3,000 r in 2–3 weeks, range 900–4,200 r in 7 to 50 days. In another group of eleven patients the treatment consisted of 740–3,500 r, mostly 2,000 r, in 2–3 weeks plus 5-fluorouracil. The chemotherapy was started on the first day of radiation aud the dosage was the same as that used by Foye and colleagues (1960). The drug was administered intravenously over a 5–10 minute period 2–6 hours prior to irradiation. Radiotherapy was also given on the drug-free days. The average survival time was 3·2 months with the combined treatment and 3·45 months with radiotherapy alone. The combined treatment resulted in increased toxicity and was therefore discontinued.

The series reported by Langdon and colleagues (1963) included 47 patients with cancer of the lung. The total tumour dose of radiation was usually slightly lower than it would have been had radiotherapy been the only method of treatment. The majority of the patients received at least 3,500 r. The 5-fluorouracil dosage was 15 mg/kg body weight for a total of three to five doses, the maximum dose being 1·0 g/day. Thereafter 7·5 mg/kg was administered once or twice a week. The total dose was at least 3·0 g. The average survival did not deviate from the average of 6·2 months achieved with x-ray therapy alone. The series lacked controls given radiotherapy only.

Benninghoff and Alexander (1968) carried out a randomized study involving 55 patients. Thirty patients were treated by radiotherapy alone. The dose was 3,000 r (250 kV) in three weeks; later, cobalt treatment was administered in a dose of 4,000 r in three weeks. The remaining 25 patients received combined treatment consisting of radiotherapy as indicated above plus 5-fluorouracil in a daily dose of 500 mg intravenously on five days during the first week of irradiation, or a total dose of 2·5 g. The survival time was the same in both groups: eight months in 59 per cent of the cases, one year in 34 per cent, two years in 14 per cent, and three years in 5 per cent. Thus, patient survival was not beneficially affected by the addition of chemotherapy.

High Dosage of Chemotherapeutic Agent

Alexander and colleagues (1962) administered at the start of radiotherapy 0·4 mg/kg nitrogen mustard once intravenously, or the same dose divided into two or four daily single injections. The x-ray dose was 2,000–3,000 r in 10–30 days or 3,000–4,000 r in 30 days. In another group, methotrexate was given 2·5 mg/day orally for the first 10 days of irradiation. The total dose was 25 mg. Actinomycin D was added intravenously in a daily dose of 0·5 mg from the sixth to the tenth day of irradiation. In this group the objective response (tumour shrinkage) was superior to that obtained with radiotherapy alone (1,200–8,000 r in 8 to 90 days) or with radiotherapy (1,200–5,000 r in 8 to 50 days) plus nitrogen mustard, but this group had the shortest survival time. The survival time for 50 per cent was five months in the radiotherapy group (58 cases), four months in the radiotherapy plus nitrogen mustard group (15 cases), and two months in the radiotherapy plus methotrexate plus actinomycin D group (39 cases). Alexander's series is the only one reported in which two cytostatic drugs have been used simultaneously in combination with radiotherapy. The x-ray dose varied widely, while the chemotherapeutic dose was constant. The treatment was stopped when toxic symptoms (bone marrow depression, stomatitis, diarrhoea, extensive cutaneous epilation in the irradiated area, nausea and vomiting) appeared. Radiotherapy plus chemotherapy caused increasing though as a rule transient toxicity.

Velasco and colleagues (1964) used the cytostatic AB-132. One group of patients received 1 g/day for 5 days. Thereafter x-ray was given in a dose of 1,800 r as 10 fractions for 12–15 days concomitantly with 0·5 g/day of AB-132 10 times on the days of irradiation. Another group was treated with x-ray alone (2,000 kV), either 1,800 r as 10 fractions in 12–15 days or 1,200–3,200 r. After an interval of two weeks the radiotherapy was continued until a total dose of 3,000–5,000 r had beeen given. The tumour response was the same for AB-132 plus 1,800 r as for radiation alone with 3,000–5,000 r. The authors concluded that the cystostatic drug had a potentiating effect. The average survival time of the dead was, however, the same in both groups, namely 3·7 months.

High Radiation Dosage

Low Dosage of Chemotherapeutic Agent

In a randomized investigation, Hosley and colleagues (1962) treated a control group with 4,000 r in 30 days, using 2,000 kV x-rays. Another group was treated by radiotherapy in conjunction with 5 mg methotrexate daily, 4 μg/kg actinomycin D daily, or 5 mg/kg 5-fluorouracil daily, two days before x-ray therapy was started and then five days a week one hour prior to irradiation. The mean survival time was five months in all groups. Thus, no advantage was derived from adding chemotherapy to irradiation. However, regression of the tumour was most frequently seen in the group treated by radiotherapy plus actinomycin D.

High Dosage of Chemotherapeutic Agent

In Lochman and Morris's (1956) study of 38 patients, one group was irradiated with doses above 4,000 r and another group with doses below 4,000 r. Six patients were given 0·2 mg/kg nitrogen mustard intravenously on four consecutive days initially, while another six patients received the same dose after irradiation. Six patients received 20 mg TEM orally in 3 days, and two were given 10 mg TEPA daily for 17 days. In regard to regression of the tumour and palliation, combined radiotherapy and chemotherapy were not superior to irradiation alone.

A co-operative trial involving several hospitals was reported by Krant and colleagues (1963). This study was a continuation of an investigation with negative result reported by Chalmers (1962). In one group the radiation dosage was 4,000 r in four weeks, in some cases 5,000 r in six weeks. Another group received radiation in combination with mechlorethamine, 0·1 mg/kg body weight, on the first four nights following the start of daily radiotherapy. After a period of two weeks during which the patient received daily irradiation, 0·1 mg/kg mechlorethamine was administered once a week for four weeks. In a third group, treatment was commenced with 0·2 mg/kg mechlorethamine on the first and third days; there was then a two-week interval, after which 0·1 mg/kg of the drug was given once a week for four weeks. Radiotherapy was started a week after the administration of the last dose of mechlorethamine. The investigation demonstrated the failure of HN_2 therapy added to radiotherapy to influence favourably the response of the disease. The survival time showed no correlation with the method of treatment (*Figure 1*).

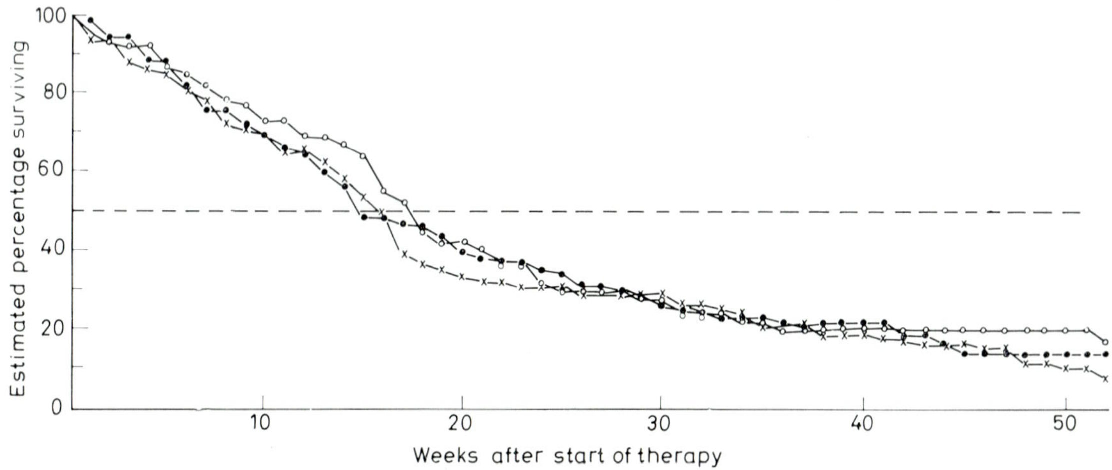

Figure 1. Treatment of bronchogenic carcinoma with 4,000 r plus nitrogen mustard in a randomized study. The survival curves indicate lack of superior treatment in any group. Median survival time 110 days. ●, *x-ray (69 patients);* ×, *x-ray + HN_2 (67 patients);* ○, *HN_2 followed by x-ray (60 patients). (Reproduced from Krant and colleagues, 1963, by courtesy of the Editor of* American Journal of Medicine)

Roswit and Kaplan (1951) and Krabbenhoft and Leucutia (1958) treated a series of patients with 0·1 mg/kg nitrogen mustard for four consecutive days; the radiotherapy dosage was not stated. They found that this combined treatment improved the early survival rates. Data concerning the dosage are also lacking in some other reports (Watson, 1956; Hughes, Pate and Campbell, 1960; Salsali and Clifton, 1965).

In a second study performed by the Eastern Co-operative Group, radiation therapy was combined with the administration of nitrogen mustard, actinomycin D or 5-fluorouracil (Hall and colleagues, 1967). The total planned irradiation dose was 5,000 r in five weeks; the daily dose was 200 r and the treatment was given five times a week. The total duration of treatment did not exceed eight weeks. The 5-fluorouracil was given by rapid intravenous injection daily for four days immediately before the start of radiotherapy and thereafter on each day of radiotherapy within three hours before irradiation. The daily dose of 5-fluorouracil was 5 mg/kg, and the total dose 7,200–7,600 mg. Actinomycin D was given by the same route and schedule as 5-fluorouracil in doses of 4 μg/kg/day, the total dose being 5,500 μg. The results indicated that the addition of chemotherapy was not of any advantage. Patient survival was not affected beneficially (*Figure 2*). The median survival time was 136 days in the group given x-ray alone, 133 days in the x-ray plus 5-fluorouracil group, and 105 days in the x-ray plus actinomycin D group. When over 50 per cent shrinkage of the tumour was used as an index, irradiation alone gave significantly better results than the other two regimens. The addition of drugs to x-ray therapy increased the incidence of gastro-intestinal toxicity and bone marrow suppression. Toxicity showed no correlation with the responses induced.

In a randomized controlled study, Gollin and colleagues (1962) compared 5-fluorouracil plus x-ray therapy with x-ray alone in a series of 26 patients with inoperable carcinoma of the lung, confined to the chest or the supraclavicular nodes. Thirteen patients received x-ray alone, the average dose being 4,075 r in four weeks. In combination with chemotherapy, the average radiation dose was 3,415 r. The 5-fluorouracil dose was 15 mg/kg/day for four days, and thereafter half the dose twice weekly until manifestations of toxicity appeared. The mean survival time was 5·0 $\pm$ 1·11 months with radiation therapy alone, and 9·8 $\pm$ 2·68 months with the combined treatment. In a non-randomized series of 80 patients, increased survival was also observed. Moreover, it was found that the best mean survival time was achieved with a tumour dose exceeding

4,000 r. By contrast, the addition of cyclophosphamide failed to enhance the effect of radiation in a non-randomized series. This drug was given in a dosage of 400 mg/day intravenously for 3–4 days; thereafter 200 mg was administered every second day until toxic manifestations appeared.

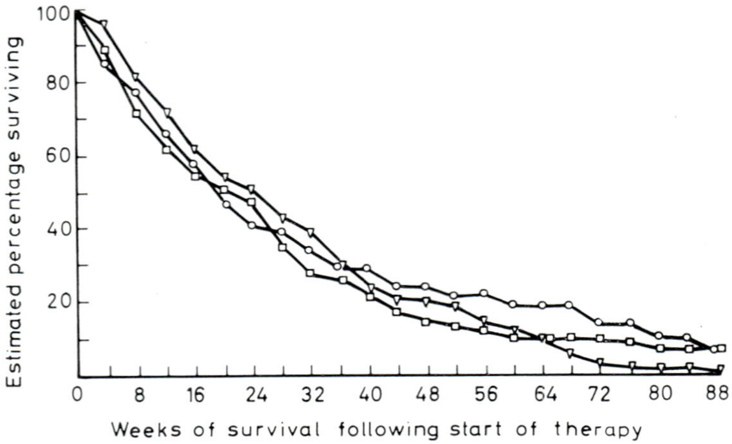

Figure 2. Radiation–chemotherapy of lung cancer in a randomized study. The survival time (mean 105–136 days) is independent of the form of treatment administered. ○, *x-ray only (115 patients);* ▽, *x-ray + 5-FU (113 patients);* □, *x-ray + actinomycin D (114 patients). (Reproduced from Hall and colleagues, 1967, by courtesy of the Editor of* American Journal of Medicine

Suppressive Chemotherapy

In a randomized clinical study, Horwitz and colleagues (1965) compared the effect of chlorambucil administered after radiation to the results achieved with radiation therapy alone. Cobalt therapy, in a dosage of 5,000 r on 4–5 days weekly, was given to both the primary tumour and the mediastinum and also, if necessary, to the supraclavicular regions. As soon as possible after completion of radiotherapy, chlorambucil treatment was instituted, the dosage being 2–8 mg/day by mouth. Fifteen patients received chlorambucil and 15 were given a placebo. The results showed that suppressive chemotherapy prolonged the mean survival time by 80 days. The effect was most conspicuous in regard to non-differentiated and oat cell carcinoma. No side effects were observed and the risk was not increased.

Periodic Fractionation

Sandison and colleagues (1967) fractionated cytostatic treatment into 5-day courses, which were repeated at 4–8-week intervals after the disappearance of toxic symptoms. This therapy was combined with similarly fractionated radiotherapy. The radiation dose was 1,000–1,200 r in 5 days, using telecobalt; the total dose was 7,200 r in 12 months. 5-Fluorouracil was given by direct intravenous injection in a dose of 15 mg/kg/day for 5 days on the same days as irradiation, the maximum daily dose being 750 mg. Natulan was administered in 250 mg doses intravenously or by mouth; the total dose was 1,250–29,850 mg in 5 to 312 days. Chromomycin (Toyomycin) was injected intravenously in 0·5 mg doses on the days of irradiation. The control patients received radiation continuously in doses ranging from 4,600 r in 4 weeks to 5,500 r in 5 weeks and 6,300 r in 6 weeks. The mean survival time in stage III was 7 months with cobalt therapy alone, 9·7 months with telecobalt plus 5-fluorouracil, and 9·6 months with telecobalt plus Natulan. These two combinations increased patient survival, while the administration of Toyomycin resulted in a decrease. The groups were not precisely comparable, however, since the fractionation of the radiotherapy varied.

Gollin, Ansfield and Vermund (1964) compared interrupted courses of 5-fluorouracil plus irradiation with courses of cyclophosphamide plus irradiation in a non-randomized study. The radiation dose was 1,500 r in 10–14 days, followed by rest periods of 4–5 weeks. The cycle was repeated until a tumour dose of 6,000 r was reached. The duration of the rest period was determined by the fact that 4–5 weeks was the time required for recovery when patients were treated to toxicity with 5-fluorouracil. The planned dose of 5-fluorouracil was 15 mg/kg/day administered by rapid intravenous injection for three days, followed by 7·5 mg/kg on the fourth day and thereafter twice weekly until signs of toxicity appeared or until completion of the course of irradiation. The planned dose of Cytoxan was 400 mg/day given by rapid intravenous injection for 3–4 days, followed by 200 mg three times weekly similarly to 5-fluorouracil. This series included no case treated with radiotherapy alone. The mean survival time was 5·8 months in the group treated by x-ray plus 5-fluorouracil (19 patients) and 6·8 months in the group given Cytoxan in conjunction with x-ray (15 patients).

In a randomized series of 20 cases, the patients treated by radiotherapy alone received a single course of 5,000 r, whereas the combined therapy was given as a split course (repeated cycles) treatment. In the combined treatment the average radiation dose was 3,823 r in conjunction with 5-fluorouracil and 4,911 r in conjunction with Cytoxan. The mean survival time of seven patients given a single course of radiation was 8·3 months. Six patients who received split course radiation and 5-fluorouracil had a mean survival time of 4·8 months, while seven patients who received radiation plus Cytoxan as split courses had a mean survival time of 7·4 months. Contrary to the results in the single course series (Gollin and colleagues, 1962; Gollin, Ansfield and Vermund, 1964), the survival time was not increased.

It seems difficult to draw any conclusions from the non-randomized split course series because there were no control patients treated with radiotherapy only. In the randomized series, radiotherapy alone was given by different fractionation from the combined treatment.

In a controlled preliminary study, Holsti (1964) compared the results of radiation plus 5-fluorouracil therapy, both administered by the split course technique, with the results obtained by split course radiation alone. The series consisted of 38 patients, 19 per group, with tumours confined to the chest. The total tumour dose was 6,400 r in 8–9 weeks in both groups. Radiotherapy was administered 15–60 minutes after intravenous infusion of 5-fluorouracil for 2–3 hours. The drug dosage was 15 mg/kg in 500 ml of 5 per cent glucose (not more than 1,000 mg in a single dose) for four consecutive days, and thereafter 7·5 mg/kg in 200 ml of 5 per cent glucose (not more than 500 mg in a single dose) every second day until the interruption of radiotherapy. The mean total dose was 12 g. The treatment was divided into two roughly equal phases separated by a rest interval of 2–3 weeks. The treatment was discontinued when a tumour dose of about 3,000 r and a 5-fluorouracil dose of about 6,000 mg had been given. After the interval, both x-ray and 5-fluorouracil administration were repeated in exactly the same way. The treatment plan was the same for the patients receiving radiotherapy alone as for those given combination therapy.

When this series was analysed in 1964, five patients in both groups had died. The average survival time of the dead was 4·6 months in the combined treatment group and 3·3 months in the radiotherapy group. Tumour shrinkage or disappearance was slightly more rapid with the combined therapy. The conclusion was drawn that the two treatments in combination were beneficial when administered by the split course method and in large doses. The final assessment was postponed, however, until it could be based on survival rates.

Enough time has now elapsed to allow the final results of the study in question to be presented. The combined treatment group finally comprised 21 patients, and the group receiving radiotherapy alone 23 patients. From the original series, 7 patients have been omitted who received continuous treatment. Randomization was applied according to the birthday method. The distribution of the cases by histology is shown in Table 1, from which it appears that there were no significant differences in this respect. The survival data are shown in Table 2. The one-year and two-year survival

TABLE 1
Distribution of Cases by Histology

Histology	*Split course radiotherapy*	*Split course radiotherapy + 5-FU*
Squamous cell carcinoma	11	7
Unclassified carcinoma	3	4
Anaplastic carcinoma	5	6
Small cell carcinoma	2	1
Cytology only	2	3
Total	23	21

TABLE 2
Survival Data

Treatment	*Number of patients*	*Survival rates* 6 months	12 months	18 months	2 years	3 years	4 years	5 years
Split course radiotherapy	23	18	13	7	4	—	—	—
Split course radiotherapy + 5-FU	21	18	10	6	4	3	2	2

rates are approximately the same in the two groups, but from three years onwards the results for the combined treatment group are more favourable. Two patients, both belonging to this group, are still alive after five years. In the group given radiotherapy alone, the longest survival time was two years and nine months. The mean survival time of the dead was 13·5 months in the radiotherapy group and 13·4 months in the irradiation plus 5-fluorouracil group. The results of split course radiation alone are about the same as those in a series in which split course was compared with continuous radiation (Holsti, 1969).

HISTOLOGY

An interesting question relates to the possibility that combined treatment is beneficial in some particular histological type of tumour. Only a few investigators have studied the possible correlation between the results of treatment and the histology of the tumour.

Velasco and colleagues (1964) observed no significant correlation between histological type and therapeutic response. On the other hand, Gollin and colleagues (1962), who noted increased patient survival with 5-fluorouracil therapy, reported that the difference compared with the group treated by radiation alone was greatest in anaplastic carcinomas. Horwitz and colleagues (1965) stated that suppressive chemotherapy with chlorambucil seemed mainly to influence the survival of patients with undifferentiated and oat cell carcinomas. Hosley and colleagues (1962) noticed that 75 per cent regression was most frequent in oat cell carcinoma, irrespective of the method of treatment. According to Hall and colleagues (1967), in all treatment groups the response of squamous cell and undifferentiated carcinomas occupied an intermediate position between the responses of the resistant adenocarcinomas and the sensitive oat cell carcinomas. This seems to be true of most series. Of the two patients with the longest survival times among those who received combined treatment in the series of Helsper and Sharp (1962), one had anaplastic and the other oat cell carcinoma. In the series of Alexander and colleagues (1962), one patient treated with x-ray plus amethopterin plus actinomycin D had a survival time exceeding two years. In this case anaplastic carcinoma was involved. Of three patients with over three years' survival described by Gollin, Ansfield and Vermund (1964), two had squamous cell carcinoma and one anaplastic carcinoma.

The available data seem to indicate that the most favourable results with combined treatment have been achieved in cases of anaplastic and oat cell carcinoma—in other words, in patients with rapidly growing undifferentiated neoplasms.

Five-year Survivors

A five-year survival time is infrequent among patients with inoperable carcinoma of the lung. However, five-year survivors have been described in series treated with x-ray alone. In studies on adjuvant chemotherapy, five-year follow-up or five-year survivors have seldom been mentioned. In the series of Salsali and Clifton (1965), comprising 137 patients, two had survived for five years. Both had been treated by irradiation plus nitrogen mustard. In one case histological verification was lacking, while the other patient had confirmed carcinoma but more precise histological data were not given. Ansfield (1966) stated that two patients in the series described by Gollin and colleagues (1962) survived for five years after treatment by x-ray plus 5-fluorouracil. Nothing was mentioned about the histology. Holsti (this paper) also had two five-year survivors, one with anaplastic carcinoma and the other with a cytologically verified malignant tumour. In the series reported by Krabbenhoft and Leucutia (1958), 5 of 393 patients had survived for five years. Three had received radiotherapy alone, while two had been treated by radiation plus nitrogen mustard. Of the former three patients, one had adenocarcinoma and two had undifferentiated oat cell carcinoma; both the patients given the combined treatment belonged to the oat cell and undifferentiated carcinoma group.

Since the five-year survivors treated by adjuvant chemotherapy amount to only eight, no conclusions can be drawn concerning the part played by the histology of the tumour. As pointed out by Horwitz and colleagues (1965), such patients may represent prognostically favourable cases in which five-year survival might have been possible without chemotherapy.

TOXICITY

Practically all authors have stated that the combination of radiotherapy and chemotherapy increases the untoward effects compared with radiotherapy alone and also compared with chemotherapy alone. With few exceptions (Fingerhut and Barnett, 1966), the side effects have been manageable and transient. In addition to gastro-intestinal, haematological and cutaneous symptoms, some authors have mentioned an increased frequency of pneumonitis. A thorough study of the side effects has been carried out, although without the use of a control group (Ottoman and colleagues, 1963).

COMMENTS AND CONCLUSIONS

Adjuvant chemotherapy has been tested in a number of very heterogeneous series in which both the methods of treatment and the radiation and drug dosages have varied. Some earlier reports have aroused enthusiasm on insufficient grounds. Only a few of the series have been adequately controlled, and the majority are too small for confident conclusions to be drawn. Moreover, in some investigations the treatment has been interrupted owing to the appearance of toxic symptoms. The criteria of toxicity have also varied considerably.

In carcinoma of the lung, which tends to metastasize easily, patient survival is the most significant and the only reasonable measure of the effect of treatment. When the results reported are analysed on this basis, the following conclusions may be drawn.

Alkylating agents used as adjuvants have offered no convincing advantages. In one retrospective series in which a small proportion of the patients had received combination therapy, patient survival was longer in this group than in a group given x-ray therapy alone, but almost the same as in a group treated by betatron radiation alone. The results of controlled studies have been unfavourable throughout. Four five-year survivors have been reported.

Actinomycin D and methotrexate in combination with radiation have not prolonged survival to any appreciable degree.

Natulan has been tested as an adjuvant in only one study (Sandison and colleagues, 1967). In this the mean survival time was slightly longer with radiotherapy plus Natulan than with radiation only, but the x-ray dose and fractionation were different in the group which received radiotherapy alone.

5-Fluorouracil as an adjuvant has been used in very different combinations, and the results reported are contradictory. It appears that a low radiation dose (below 4,000 r) and a small dose of 5-fluorouracil (90 mg/kg) have not increased the survival time. In an extensive randomized study, the Eastern Cooperative Group found that 5,000 r in five weeks plus 7,200–7,600 mg 5-fluorouracil did not lead to prolonged survival. On the other hand, in a small randomized investigation 5-fluorouracil increased the survival time, especially in anaplastic carcinomas (Gollin and colleagues, 1962).

Using periodic fractionation, Sandison and colleagues (1967) found that the addition of 5-fluorouracil to radiotherapy resulted in a slight increase of the mean survival time, whereas Gollin, Ansfield and Vermund (1964) obtained a contrary result by almost the same method. In both studies the control group was inadequate. The interval between the courses (4–5 weeks) was obviously too long, the radiation dose per course was too small, and the total duration of treatment was too long. The present author used a split course technique in a series in which the groups were clinically and histologically comparable, the only difference being whether or not

5-fluorouracil therapy was added. The average survival time of the dead did not differ in the two groups, but in the combined treatment group two patients survived for five years. The role of 5-fluorouracil as an adjuvant is not yet fully understood. Four five-year survivors have been reported. Giving the drug by rapid intravenous injection increases its toxicity, but in the light of the available results this mode of administration does not seem to differ definitely from slow infusion in its effect on survival.

So far the results of adjuvant chemotherapy of lung cancer have been disappointing. The final answer to the question of its possible importance can be obtained only with the aid of well-planned, extensive clinical trials.

Suppressive chemotherapy seems to be a method worthy of further investigation.

The best palliation has been achieved in the types of tumour with the most rapid growth rate, that is, undifferentiated tumours (Brenner, Holsti and Perttala, 1967; Garland, Coulson and Wollin, 1963). Both radiation and the chemotherapeutic agents influence DNA, and they affect rapidly proliferating tissues the most. The difference in effect between radiotherapy and cytostatics is insignificant. As pointed out by Deeley (1967), 'dramatic improvements in survival rates will only be made when some method of dealing with the metastases can be found'. Much more attention should be devoted to the invasiveness of cancer cells (Roe and Ambrose, 1966).

The modern models of tumour growth have also influenced the strategy of treatment. It has been stated that in order to affect all the tumour cells, the chemotherapeutic agents must be administered for an entire generation time (Mendelsohn, 1966). However, the administration of cytostatics in short repeated courses has many advocates, and this regimen may be compared with the modern trends in radiation therapy. As long as no drugs are available other than those employed today, it is advisable to test the cytostatics, principally 5-fluorouracil, as adjuvants by fractionation techniques which differ from the conventional routine methods. Synchronization of the tumour cell population before radiation, for example by 5-fluorouracil, also seems to offer a significant possibility. This was suggested by Kaplan in 1965, but lately this aspect has attracted increasing attention.

ADDENDUM

Since the submission of this chapter, Cook, West and Kraft (*Am. J. Roentg*. 1968, **103,** 772) have concluded that nitrogen mustard does not increase the life expectancy in irradiated lung cancer. Vermund,

Gollin and Ansfield (*Front. Radiat. Ther. Oncol.* 1969, **4,** 132) found in a randomized study that low doses of 5-fluorouracil in a single course were not effective and that the initial favourable results from repeated courses of 5-FU as an adjuvant to radiotherapy had not yet been corroborated in larger series.

REFERENCES

Alexander, L. L., Causing, J., Schwinger, H. N. and Li, M. C. (1962.) 'Bronchogenic carcinoma: a comparative study of the palliative effects of radiation therapy, radiation therapy plus nitrogen mustard, and radiation therapy plus amethopterin and actinomycin D in combination.' *Am. J. Roentg.* **87,** 375.

Ansfield, F. J. (1966). *Chemotherapy of Disseminated Solid Tumours.* Springfield, Ill.: Thomas.

Bagshaw, M. A. (1963). 'Approaches for combined radiation and chemotherapy.' *Laval méd.* **34,** 124.

Bagshawe, K. D. (1968). 'Tumour growth and anti-mitotic action: the role of spontaneous cell losses.' *Br. J. Cancer* **22,** 698.

Benninghoff, D. L. and Alexander, L. L. (1968). 'Treatment of lung carcinoma: radiation versus radiation combined with 5-fluorouracil' *N.Y. St. J. Med.* **68,** 532.

Brenner, M. W., Holsti, L. R. and Perttala, Y. (1967). 'The study by graphical analysis of the growth of human tumours and metastases of the lung.' *Br. J. Cancer* **21,** 1.

Chalmers, T. C. (1962). 'Combination of radiotherapy and chemotherapy in the treatment of carcinoma of the lung.' *Cancer Chemother. Rep.* **16,** 463.

Deeley, T. J. (1967). 'The treatment of carcinoma of the bronchus. Review article.' *Br. J. Radiol.* **40,** 801.

Doggett, R. L., Bagshaw, M. A. and Kaplan, H. S. (1967). 'Combined therapy using chemotherapeutic agents and radiotherapy.' In *Modern Trends in Radiotherapy—1*, p. 107. Ed. by T. J. Deeley and C. A. P. Wood. London: Butterworths.

Fingerhut, A. G. and Barnett, M. B. (1966). 'X-ray therapy and combined therapy (x-ray and 5-fluorouracil) in the treatment of cancer of the lung.' *Dis. Chest* **49,** 393.

Foye, L. V. (1963). 'The modification of radiosensitivity.' In *Cancer Progress 1963*, p. 203. Ed. by R. W. Raven. London: Butterworths.

— Willett, F. M., Hall, B. and Roth, M. (1960). 'The potentiation of radiation effects with 5-fluorouracil.' *Cancer Chemother. Rep.* **6,** 12.

Garland, L. H., Coulson, W. and Wollin, E. (1963). 'The rate of growth and apparent duration of untreated primary bronchial carcinoma.' *Cancer, N.Y.* **16,** 694.

Gollin, F. F., Ansfield, F. J. and Vermund, H. (1964). 'Clinical studies of combined chemotherapy and irradiation in inoperable bronchogenic carcinoma.' *Am. J. Roentg.* **92,** 88.

Gollin, F. F., Curreri, A. R., Heidelberger, C. and Vermund, H. (1962). 'Combined chemotherapy and irradiation in inoperable bronchogenic carcinoma.' *Cancer, N.Y.* **15,** 1209.

Hall, B. E. and Good, J. W. (1962). 'Treatment of far-advanced cancer with 5-fluorouracil, used alone and in combination with irradiation. Incidence and duration of remission and survival-time data in 223 patients.' *Cancer Chemother. Rep.* **16,** 369.

— Foye, L. V., Roth, M., Willett, F. M., Hales, D. R., Ward, J. H., Butler, H. T. and Godfrey, M. H. (1960). 'Treatment of inoperable cancer with 5-fluorouracil and irradiation.' *Lancet* **1,** 115.

Hall, T. C., Dederick, M. M., Chalmers, T. C., Krant, M. J., Shnider, B. I., Lynch, J. J., Holland, J. F., Ross, C., Koons, R., Owens, A. H., Frei, E., Brindley, C., Miller, S. P., Brenner, S., Hosley, H. F. and Olson, K. B. (1967). 'A clinical pharmacologic study of chemotherapy and x-ray therapy in lung cancer.' *Am. J. Med.* **43,** 186.

Helsper, J. T. and Sharp, G. S. (1962). 'Combination therapy with 5-fluorouracil and cobalt-60 for inoperable carcinoma of the lungs.' *Cancer Chemother. Rep.* **20,** 103.

Holsti, L. R. (1964). 'Combined split-course therapy with 5-fluorouracil and megavoltage irradiation.' *Annls Med. intern. Fenn.* **53,** 79.

— (1969). 'Clinical experience with split-course radiotherapy: a randomized clinical trial.' *Radiology* **92,** 591.

Horwitz, H., Wright, T. L., Perry, H. and Barrett, C. M. (1965). '"Suppressive" chemotherapy in bronchogenic carcinoma: a randomized prospective clinical trial.' *Am. J. Roentg.* **93,** 615.

Hosley, H. F., Marangoudakis, S., Ross, C. A., Murphy, W. T. and Holland, J. F. (1962). 'Combined radiation–chemotherapy for bronchogenic carcinoma—pilot study.' *Cancer Chemother. Rep.* **16,** 467.

Hughes, F. A., Pate, J. W. and Campbell, R. E. (1960) 'Bronchogenic carcinoma: comparison of natural course and treatment with resection, x-radiation, and nitrogen mustard.' *J. thorac. cardiovasc. Surg.* **39,** 409.

Kaplan, H. S. (1965). 'Clinical potentialities of recent advances in cellular radiobiology.' In *Cellular Radiation Biology*, p. 584. Baltimore: Williams & Wilkins.

Kligerman, M. M. (1965). 'Present status of combined radiation therapy and chemotherapy.' In *Progress in Radiation Therapy*, Vol. III, p. 183. Ed. by F. Buschke. New York: Grune & Stratton.

Krabbenhoft, K. L. and Leucutia, T. (1958). 'Combined roentgen therapy and nitrogen mustard in carcinoma of the lung as compared to other methods.' *Am. J. Roentg.* **79,** 491.

Krant, M. J., Chalmers, T. C., Dederick, M. M., Hall, T. C., Levene, M. B., Muench, H., Shnider, B. I., Gold, G. L., Hunter, C., Bersack, S. R., Owens, A. H., de Leon, N., Dickson, R. J., Brindley, C., Brace, K. C., Frei, E., Gehan, E. and Salvin, L. (1963). 'Comparative trial of chemotherapy and radiotherapy in patients with non-resectable cancer of the lung.' *Am. J. Med.* **35,** 363.

Langdon, E. A., Ottoman, R. E., Rochlin, D. B. and Smart, C. R. (1963). 'Early results of combined radiation and chemotherapy in treatment of malignant tumours.' *Radiology* **81,** 1008.

Lochman, D. J. and Morris, R. S. (1956). 'The treatment of lung cancer with radiation and radiomimetic drugs.' *Radiology* **66,** 842.

Mendelsohn, M. M. (1966). 'Some clinical implications of models of tumour growth.' In *Current Perspectives in Cancer Therapy*, p. 10. Ed. by W. S. Blakemore and I. S. Ravdin. New York: Harper & Row.

Ottoman, R. E., Langdon, E. A., Rochlin, D. B. and Smart, C. R. (1963). 'Side-effects of combined radiation and chemotherapy in the treatment of malignant tumours.' *Radiology* **81,** 1014.

Rissanen, P. M., Tikka, U. and Holsti, L. R. (1968). 'Autopsy findings in lung cancer treated with megavoltage radiotherapy.' *Acta radiol. ther.* **7,** 433.

Roe, F. J. C. and Ambrose, E. J. (1966). 'Future strategy.' In *The Biology of Cancer*, p. 223. Ed. by E. J. Ambrose and F. J. C. Roe. London: Van Nostrand.

Roswit, B. and Kaplan, G. (1951). 'Nitrogen mustard as an adjunct to radiation in the management of bronchogenic cancer.' *Radiology* **57,** 384.

Salsali, M. and Clifton, E. E. (1965). 'Superior vena caval obstruction with carcinoma of the lung.' *Surgery Gynec. Obstet.* **121,** 783.

Sandison, A. G., Falkson, G., Fichardt, T. and Savage, D. J. (1967). 'A statistical evaluation of the treatment of 215 patients with advanced bronchial cancer managed by telecobalt therapy alone, and in combination with various cancer chemotherapeutic agents.' *S. Afr. J. Radiol.* **5,** 21.

Tarnowski, G. S., Bane, H. N., Conrad, J., Nickson, J. J., Stock, C. C. and Sugiura, K. (1958). 'Effect of combinations of radiation and chemotherapeutic agents against experimental animal tumours.' *Cancer Res.* **18,** 225.

Velasco, H. A., Ross, C. A., Webster, J. H., Sokal, J. E., Stutzman, L. and Ambrus, J. L. (1964). 'Combined use of AB-132 (Meturedepa, Turloc) and x-irradiation in the management of advanced bronchogenic carcinoma.' *Cancer, N.Y.* **17,** 841.

Vermund, H. and Gollin, F. F. (1968). 'Mechanisms of action of radiotherapy and chemotherapeutic adjuvants: a review.' *Cancer, N.Y.* **21,** 58.

Watson, T. A. (1956). 'Supervoltage roentgen therapy in cancer of the lung.' *Am. J. Roentg.* **75,** 525.

Willett, F. M., Foye, L. V., Roth, M. and Hall, B. E. (1961). 'Combined therapy of inoperable lung carcinoma with 5-fluorouracil and irradiation.' *Dis. Chest* **39,** 38.

IV—Hyperbaric Oxygen

J. B. McEwen

INTRODUCTION

'The theoretical prospect of therapeutic advantage from the inhalation of oxygen under high pressure (HPO) during irradiation of clinical tumours is derived from three considerations which do not appear to be seriously questioned: that a proportion of the proliferating cells in many tumours are under severely hypoxic, or anoxic, conditions; that the reproductive integrity of such cells is substantially more resistant to damage by radiation than cells oxygenated to normal physiological levels; and that the chance of local radical cure is better, or more palliation is achieved, the greater the proportion of tumour cells which have lost their reproductive capacity following the largest dose of radiation which can be tolerated by the normal tissues' (Hewitt, 1966).

The history of the oxygen effect in radiotherapy has recently been comprehensively reviewed (Churchill-Davidson, 1968).

The clinician may regard patients with carcinoma of the lung as classifiable into three categories. First, those in whom the lesion is sufficiently localized in the chest to be regarded as fit for resection. Secondly, those whose pulmonary condition contra-indicates resection, but in whom the tumour appears to be confined to a reasonable volume in the chest and whose general condition is good. Thirdly, a large group in poor health who have an extensive pulmonary lesion or extrathoracic metastases and are fit only for palliative measures.

This chapter is concerned with the management of the second group—about 25 per cent of the total—in whom adequate local treatment may be expected to offer some hope of cure. Except for one outstanding series (Hilton, 1955), the results achieved by radiotherapy have been uniformly disappointing. In January 1964, we in Portsmouth initiated a clinical trial of radiotherapy in hyperbaric oxygen designed to answer the following question:

Is the survival time of certain patients with carcinoma of the lung treated with megavoltage radiotherapy in oxygen at a pressure of

3 ATA as good as, better than or worse than that of a similar group of patients treated in the same way in air at atmospheric pressure?

All patients fulfilling the following criteria are included in the trial:

(1) Age not over 75 years.

(2) Diagnosis histologically or cytologically proven before treatment.

(3) Known extent of disease able to be included in a field size of 150 cm^2.

(4) No previous radiotherapy or surgery with the exception of thoracotomy. Previous chemotherapy permissible.

(5) Patient able to lie flat—both prone and supine.

(6) No superior vena caval obstruction.

(7) No pleural effusion other than a trivial or post-operative one.

We have found it necessary to obtain a radiological skeletal survey to exclude occult bone metastases.

Patients fitting the criteria are randomly selected for treatment in air or in oxygen by drawing a card from a series of sealed envelopes provided by the Medical Research Council's statistical division.

TECHNIQUE OF TREATMENT

Both groups receive identical radiotherapy on a cobalt teletherapy unit. Two opposed parallel fields are used of a size likely to include all known tumour, with a margin. Neither anaesthesia nor myringotomy is employed for the hyperbaric series. Sedation is rarely required. Almost all cases are treated as out-patients. All clothing is removed, and the patient is dressed in a non-inflammable cotton gown to reduce the fire hazard; rings, watches and jewellery are left off in order to avoid scratching the cylinder wall. In warm weather it is desirable to cool the incoming oxygen to minimize the rise of temperature within the chamber which accompanies the rise in pressure.

It is wise to offer the patient a careful and leisurely explanation of the method before he undresses so to avoid losing patients from the trial due to alarm or intolerance. At the same time he should be taught Valsalva's manoeuvre in case swallowing is insufficient to equalize middle ear pressure. He should be kept talking during pressurization, which, once confidence has been gained, takes about 10 minutes to 3 ATA. Before pressurizing, the ears must be examined with an auriscope and wax removed. We have not found scarring of the drums to be a contra-indication.

We use the standard Vickers transparent-walled chamber. At the first exposure the pressure is increased slowly at about 2 lb/in^2/min, being held in steps if the patient complains of any discomfort. Sinus or ear pain can be relieved by temporarily lowering the pressure by a few pounds. The patient's tolerance improves with experience. Oxygen toxicity has been observed in only one patient in this series, who developed generalized convulsions during decompression at the end of his thirty-fifth and last exposure. The patient must be closely observed during compression and decompression for twitching of the lips or other sign of toxicity.

A standard period of 15 minutes at 3 ATA is allowed for tissue oxygen saturation. During this time the chamber is wheeled into the cobalt treatment room for the setting-up procedure. We use a light beam to define the field and optical measurement of the source skin distance. The output of our 8,000 curie cobalt source is now 150 r per minute at 80 cm. Treatment to two fields daily requires 10–12 minutes, which includes the time necessary to set up the second field. Decompression takes about 3 minutes. If the total time of exposure to hyperbaric oxygen can be limited to 40 minutes, the risk of oxygen convulsions is negligible.

RADIATION DOSE

For the first three years of the trial, a tumour dose of 6,000 r was given in daily fractions on five days a week for eight weeks. In the fourth year the dose was modified to 4,500 r in six weeks because the results achieved after 40 compressions per patient did not seem to justify the stresses of the method.

At the end of the fourth year, when we had included 79 patients in the trial, there appeared to be no difference in survival time on either side. Most authors claiming beneficial results from the method had been using 'unorthodox' fractionation of dose, for example 6 × 500 rads, 3 × 800 rads, or 6 × 600 rads. We therefore decided, with the approval of the Medical Research Council's Working Party on Radiation and Hyperbaric Oxygen, to adopt Dr. Ian Churchill-Davidson's dose scheme as from 1 January, 1968. We now give 600 r maximum tissue dose twice weekly for 3 weeks. The central dose is about 3,200 r and the maximum tissue dose 3,600 r in 18 days. Only 15 patients on this regimen are included in this report. Both fields are treated at each session, the patient turning over in the chamber for the treatment of the posterior field.

COMPLICATIONS

Complications have been minimal. Failure to complete treatment in the trial is most commonly due to extension of the tumour beyond the treatable volume. Six patients did not complete treatment in oxygen because of dislike of the method or because of claustrophobia. Barotrauma has been seen in five cases and consists of bleeding from or an effusion into the tympanum followed by spontaneous recovery. In only one patient did this prevent completion. Although there are physical and biological reasons for expecting increased skin reactions, these are not observable clinically except in the obese patient whose skin lies within 10 cm of the chamber wall and is exposed to electron contamination by the beam: above 8 cm from the wall this can be neglected.

SUMMARY

The clinical trial of radiotherapy with hyperbaric oxygen in carcinoma of the bronchus is summarized in Table 1. Ninety-three patients

TABLE 1

Clinical Trial of Radiotherapy with Hyperbaric Oxygen

	Oxygen	*Air*
Number of patients:	45	48
Male	39	45
Female	6	3
Histology:		
Squamous cell	29	32
Oat cell and undifferentiated	15	12
Adenocarcinoma	1	4
Treatment within the trial completed	32	41
Treatment incomplete because of:		
Spread of disease	6	7
Intolerance	6	—
Barotrauma	1	—
Minor complications not preventing completion:		
Intolerance and claustrophobia	3	—
Barotrauma	4	—
Convulsions	1	—
Skin reaction	2	—
Patients surviving at:		
6 months	22/45 (49%)	28/48 (55%)
12 months	14/39 (36%)	14/40 (36%)
18 months	5/37 (13%)	7/38 (18%)
2 years	4/30 (13%)	3/32 (9%)
3 years	2/25 (8%)	1/24 (4%)
Autopsies	14	16
Local clearance at autopsy	2	3

were entered in the trial and followed up till death or for at least six months. It can be seen that there is as yet no significant difference in survival time between the two groups of patients.

ACKNOWLEDGEMENTS

The project has been supported by the British Empire Cancer Campaign for Research, the Medical Research Council and the Wessex Regional Hospital Board. The day-to-day work of the trial has been done by my successive Research Assistants Dr. Edith Wilson, Dr. Patricia Golding and Dr. Hilary Milward-Sadler, to all of whom, as well as to my colleague Miss Irene Cade, I wish to acknowledge my gratitude.

REFERENCES

Churchill-Davidson I. (1968). In *Proceedings of 1st Annual San Francisco Cancer Symposium*. Basel and New York: Karger.

Hewitt, H. B. (1966). *Br. J. Radiol.* **39,** 19.

Hilton, G. (1955). In *British Practice in Radiotherapy*. London: Butterworths.

13—Dose Distribution in Lung Treatments

J. G. Stewart and D. Greene

INTRODUCTION

In planning and discussing the dose distribution used in radiation therapy, it is usual to simplify the situation by assuming that the relevant body section is made of unit density material, usually water. The next stage, bringing this assumption closer to reality, is to assume that the body section consists of water, air gaps, bone and lung arranged in accordance with some assumed standard anatomy. The further stage of considering the effect of soft organ boundaries has not to our knowledge been discussed in the literature, but it is unlikely that this will produce changes of any clinical significance. It would be ultimately desirable, of course, to consider all this in relation to the anatomy of the individual patient, but the possibility of doing this is limited by the difficulties in determining the patient's anatomy as well as by the more obvious physical difficulties which are considered in this chapter.

In treatment of lesions of the lung, dosimetry problems associated with transit of the radiation fields through bone are usually not serious. For clinical reasons, the beam directions in a small field treatment are usually chosen to avoid the spine, so that the only bones involved are the ribs and the transmitted dose will be changed by only 1 or 2 per cent for megavoltage x-rays. Regional treatments of the chest may, however, involve irradiation through the spine; but as such treatments are either directed at sensitive tumours or given with only palliative intent for other tumours, variations within the field are of lesser clinical importance.

Although the lung is a complex structure of soft tissue and air spaces, no individual air space is sufficiently large to produce a gross local disturbance in the radiation field. For this reason it is usual to make the simplifying assumption that lung consists of uniform soft tissue of low density. This chapter is thus concerned mainly with the effect of such tissue on the dose given to tumours embedded therein. It is proposed to consider the physical methods used to determine the dose to a tumour under these circumstances and then to apply these methods to treatment planning. This chapter is intended to present our own approach to the problem, rather than to be a comprehensive review of large literature on the subject. However, we also append a small bibliography of papers on relevant topics. In the text, references are given only when the work or results of an author are being directly quoted.

EXPERIMENTAL METHODS

Measurements in Phantom

Figure 1 illustrates, in principle, the type of arrangement that has been used to study the effect of lung on the dose distribution in a phantom. The low-density slab shown in *Figure 1a* has to consist of a material of about the same atomic composition as water, in a

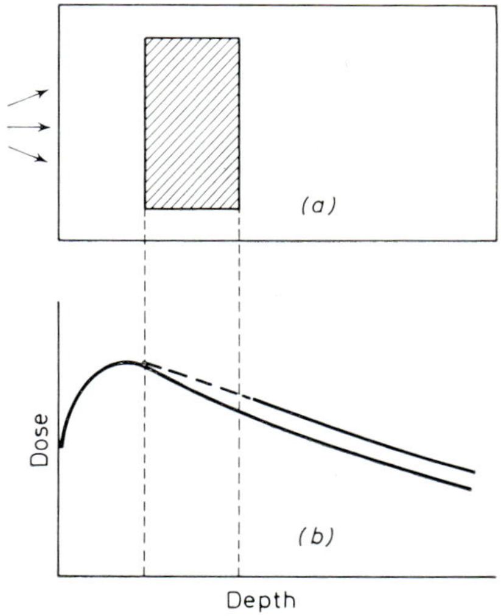

Figure 1. (a) Schematic diagram of water phantom containing slab of simulated lung. (b) Depth dose curves. Lower curve measured in uniform water phantom; upper curve measured with simulated lung in position

convenient and easily handled form. The density of lung in a living subject is by no means uniform, but it is usually assumed that its mean density is about 0·3 g/cm^3 (Fowler and Young, 1959). Cork of this density has frequently been utilized to simulate lung and, enclosed in a watertight bag, may be used in a water phantom.

Most experimenters have made measurements along the central axis of the radiation beam and have demonstrated an increased transmission through lung, as is illustrated qualitively in *Figure 1b*. Here the lower line is the depth dose curve in water, while the upper line shows the curve as measured with the cork in position. We are

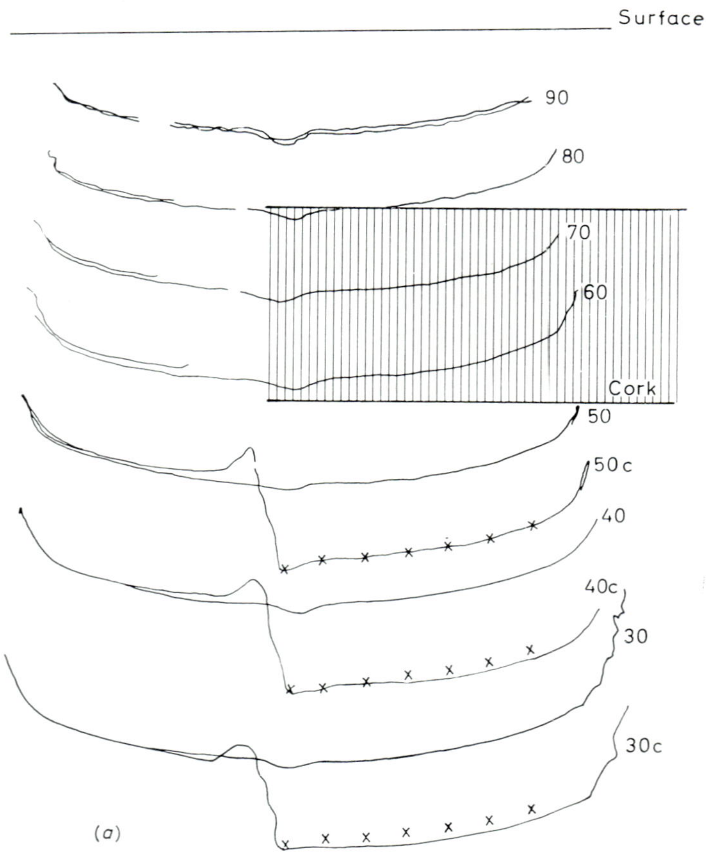

Figure 2a

not aware of any measurements made in the simulated lung or at the interfaces. Since lung is of the same atomic composition as tissue, if electronic equilibrium has been established in front of the slab it will be maintained within it and there are no discontinuities in dose ('build-up' or 'build-down' effects) at the interfaces. For this reason, the dose in the simulated lung will vary continuously along the dotted line interpolated between the measured depth dose curves in front of and behind the lung in *Figure 1b*. The situation discussed here for lung is thus less complex than that arising at a bone–tissue interface, where the change in atomic number results in loss of electronic equilibrium (Spiers, 1949; Deutreix and Bernard, 1966).

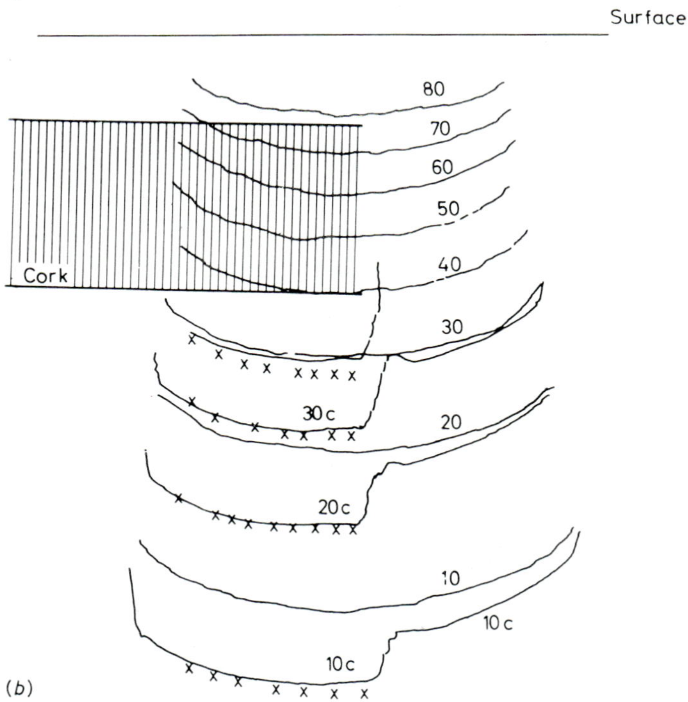

Figure 2. Isodose curves. (a) For cobalt-60 radiation. Those marked 80, 70, 60 etc. were measured in water phantom. Those marked 30c, 20c etc. were measured with cork slab in position shown. The points marked were determined by the isodose displacement method discussed in the text. (b) For 250 kV x-rays. Curves labelled as above. (Reproduced from Greene and Stewart, 1965, by courtesy of the Editor of British Journal of Radiology)

Experiments have been carried out to study the effect of simulated lung on the whole isodose chart (Greene and Stewart, 1965), and this is illustrated in *Figure 2a* for cobalt-60 γ-rays. The cork slab extended half-way across the beam, and in this presentation the increased transmission results in a forward displacement of the isodose lines. An equivalent result for 2·5 mm Cu HVL radiation is shown in *Figure 2b*.

Measurements *in vivo*

Three methods of making experimental measurements on patients with a view to determining the dose to regions in the lung have been considered by various authors: (1) measurement of exit doses, (2) measurements in the oesophagus, and (3) measurements in the bronchus. Exit doses have usually been measured on the central axis of therapy beams with a suitable instrument placed on the patient's skin. Alternatively, the patient may be exposed to a series of narrow beams (Holt and Laughlin, 1969) covering the region to be treated by the therapy beam, and the information used to estimate the cross-field variation due to non-unit-density tissues. Neither of these methods will give direct information about the dose at the tumour. Measurements made with an instrument introduced into the oesophagus or the bronchus provide more direct information about the tumour dose, but these techniques are very time-consuming, are uncomfortable for the patient, and require the taking of stereo pairs of x-rays films if the position of the measuring instrument is to be known.

Results

The results of phantom measurements are usually expressed in terms of correction factors to be applied to the doses estimated for a unit density phantom. For any particular field size and thickness of simulated lung, the correction increases slightly with distance from the lung–tissue interface. This happens because while immediately behind the lung there is an increased radiation transmission, there is also a loss of photon scatter which builds up again as the distance from the lung increases. This is illustrated in *Figure 3* (Massey, 1962), which shows the correction factor to be applied for 4 MV radiation for an 8 $\times$ 8 cm field at 100 cm FSD as a function of lung thickness and distance beyond lung. From data such as these it is also possible to draw up a table of typical lung corrections. These are given in Table 1.

Greene and Stewart (1965) have shown that the dose at a point in a unit density medium irradiated through simulated lung may be determined by shifting the normal isodose curves forward by 0·4 times the thickness of lung traversed for cobalt-60 and 4 MV radiations.

As can be seen in *Figure 2a*, for megavoltage radiation the doses at points along rays not intersected by lung or at points on the proximal side of the lung are not significantly changed from those in a unit density medium. For megavoltage quality radiation, corrections to the dose at points irradiated through simulated lung by either of the methods described are in accordance with measured values to

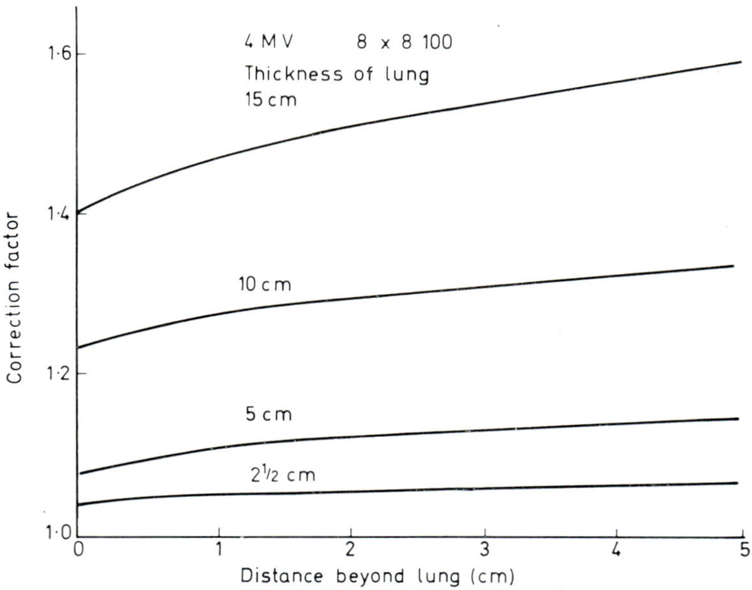

Figure 3. Measured increase in dose beyond lung for 4 MV x-rays. When a slab of simulated lung is placed in the phantom, the standard depth dose values are increased by the factor shown. (Reproduced from Massey, 1962, by courtesy of the Editor of British Journal of Radiology)

TABLE 1

Corrections to be Applied to the Dose in a Tumour Irradiated through 6 cm of Lung Tissue: Correctors are to be Applied to Central Axis Data Read from Standard Tables

Radiation	*FSD (cm)*	*Correction for 6 cm of lung (per cent)*
300 kV	50	+40
Cobalt-60	80	+20
4 MV	100	+15
8 MV	100	+10

an accuracy of $\pm$ 2 per cent. The doses at points in the simulated lung can be estimated by interpolation to about the same accuracy. The assumption that the doses at points not irradiated through lung are as given by the ordinary isodose chart is also accurate to about $\pm$ 2 per cent.

For conventional quality x-rays, the isodose lines are shifted forward by 0·5 times the thickness of lung traversed. Since at this quality a much higher proportion of the dose at a point is due to side and back scattering radiation, the dose at all points in the irradiated volume is changed by the presence of lung in the field, as shown in *Figure 2b*. The doses at points irradiated through lung can be predicted to an accuracy of about $\pm$ 5 per cent. The change in dose at those points in the field not irradiated through lung is not predictable by a simple rule as it is a function of field size and of the volume of lung in the field. The error in ignoring the change in dose at these points may be as much as 10 per cent.

As stated above, *in vivo* measurements rarely give direct information about the tumour dose for the patient, but they are useful as a means of checking the predictions made from phantom measurements. Detailed comparisons between measurements made *in vivo*, as reported in the literature, and phantom measurements are difficult for two reasons:

(1) Even in an individual patient, measurements of exit dose or dose in the oesophagus show very wide variations.

(2) Often the anatomical information about the individual which is needed to make a prediction from the phantom measurements is lacking.

It can be said that while in general there is reasonable agreement between the two types of estimate of dose to tumour in the lung, it is difficult to find sufficient information to discuss this question in quantitative terms. The marked differences in exit doses measured in patients with similar external dimensions may arise from (*a*) differences in the tissue-to-lung ratio in the beam through the patient or (*b*) the presence of fluid, fibrosis or tumour in the lung.

The problems of dose distribution in lung irradiated with electrons seem to have been discussed in the literature mainly in terms of chest wall irradiations rather than in connection with the treatment of lung cancer. It is well established that the 'tail' of an electron beam is extended in lung over a length which is large compared with its length in water. As a result, in a chest wall treatment the dose to points in the lung behind the treatment area may be twice the estimated dose if no correction for the presence of lung is applied.

However, if the electron energy is chosen to put a lesion of the lung on the plateau of the depth dose curve, then the effect of the lung will be to lengthen the plateau with no significant change in the dose to the region to be treated. Here again the region beyond the treatment zone will receive a very high dose compared with that estimated from an isodose chart measured in unit density material. Cova and colleagues (1965) have demonstrated this effect by making measurements in thorax phantoms.

From the foregoing paragraphs we conclude that the results of phantom measurements can be used with reasonable confidence to calculate the effect of lung on the dose distribution produced in patients for megavoltage quality x-rays or γ-rays, and the rest of this chapter is mainly concerned with this aspect. It is clearly less useful, however, to carry out this type of detailed calculation for conventional quality radiation or for electron beam treatments because of the limited accuracy of the results.

APPLICATION OF EXPERIMENTAL RESULTS

Effect of Lung Corrections on Single Field Isodose Curves

We will now consider the use of the isodose shift method to determine the effect of lung tissue on single field isodose curves for 4 MV radiation. For this quality it is clear that electronic equilibrium is always established in the chest wall, and therefore in all cases the build-up region of the isodose chart is not significantly affected by the presence of lung.

Some ideally simple situations in which there is a plane parallel slab of low-density lung with unit density material on either side are illustrated in *Figure 4*. In *Figure 4a* the central axis of a plain field is normally incident on the surface, and here each isodose line is displaced forward by 0·4 times the thickness of lung. In *Figure 4b*, where there is oblique incidence, the normal incidence isodose lines, those corrected for oblique incidence and those corrected for oblique incidence and the presence of lung are shown. In *Figure 4c* there is a wedged field at normal incidence, and the ordinary isodose lines and those corrected for the presence of lung are shown. In each of these situations, the isodose lines are displaced forward parallel to their normal positions in the unit density region beyond the lung, and thus the distribution of relative dose across the beam is unchanged. This will also be true where the beam is incident on a curved surface and where the lung slab is parallel to the surface. It may be noted in *Figure 4c* that the isodose lines become steeper

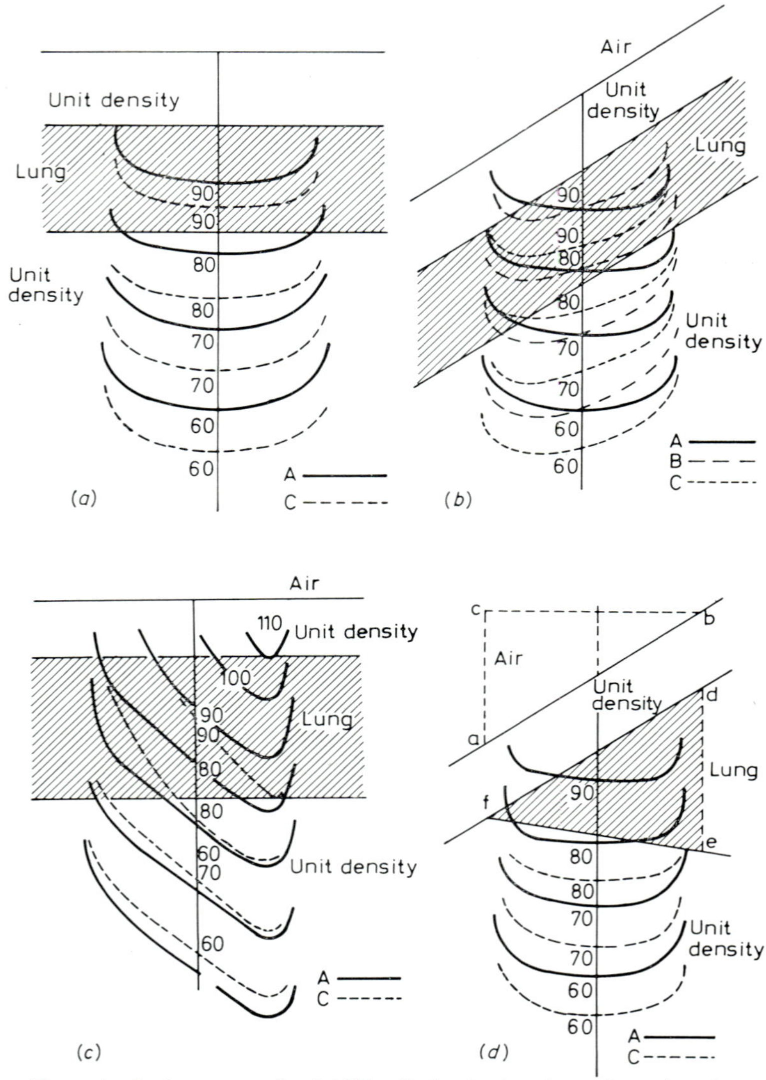

Figure 4. Isodose curves for 4 MV radiation in situations where there is a slab of simulated lung in a phantom. The curves in each diagram are labelled A, ordinary isodose curves; B, isodose curves corrected for oblique incidence; C, isodose curves corrected for oblique incidence and for presence of lung. (*a*) *Plain field, normal incidence.* (*b*) *Plain field, oblique incidence.* (*c*) *Wedged field, normal incidence.* (*d*) *Plain field, 'lung wedge', oblique incidence*

in the lung tissue but return to their normal wedge angle in the region beyond the lung. In *Figure 4d* there is a parallel slab of 'chest wall' followed by a wedge-shaped section of lung, beyond which is unit density material. The beam is obliquely incident as shown by the central axis marked. This diagram has been chosen such that the distance DE is 5/4 the distance AC. In this situation the effect of the 'air wedge' (abc) is exactly compensated by the 'lung wedge' (def), and again the cross-field dose distribution is unchanged.

Figure 5 illustrates the dose distributed produced by plain fields in a thorax section. The section is taken from Eycleshymer and Schoemaker (1911), and it is assumed that a unit density tumour is situated in the centre of the lung at the position shown. In *Figure 5a* the beam direction has been chosen to give normal incidence and is such that the inside of the chest wall and the adjacent edge of the tumour are almost parallel. It can be seen that in the tumour there is no cross-field variation in the relative dose, but that the absolute dose has been increased by the presence of lung. In *Figure 5b* the field is directed obliquely at the surface and the normal isodose lines, those corrected for oblique incidence and those corrected for oblique incidence and lung are shown. Here the latter lines within the tumour are nearly parallel to the lines corrected for oblique incidence only, and this is so because the chest wall section and the lung section traversed by the beam are again approximately parallel. Outside the tumour it can be seen that the isodose lines are symmetrically deflected forward, and this tendency of the lines to 'flow around' the tumour appears in all the diagrams. In *Figure 5c* the beam direction is the same as in *Figure 5b* but a unit density compensator has been used to correct for oblique incidence at the surface. Here the corrected isodose lines within the tumour are less parallel to the lines uncorrected for lung than in *Figure 5b* and there is more asymmetry of the lines outside the tumour. In *Figure 5d* the beam direction has been chosen to make the lung section traversed as irregular in shape as possible, and it can be seen here that in the tumour the cross-field distribution has been considerably distributed.

The illustrations in *Figures 4* and *5* are given in some detail because it is possible to use them to justify certain generalizations which are useful in planning multifield treatments. These are as follows:

(1) Where the beam traverses a parallel chest wall section and the lung section between the inner edge of the chest wall and the proximal edge of the tumour are parallel, the relative cross-field dose distribution will be the same in tumour as it would be in a unit density section of the same outline.

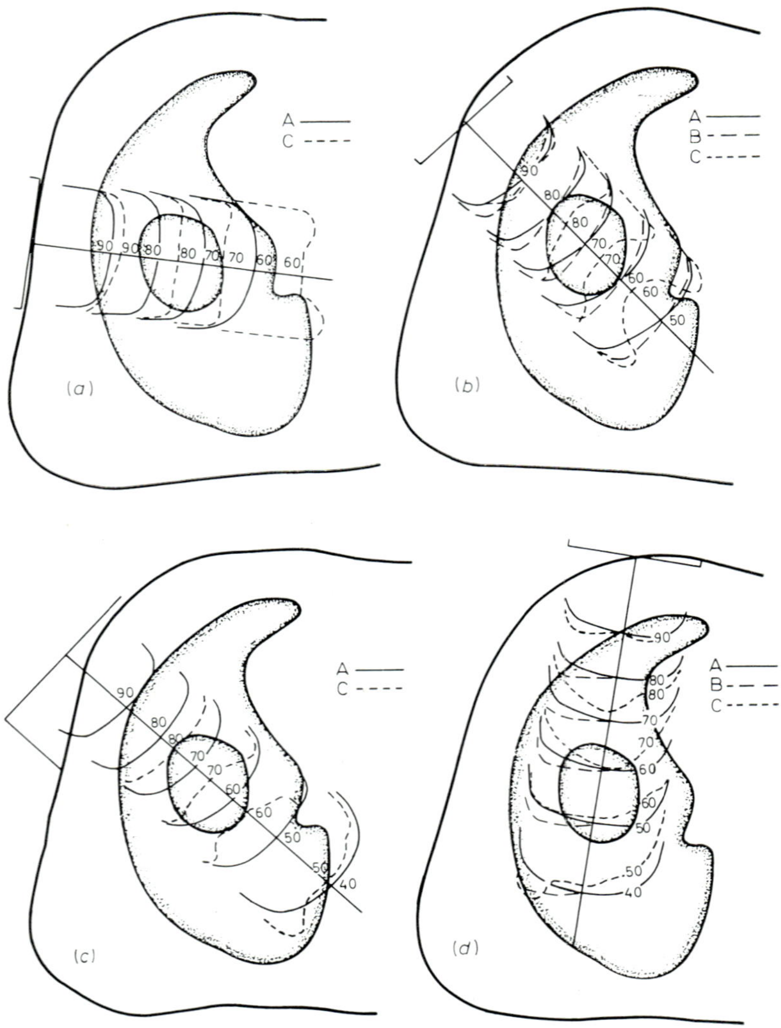

Figure 5. Single field isodose curves for 4 MV radiation applied to a tumour in a thorax section. The lung and tumour outlines are shaded. The curves are labelled as in Figure 4. (a) Plain field, normal incidence. (b) Plain field, oblique incidence. (c) Plain field, beam direction as in Figure 5b, wax compensator giving normal incidence. (d) Plain field, normal incidence

(2) It follows from (1) that if a surface compensation is used to correct for oblique incidence, it may change the cross-field dose distribution unfavourably by making the 'effective chest wall' non-parallel. This will still be true if the compensator is withdrawn from the surface in the interest of skin sparing.

(3) If it is not possible to select a beam direction in which the conditions in (1) are satisfied, it may be possible to utilize a non-parallel section of chest wall where the 'air wedge' due to oblique incidence is balanced by a 'lung wedge' as illustrated in *Figure 4d*.

(4) If compensators are used to correct the cross-field distribution for oblique incidence and lung, these will tend to be in opposite senses, as previously pointed out by Ellis, Feldman and Oliver (1964).

(5) If it is necessary to traverse a very irregular section of lung as in *Figure 5d*, then the only way to achieve a desirable cross-field distribution is to use an external compensator. Alternatively, it may be possible to 'balance' the cross-field distribution by a suitable choice of direction of other fields.

(6) All these considerations have only been applied in two dimensions. However, for small field beam directed treatments the body section is usually sufficiently uniform in the longitudinal section for two-dimensional planning to be adequate. This will not be the case for treatments involving the apex of the lung, and here three-dimensional compensators may be necessary.

For simplicity, all the examples in *Figure 5* have been given in terms of the use of plain fields. However, since the same rules apply to the correction of plain and wedged fields, the same generalizations must apply.

Although it has been shown that by suitable choice of field directions the cross-field variations in tumour may be minimized, it must be emphasized that in all cases the dose at the tumour centre will be increased by a factor which may be determined either by the isodose shift method or by the use of data such as those in Table 1.

Effect of Lung Corrections on a Two-field Treatment Plan

The use of a two-field treatment for the tumour already illustrated in *Figure 5* will next be considered. Since this tumour is peripherally situated in the body section, a two-field treatment using wedge filters is indicated. The availability of wedged fields of various angles affords the prescriber a choice of beam directions, and it is therefore practicable to look for directions meeting the criteria already discussed.

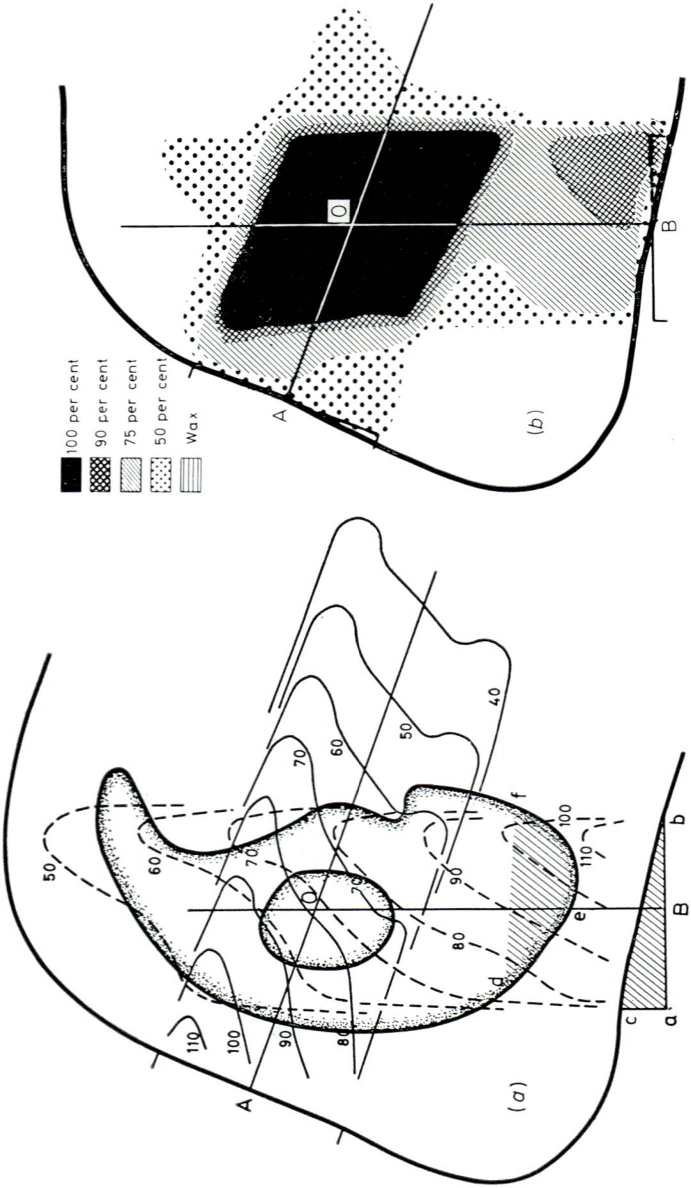

Figure 6. Two-field treatment plans for the lung tumour illustrated in Figure 5. (a) Corrected isodose lines for wedged fields applied along central axis AO and BO. (b) Treatment plan for two wedged fields applied to a unit density phantom and balancing to give equal contributions at 0

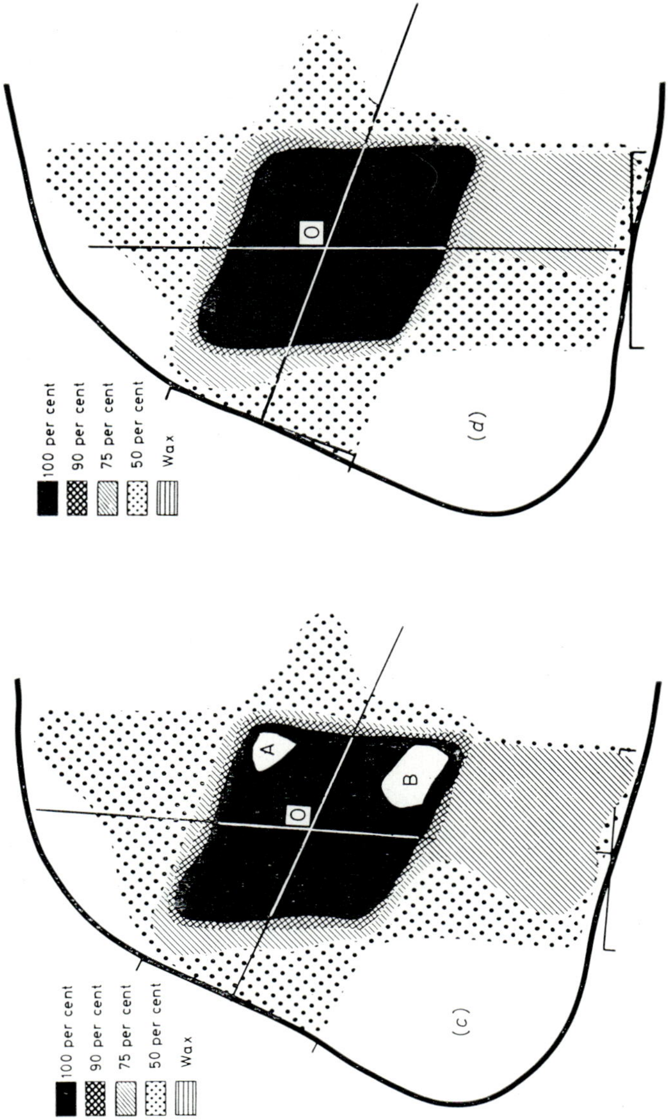

Figure 6. (c) *Treatment plan based on corrected isodoses shown in Figure 6a and giving same contributions as in Figure 6b. The regions marked A and B are 'hot', their relative dose levels being 108 per cent.* (d) *Treatment plan based on corrected isodoses and balancing to give equal contributions at 0 after correcting for lung*

Such an arrangement is illustrated in *Figure 6a*. Beam direction AO has been chosen to give normal incidence, to send the beam through an approximately parallel section of chest wall, and so that the lung section between the chest wall and the tumour is also nearly parallel. Field direction BO has been chosen such that the wedged isodose lines in unit density material would be parallel to those of the field delivered in the direction of AO. It can be seen that the oblique incidence (air wedge abc) is partly compensated by the lung wedge def. From previous discussion, the isodose lines in the tumour should remain nearly parallel to their positions in the solid phantom. This is illustrated in *Figure 6a*, where the corrected lines for each field are drawn in. It can be seen also that these lines 'flow around' the tumour in the way already discussed, and this may tend to create a 'hot spot' where the forward bulging sections of the curves from the two fields overlap.

Figure 6b shows the treatment plan obtained when the fields A and B are applied to a unit density phantom of the same outline as in *Figure 6a*. In order to achieve uniformity in the high-dose zone, the given doses from the two fields have been weighted to give equal contributions at the point O. If this plan is now recalculated, using the 'lung-corrected' isodose curves shown in *Figure 6a* but maintaining the same relative weighting as in *Figure 6b*, the plan shown in *Figure 6c* is obtained. There are now two hot spots, marked A and B, in the high-dose zone where the relative dose rises to 108 per cent. If, however, the given doses are reweighted to give equal contributions at O after correction for the presence of lung, the hot spots disappear (*Figure 6d*). It can be seen from either *Figure 6c* or *Figure 6d* that correction for lung results in a considerable increase in the area of the 50 per cent zone beyond the tumour, but this is probably not of any clinical significance.

It is thus demonstrated by suitable choice of beam directions, and by 'balancing' the relative contributors from each field after connection of the central axis doses for the presence of lung, that the relative dose distribution in the neighbourhood of the tumour is not significantly different from that calculated for a unit density phantom.

Effect of Lung Corrections on a Three-field Treatment Plan

For a centrally placed tumour, a three-field treatment plan is more appropriate. The section in *Figure 7* is again taken from Eycleshymer and Schoemaker (1911). *Figure 7a* shows a treatment plan, assuming a unit density body section, in which the posterior fields are corrected for oblique incidence. *Figure 7b* shows the plan obtained when the fields are also corrected for lung, and it can be seen that the differences between the size and shape of the high-dose zone are negligible in these two cases. It is of interest to compare

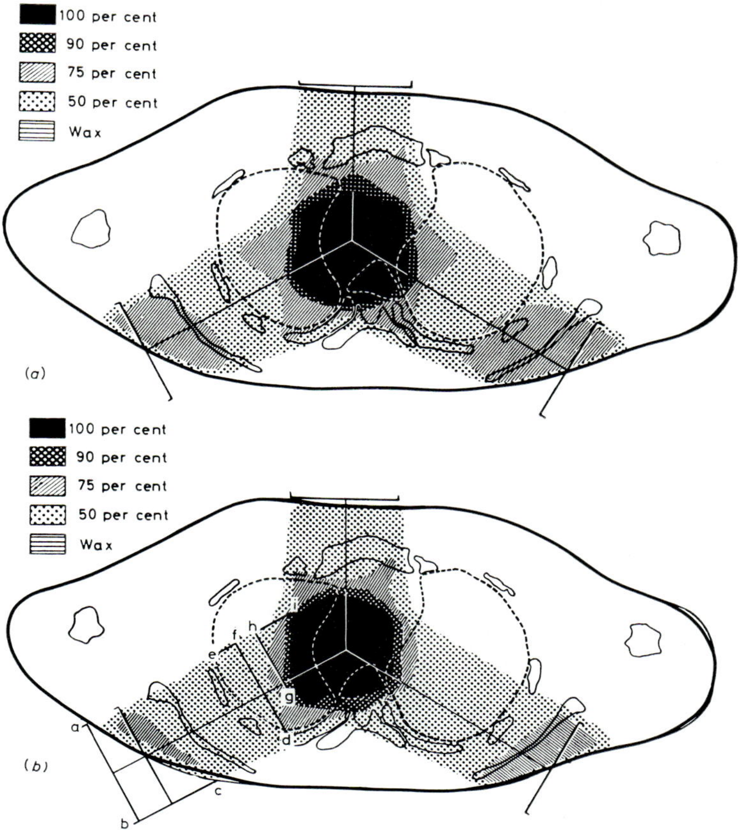

Figure 7. Three-field treatment plans for a lung tumour. (a) Assuming a unit density phantom. (Reproduced from Greene and Stewart, 1965, by courtesy of the Editor of British Journal of Radiology.) *(b) Isodoses corrected for lung penetration*

these plans with those obtained when wax compensators are used to achieve normal incidence for the posterior fields. *Figure 7c* shows the unit density plan obtained under these conditions, and *Figure 7d* illustrates the plan obtained after correcting for lung. It can be seen that there is a significant difference in the dose distribution in the high-dose zone in *Figures 7c* and *d*. The chest wall traversed by the posterior fields is not parallel, and one might conclude that the introduction of wax compensators might be helpful. However, the

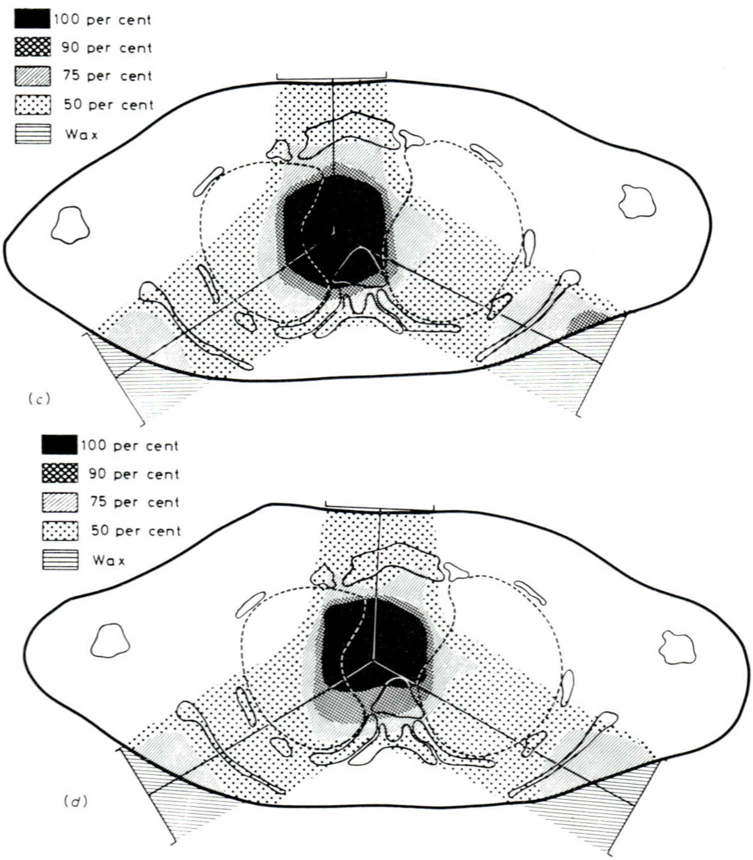

Figure 7. Three-field treatment plans for a lung tumour. (c) Assuming a unit density phantom and wax compensators to correct for oblique incidence of posterior fields. (d) As in Figure 7c, but correcting for lung

obliquity of the required high-dose zone (which we assume to be of unit density material) to the central axis is further accentuating the effect of the 'lung wedge'. In *Figure 7b* the air wedge (abc) is now

In cases of early mediastinal obstruction, the diagnosis may be difficult. In 14 patients who were seen when this procedure was first adopted and in whom the diagnosis was in doubt, it was confirmed in six. One of the other eight had a raised venous pressure following a lobectomy: the phlebogram showed no evidence of obstruction of the great veins, but the venous pressure remained raised until the patient's death six months later from cerebral metastases, the primary being apparently cured.

The site of the obstruction to the great veins was revealed by phlebography. In the first 45 phlebograms it was shown not only that the obstruction could be proximal to the superior vena cava, even involving the subclavian veins, but that this was a frequent finding (Table 1). So frequently, indeed, is the obstruction outside the superior vena cava that the term superior vena caval obstruction is too restricted and inaccurate and should be discarded. As suggested elsewhere (Howard, 1961, 1963, 1967), a more suitable term is 'mediastinal obstruction'. This places the obstruction in the great veins in the mediastinum without defining its site too closely. This comprehensive descriptive term is more desirable because the obstruction may obstruct not merely one segment of the great veins but two or even all three segments—superior vena cava, innominate and subclavian veins. It is reasonable to suppose that the more extensive the obstruction, the worse the prognosis. This has been difficult to prove, but certainly both the patients I have seen, in whom all three segments were obstructed, responded only partially to radiotherapy and failed to survive the course of treatment.

Phlebography establishes whether or not a collateral circulation is present and whether it is effective. It seems probable that the better the collateral circulation, the greater the likelihood of response to radiotherapy and the better the prognosis. In a series of 48 patients, 21 had no such circulation; in 14 patients it was present but not extensive; and in the remaining 10 it was good. Of those with no collateral circulation, 50 per cent were dead within three months, whereas 80 per cent of those with a good collateral circulation survived for more than three months. Moreover, only one patient with a good collateral circulation failed to respond completely to radiotherapy, whereas 50 per cent of those without such a circulation failed to show a complete response. The pattern of this collateral circulation varies considerably, although this is not reflected in the clinical presentation. In other words, the clinical picture does not reflect the site of the obstruction, but only its severity. The site determines the way in which the collateral circulation is opened up.

A common finding is an obstruction of the superior vena cava distal to the azygos vein. As result, this vein becomes considerably dilated, and blood is shunted to the right atrium via the azygos system of veins to the inferior vena cava (*Figure 1*). Less frequently, gross obstruction of the left subclavian, the right and left innominate veins and the superior vena cava opens up an effective collateral circulation via the hemiazygos vein (*Figure 2*). An unusual pattern was seen in a young woman with obstruction of the left innominate vein when collateral circulation was provided by way of the arcus venosus jugulare, thus shunting blood from left to right (*Figure 3*). The massive increase in the volume of blood deviated into the inferior vena cava can sometimes be gauged from the greatly enlarged and tortuous veins over the anterior abdominal wall—the superficial epigastric veins.

TABLE 1

Frequency of Sites of Obstruction to Great Veins in 45 Phlebograms

Site of obstruction	*Number of patients*	
Superior vena cava	16	(36%)
Innominate veins	12	(27%)
Subclavian veins	8	(18%)
Superior vena cava and innominate veins	3	(6%)
Innominate and subclavian veins	4	(9%)
All three segments	2	(4%)

Phlebography has demonstrated that in some patients the wall of the vein is involved by tumour. This mural involvement would also appear to be a bad prognostic finding. One such patient completely failed to respond to radiotherapy and died during treatment, while another responded only partially and died at the end of treatment (*Figure 4*). Three other patients responded to radiotherapy but died within three months.

It has been interesting to repeat phlebography following a course of radiotherapy when the patient has responded completely to treatment. In some cases there is surprisingly little change in the picture. Presumably slight changes in the haemodynamics have been sufficient to compensate for the obstruction and restore the patient to his previous condition. In many cases a phlebogram at the end of treatment shows a normal circulation through the great veins. Clinically it makes no difference to the care of the patient

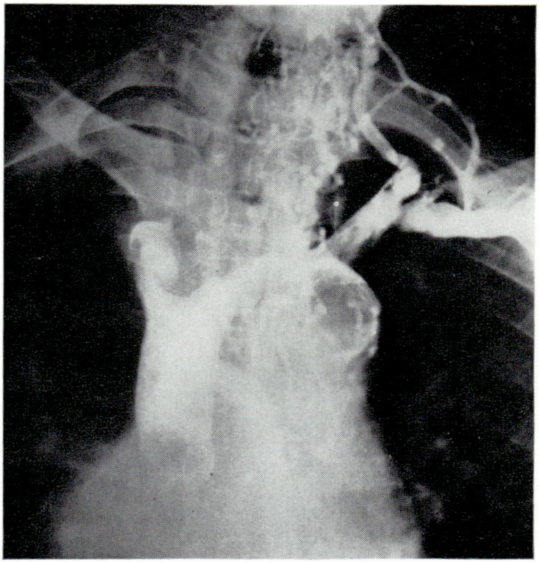

Figure 1. Phlebogram showing obstruction of the superior vena cava, with a good collateral circulation via the azygos vein

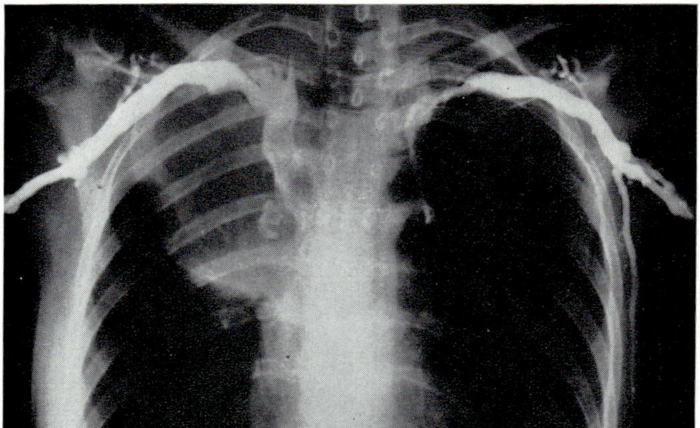

Figure 2. Phlebogram showing obstruction of the left subclavian vein, the right and left innominate veins and the superior vena cava. There is a good collateral circulation via the hemiazygos vein

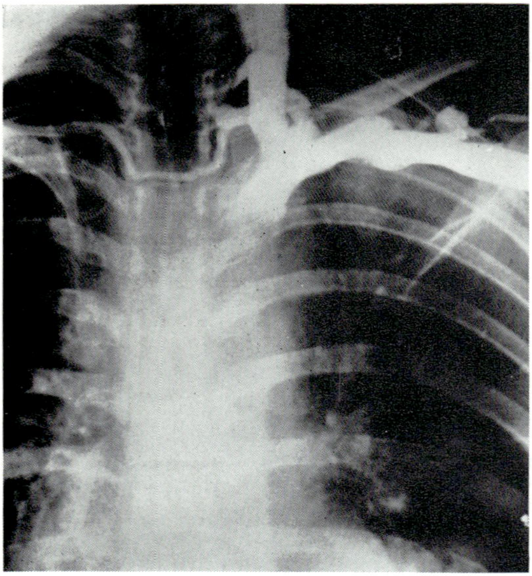

Figure 3. Left-sided phlebogram showing obstruction of the left innominate vein. The collateral circulation is via the arcus venosus jugulare and there is reflux into the left internal jugular vein

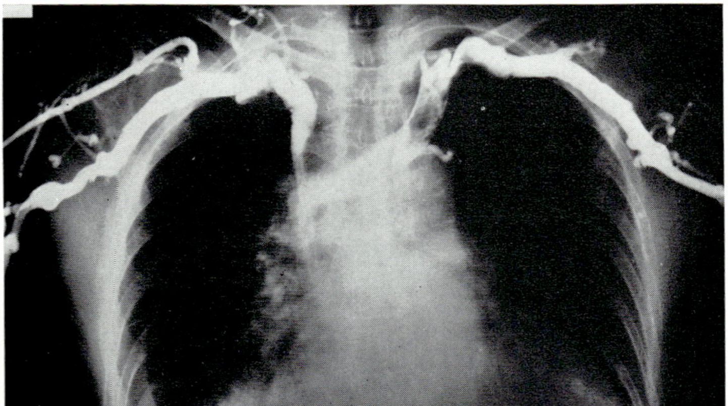

Figure 4. Phlebogram showing mural involvement. There is a gross filling defect in the left innominate vein in a patient with gross signs of mediastinal obstruction. The superior vena cava itself is only partially obstructed

whether the phlebogram shows a return to the normal circulation or not. Consequently, phlebography is no longer repeated routinely or without some special indications.

APPLICATIONS

Some of the applications of phlebography are implicit in the foregoing discussion. The most obvious application is in the diagnosis of mediastinal obstruction. The diagnosis is easy when the obstruction is moderate or severe, but may be difficult when it is mild. It may be suspected but hard to prove, or may be hard to distinguish from congestive cardiac failure. Phlebography can save the patient from days or even weeks of discomfort by defining the situation and allowing the appropriate treatment to be initiated rapidly.

It has been generally agreed that radiotherapy is the treatment of choice for mediastinal obstruction (Price Thomas, 1950; Brooks and colleagues, 1951; Roswit, Kaplan and Jacobson, 1953; Hilton and Pilcher, 1955; Smithers 1958; Howard, 1961, 1967). The radiotherapeutic approach has always been empirical with regard to treatment volume (and thus to field size and position) as well as to dosage. Phlebography, because it defines the site and extent of the obstruction, allows a rational basis for radiotherapy. It is the only way of defining the volume which must be treated, and hence the field size and position. In the past these have been decided from the radiological appearance and from experience, and phlebography has shown that these are by no means infallible guides. The field size may be too small or unnecessarily large, or the positioning of the fields may be such that the obstruction and tumour are only partially treated and uninvolved tissues are irradiated unnecessarily.

In the patients originally investigated by phlebography, treatment was initially applied empirically and immediately to ensure rapid relief of symptoms. Phlebography was carried out after a few days and the treatment volume reassessed. In 40 per cent of these patients the treatment volume was altered—the fields most often being enlarged and moved, but also occasionally being reduced. It is obviously preferable to perform phlebography before radiotherapy is intitiated, but the pressure of work in most radiology departments makes this difficult, and radiotherapy is urgent.

It has already been suggested that the *routine* repetition of phlebography at the end of a course of radiotherapy is unlikely to be helpful. On occasion, such repetition may be essential. Thus, a recently treated patient developed a recurrence of his mediastinal obstruction in spite of a carefully planned course of radiotherapy giving 4,000 r with telecobalt therapy in one month. Phlebography was repeated to define the site of the obstruction, this time confined to the left innominate vein, and a second but localized course of treatment, using small fields, was given. The patient in fact failed to respond and died within three weeks, but a second attempt at palliation would scarcely have been contemplated without phlebography.

In the past little effort has been made to improve the treatment of mediastinal obstruction because, as Adler said of lung cancer in 1912, 'it is not to be wondered at that the Physician takes little interest in types of disease that offer not the slightest hope of therapeutic success'. The need to define the treatment volume even in a palliative treatment for such hopeless cases is not entirely academic. Although survival rates in mediastinal obstruction are never good, some patients undoubtedly fare worse because their treatment is inadequate. Thus in a series of 253 cases previously studied (Howard, 1967) who were treated empirically, only 14 per cent of those who responded to radiotherapy survived for more than one year. In contrast, in a series of patients who were investigated by phlebography and whose treatment volume was accurately defined, 22 per cent survived for over a year.

The recurrence rate is also an important measure of the effectiveness of treatment; the aim of radiotherapy should be the complete and lasting relief of mediastinal obstruction and, if this is relieved for a short time only and then recurs, the treatment has achieved only a partial and limited success. It is the quality of life which is perhaps of the greatest importance, not merely the length of survival. Phlebography helps to reduce the recurrence rate. In a series of 183 patients who responded completely to irradiation, 10 per cent had a recurrence of their mediastinal obstruction. In a series of patients investigated by phlebography, where the treatment was accurately planned, only 3 per cent recurred.

REFERENCES

Abbott, O. A., Hopkins, W. A. and Leigh, T. D. (1949). *J. thorac. Surg.* **18,** 869.

Barrett, N. R. (1958). *Br. J. Surg.* **46,** 207.

Brooks, W. D. W., Davidson, M., Price Thomas, C., Robson, K. and Smithers, D. W. (1951). *Thorax* **6,** 1.

Dougherty, J. and Homans, J. (1940). *Surgery Gynec. Obstet.* **71,** 697.

Hilton, G. and Pilcher, R. S. (1955). In *British Practice in Radiotherapy*, p. 271. Ed. by E. R. Carling, B. W. Windeyer and D. W. Smithers. London: Butterworths.

Howard, N. (1961). *Clin. Radiol.* **12,** 295.
— (1963). *Radiology* **81,** 380.
— (1967). *Mediastinal Obstruction in Lung Cancer.* Edinburgh: Livingstone.
— and Pick, E. J. (1961). *Clin. Radiol.* **12,** 290.
Hudson, G. W. (1957). *Radiology* **68,** 499.
Katz, S., Hussey, H. H. and Veal, J. R. (1947). *Am. J. med. Sci.* **214,** 7.
Maruyama, Y., Wilkins, E. W. and Wyman, S. N. (1962). *Radiology* **79,** 617.
Price Thomas, C. (1950). In *Malignant Disease and its Treatment by Radium*, Vol. III, p. 157. 2nd ed. Ed. by Sir Stanford Cade. Bristol: Wright.
Robb, G. P. and Steinberg, I. (1938). *J. clin. Invest.* **17,** 507.
Roberts, D. J. Jnr., Dotter, C. T. and Steinberg, I. (1951). *Am. J. Roentg.* **66,** 341.
Rosenbloom, S. E. (1949). *Ann. intern. Med.* **31,** 470.
Roswit, B., Kaplan, G. and Jacobson, H. G. (1953). *Radiology* **61,** 722.
Sammons, B. P., Lund, R. R. and Pischnotte, W. O. (1961). *Am. J. Roentg.* **86,** 718.
Sanders, D. E., Delarue, N. C. and Lau, G. (1962). *Am. J. Roentg.* **87,** 884.
Seldinger, S. I. (1953). *Acta radiol.* **39,** 368.
Smithers, D. W. (1958). In *Carcinoma of the Bronchus*, p. 245. Ed. by J. R. Bignall. Edinburgh: Livingstone.
Steinberg, I. and Dotter, C. T. (1952). *Archs Surg., Lond.* **64,** 10.
— and Finby, N. (1959). *Am. J. Roentg.* **81,** 807.
Szur, L. and Bromley, L. L. (1956). *Br. med. J.* **2,** 1273.

II—High Daily Dose for Rapid Decompression

Philip Rubin and Samuel Ciccio

INTRODUCTION

There is an urgent need to institute effective treatment in cases of superior vena caval obstruction (SVCO). What is at issue is whether there is an optimal dose rate of irradiation and whether chemotherapy in combination with radiotherapy can give consistently better results. When obstruction occurs rapidly, the acute onset of swelling of the face and upper torso is alarming to the patient and can be perplexing to the physician unless he has a well-defined treatment plan. The clinical variations in the onset and progression of this syndrome have allowed for different principles of management, depending upon the specialty of the physician encountering the patient on presentation.

Our programme of radiotherapeusis has evolved on the basis of sound experimental radiobiological and pathological observations (Green, Rubin and Holzwasser, 1963), and has led to a very effective clinical regimen (Rubin and colleagues, 1963) to cope with this problem. The myth of 'radiation oedema', necessitating the use of small doses of radiation, has been supplanted by the concept that rapid resolution of the oedema follows prompt tumour decompression and is best achieved by high daily doses of radiation. Experimental evidence on this point is presented in this chapter. A current statement of our approach is offered, with reassessment of the experience at the University of Rochester Medical Center from 1957 to 1969, based on 48 cases of whom 29 were treated by this rapid dose regimen.

DIAGNOSTIC PRINCIPLES

The first step in the treatment of acute SVCO is accurate diagnosis. Unlike most other clinical situations in which pathological confirmation is required prior to instituting radiation treatment, histological diagnosis is waived. The essential features of the diagnostic study are first to determine the presence of SVCO and secondly to discover its aetiology. Diagnostic studies and therapy are allowed to proceed simultaneously and quickly.

Initial Studies

The history and physical examination in the emergency department often permit a working diagnosis. The classical presentation of swollen facies and arms and prominent venous collaterals on the chest wall, aggravated by recumbency, is indicative of the syndrome of SVCO (*Figures 1* and *2*). In the tabulation of clinical findings on presentation, venous obstructive symptoms occur more frequently than respiratory complaints and often are unassociated with or obscure the latter (Table 1).

TABLE 1
Frequency of Various Presenting Symptoms

Symptom	*Number of patients*	*Percentage of patients*
Swelling:		
Face	36	75
Neck	32	67
Peri-orbital	30	63
Extremities	15	31
Dyspnoea	28	58
Chest pain	16	33
Cough	25	52
Haemoptysis	6	13
Hoarseness	6	13
Cyanosis	15	31
Dysphagia	5	10
Headache	3	6
Vertigo	1	2
Tinnitus	3	6
Disturbed mentation	4	8
Prominent venous patterns	35	73
Palpable liver	6	13
Weight loss	15	31

The following procedures should be carried out immediately.

Chest Film

A mass (*Figure 2*), most often right-sided, was identified in 97·9 per cent of all patients studied (47 out of 48). The presumptive diagnosis was either bronchogenic carcinoma or lymphoma, and eventually the former was confirmed in the majority of our patients.

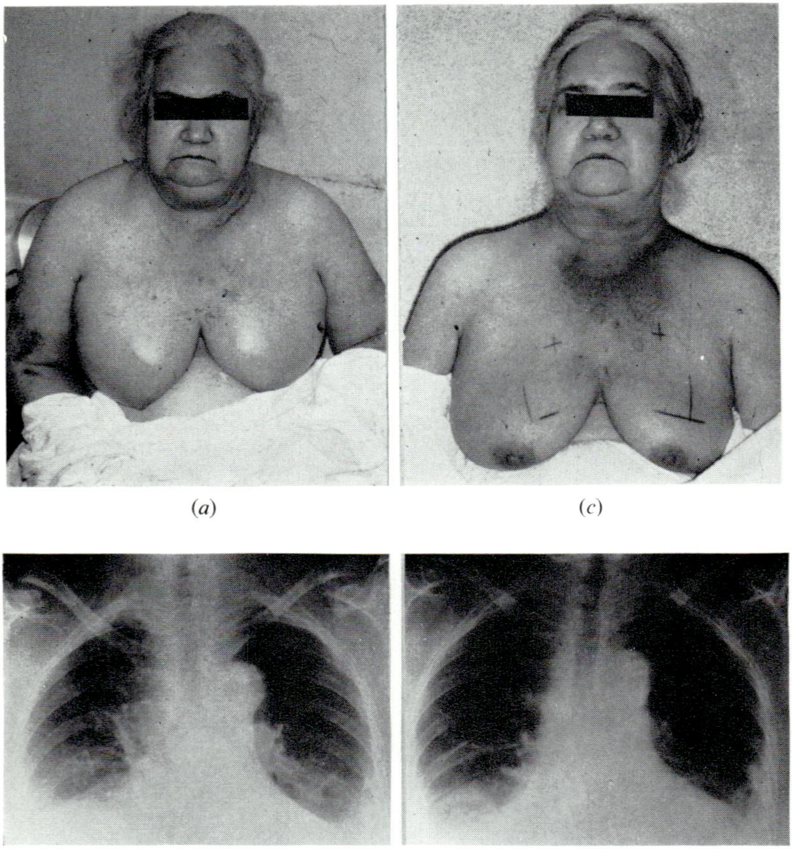

Figure 1. Slow low daily dose treatment for superior vena caval obstruction. R.M., a 64-year-old white woman with anaplastic carcinoma of the lung, had 2 weeks' history of increasing dyspnoea and oedema of neck, face and breasts. (a) Photograph shows condition before treatment. (b) Radiograph showed large superior mediastinal mass with bilateral fluid at bases. Thoracotomy revealed inoperable carcinoma; patient referred for radiotherapy. Oedema had increased since admission, and sensorium was dulled. Venous pressure in left arm was over 300 mm saline. Irradiation (1 MeV) was initiated to the mediastinum through 10 × 10 cm port with 180 degrees anterior oscillation. Tumour dose was 100 r/day for the first 12 treatments. (c) There was no appreciable clinical improvement until after 3,000 r in 26 days, with subsequent rapid relief of symptoms. (d) Radiograph showed tumour regression. A total tumour dose of 6,000 r was given in 42 days. Patient died 6 months after therapy without recurrence of caval obstruction

Venous Pressure

Demonstration of an elevated venous pressure is conclusive proof of obstruction and is obtained simply by means of a spinal fluid manometer in an arm vein 10 cm below the anterior chest wall. Values from 150 to 400 mm saline have been observed (*Figures 1* and *2*). Both arms can be tested to determine innominate vein obstruction; femoral vein pressures are rarely taken unless one is interested in ascertaining whether the obstruction is caudal to the azygous vein.

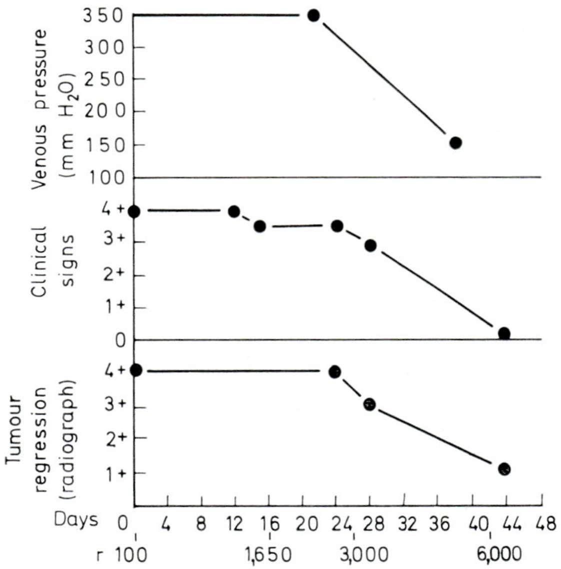

Figure 1e

Scintiphlebogram

This isotopic procedure has supplanted phlebograms since it is accurate in demonstrating the actual site of caval obstruction and is without hazard, easy to repeat and lower in cost. The detail of collateral vessels is lacking compared with phlebography (Farrer, Ciccio and Rubin, 1969) (*Figure 3*). A bolus of 10–12 mc technetium (^{99m}Tc), using the same needle as for the venous pressure study, quickly demonstrates the slow circulation in the subclavian vein and pin-points the venous obstruction (Farrer, Ciccio and Rubin, 1969).

(*a*) (*c*)

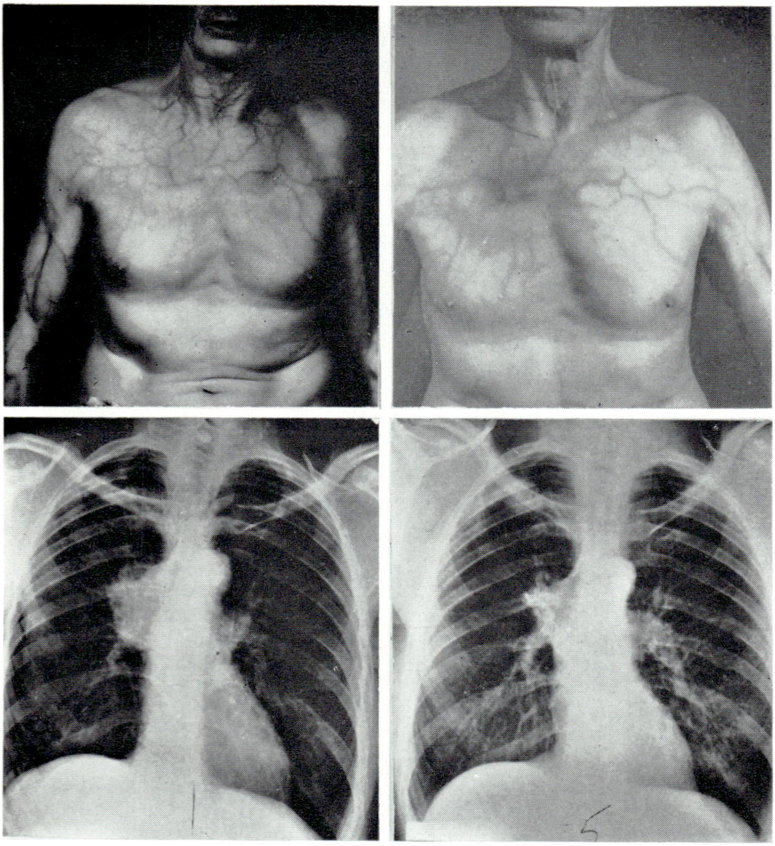

(*b*) (*d*)

Figure 2. Rapid high daily dose treatment for SVCO. N.B., a 58-year-old white man with anaplastic carcinoma of the lung, had 5 weeks' history of progressive dyspnoea and oedema of head and neck. He was in moderately severe distress when first seen. (a) *Infra-red photograph shows condition before treatment.* (b) *Chest radiograph revealed large right mid-mediastinal mass. Venous pressure in right arm was 250 mm saline. Mediastinal irradiation (2 MeV) was started at once, 400 r/day tumour dose through opposed 13 × 18 cm ports. Clinical improvement was first noted on fourth day and was quite rapid thereafter. A dose of 2,800 r was given in 7 days. (c and d) Infra-red photograph and radiograph after 2,800 r. Bronchoscopy and scalene node biopsy were both negative. Thoracotomy was performed after 2 weeks' wait, but inoperable carcinoma was found. Radiotherapy was subsequently resumed and the tumour dose was carried to a total of 5,600 r. The patient is now 7 months post-therapy without evidence of caval obstruction*

An associated finding of some interest is the failure to perfuse the right lung, suggesting that the pulmonary arterial circulation can be compromised as well. The severe thrombophlebitis occasionally encountered after contrast media phlebograms is not seen with ^{99m}Tc scintiscans. The most valuable feature of this method is the ease with which the patient can be serially followed during treatment and the relief of caval obstruction clearly shown (Farrer, Ciccio and Rubin, 1969) (*Figure 4*).

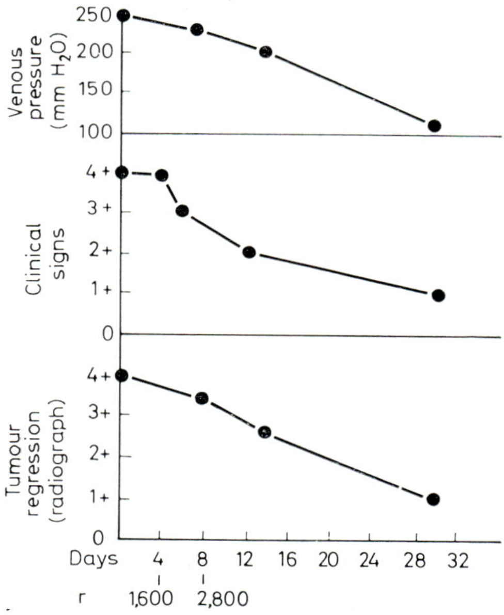

Figure 2e

Blood Chemistry and Blood Counts

Electrolyte studies, liver chemistry tests and a routine haemogram complete the initial investigations. Abnormal serum sodium, chloride and CO_2 levels can occur and need to be documented. Anaemia may also be present.

Photographs

Photographs are helpful to complete the record. In addition to colour photographs, infra-red photography of collateral venous patterns is of interest. It is important to standardize the procedure if one desires to follow patients serially after treatment has been instituted, and this method proved too difficult to standardize to be of value in such cases.

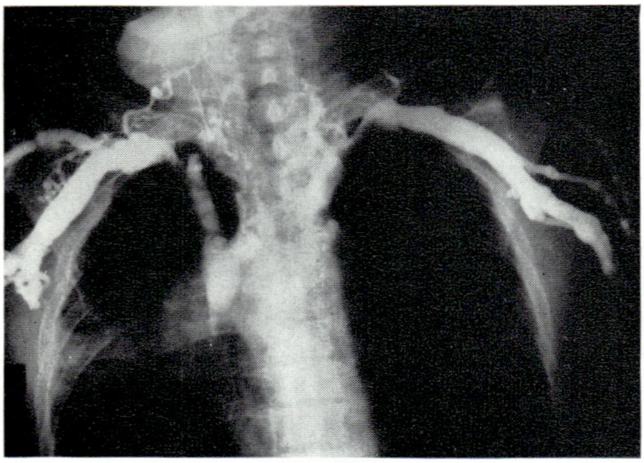

(*a*)

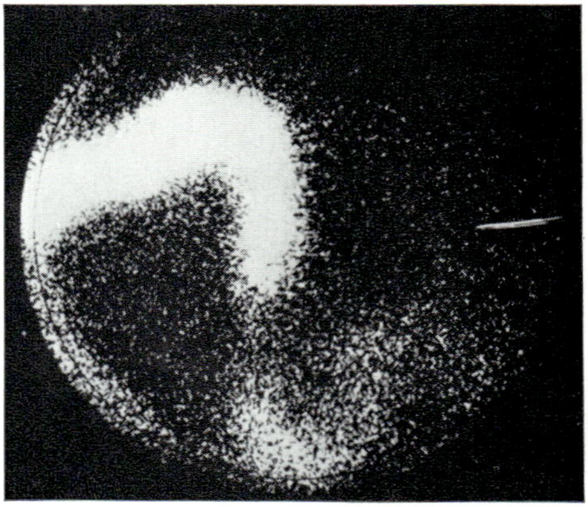

(*b*)

Figure 3. Phlebogram v. scintiphlebogram in SVCO. (a) Bilateral venous phlebogram shows complete obstruction of superior vena cava with collateralization taking place about the subclavian veins bilaterally. (b) Scintiphlebogram with ^{99m}Tc shows radioactive bolus blocked at point of obstruction, with very small trickle through to right auricle

Later Studies

Once the superior vena caval obstruction has been relieved, pathological diagnosis should be attempted. From earlier review of the literature, a large variety of causes of superior vena caval obstruction has been listed and includes chronic inflammatory nodes, tuberculosis and syphilitic aortitis in addition to thoracic neoplasm. The clinical evidence currently is that 80–90 per cent of all admissions for SVCO are due to bronchogenic carcinoma, another 10–20 per cent are due to lymphoma and Hodgkin's disease, and as few as 5–10 per cent are due to benign conditions (Rubin, 1963). The diagnostic work-up is then similar to that of bronchogenic carcinoma.

(*a*)

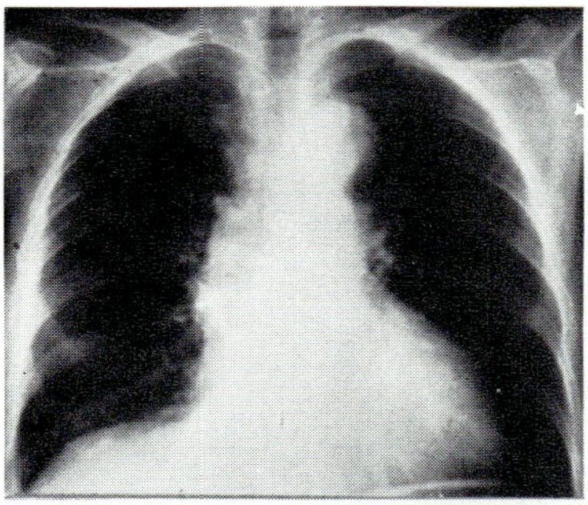

Figure 4. Serial scintiphlebogram taken in following relief of SVCO. (*a*) *Nodes in right hilar region and paratracheal area due to metastatic carcinoma of the breast.* (*b*) *On the 0–8-second isotope angiogram, complete obstruction to flow into right auricle is shown. Obstruction is in region of superior vena cava.* (*c*) *At 4,600 rads, repeat isotope angiogram after irradiation shows relief of obstruction and flow of radioactive bolus into right auricle and right ventricle*

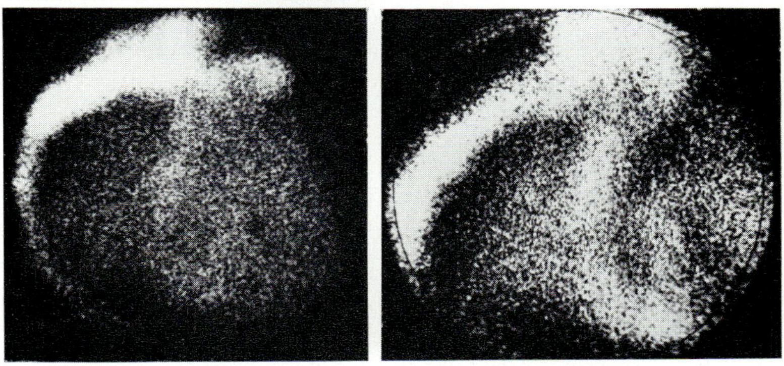

(*b*) (*c*)

Pathological Diagnosis

Although it is important to establish whether the patient has a carcinoma or a lymphoma, this is of secondary importance to relieving the venous obstruction. Occasionally house officers proceed to obtain repeated cytology studies, bronchoscopy and scalene node biopsy and await pathology reports before sending the patient for radiotherapy. In our experience, a successful diagnosis is made in only 50 per cent of our cases prior to therapy, and such delays are unjustified and can endanger the patient's life. Thoracotomy is justified only in selected cases where other measures have failed to yield a diagnosis and a non-neoplastic origin is suspected. Mediastinoscopy and biopsy are at present being used more often and have proved as effective as thoracotomy in obtaining tissue for histological study. A diagnosis of carcinoma was made in 83 per cent of our patients, and the ratio of cancer to lymphoma was 5:1.

Associated Syndromes

There are in bronchogenic carcinoma a variety of associated syndromes of a non-neoplastic nature which have been summarized by Knowles and Smith (1960). Of particular note are some clinical manifestations associated with SVCO which require special attention.

Wet Brain Syndrome

Severely disturbed mentation, headache, drowsiness, lethargy and vertigo may be found on presentation. An elevated intracranial pressure may be manifest, and the fundi may show evidence of papilloedema and venous engorgement. A brain scan is indicated to rule out metastases but will often be negative, confirming a 'wet brain' condition. Relief of the central nervous system signs follows the relief of the caval obstruction and can be dramatic. Extensive diagnostic tests for cerebral metastases should always await relief of venous obstruction.

Salt-losing Syndrome

Profound weakness and mental confusion may also be associated with hyponatraemia without elevation of CO_2-combining levels. This entity was first described by Schwartz and colleagues in 1957. The pathophysiology may be untoward secretion of an anti-diuretic hormone. It is difficult to correct the salt loss unless the caval obstruction is relieved by radiotherapy bringing about tumour regression.

Spinal Cord Compression

The association of spinal cord compression with SVCO in 5 of 48 cases suggests a relationship between the two processes. Cord compression has most often been heralded by severe unremitting back pain, and this should alert the clinician to this complication. In bronchogenic carcinoma, vertebral destruction is readily observed, but the radiographs are often negative in cases of lymphoma (*Figure 5*). Bone scans are of value in detecting a reactive process to neoplasia and are indicated when radiographs of the spine are

(*a*) (*b*)

(*c*)

(*d*)

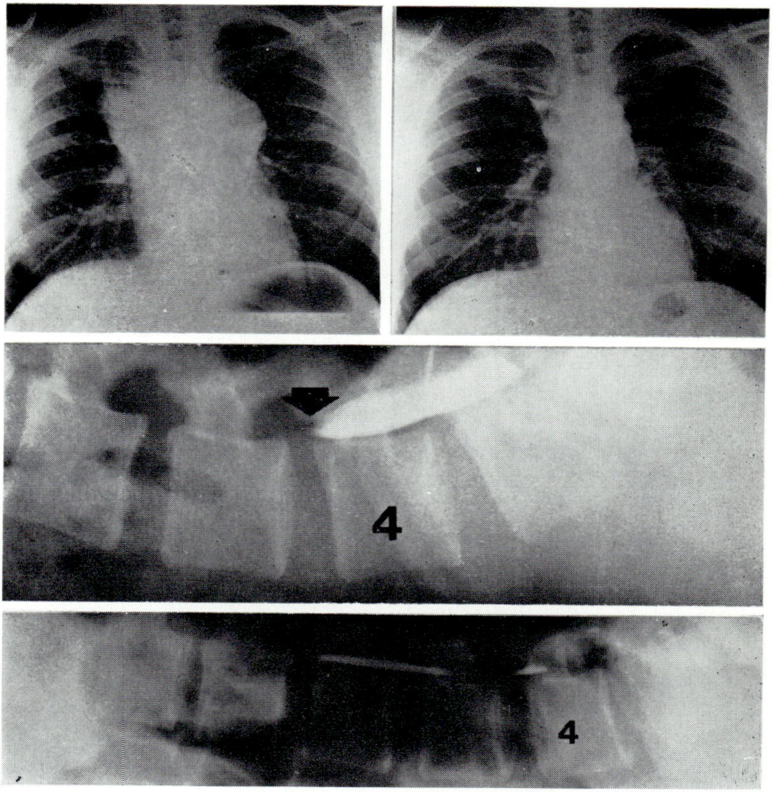

Figure 5. Association of spinal cord compression with SVCO. R.M., a 24-year-old white man with reticulum sarcoma, had 1 month's history of increasing facial and neck oedema, most pronounced upon rising in the morning. He was in moderate distress on admission. (*a*) *Chest radiograph revealed huge right-sided mediastinal mass. Venous pressure in right arm was 190 mm saline. Diagnosis made by scalene node biopsy. Irradiation (2 MeV) was started immediately—400 r/day tumour dose through opposed 15 × 15 cm ports. Relief was noted on first day and patient was relatively asymptomatic by fourth day.* (*b*) *Radiation schedule was modified after 1,600 r had been delivered in 4 days, and a total dose of 3,500 r was given in 19 days. In subsequent follow-up 2 years later, patient developed two bouts of spinal cord compression manifested by varying degrees of pain, sphincter loss, sensory defects and motor impairment. Rapid relief of the compression took place with a high daily dose of radiation.* (*c and d*) *Myelograms show relief of cord compression and flow of contrast media past superior border of L.4 after one radiation dose of 400 rads.*

negative. Myelograms should always be done if neurological changes are found. The radiation treatment of spinal cord compression is similar to that of SVCO (Rubin and colleagues, 1971) and is likewise a medical emergency. The underlying mechanism may be in the collateral circulation formed as a result of SVCO in bronchogenic cancers. The extensive intercommunication between the vertebral plexus of veins and the azygous system is described by Okay and Bryk (1969), particularly where the block extends to the azygos vein. By contrast, in lymphomas a retrograde flow in the thoracic duct due to mediastinal obstruction may lead to retroperitoneal involvement and spinal cord extension. This subject will be reported in more detail in a separate publication (Rubin, 1971).

THERAPEUTIC PRINCIPLES

Superior vena caval obstruction of rapid onset is a medical emergency. The treatment should be aimed first at relieving the obstruction and secondly at definitive treatment of its cause. If this sequence is followed, a high degree of therapeutic effectiveness will be achieved with the lowest morbidity and mortality. The prime principle is to produce *rapid* decompression by bringing about immediate regression of the mediastinal neoplasm. The underlying assumption in our philosophy of management is that acute and subacute SVCO are invariably due to a rapidly growing neoplasm causing venous compression without allowing for collateralization.

This distinction between acute, subacute and chronic obstruction is clinically important. Chronic obstruction can be due to non-neoplastic disease or to slowly growing tumours. Patients with chronic SVCO are not a medical emergency since they are usually well compensated with a collateral circulation, and a full diagnostic work-up can proceed to completion and pathological diagnosis without risk. On the other hand, *acute superior vena caval obstruction, once diagnosed, demands immediate attention.*

Diuresis

Diuresis is the most effective measure to relieve the accumulated fluid and oedema of the face, arms and upper torso. It will not relieve the obstruction. Ethacrynic acid has supplanted intravenous urea or mannitol where rapid relief is desired. Diuril is often used in subacute conditions where an immediate effect is not needed. All intravenous medication and infusions are preferably given in leg veins. No attempt at transfusion or electrolyte replacement should be made in the arm veins. The iatrogenic induction of SVCO syndrome has been precipitated by an arm intravenous infusion or transfusion when incipient caval obstruction was suspected.

Rapid High Daily Dose Schedule

In 1960, a rapid high daily dose schedule was initiated, based on the experimental evidence in our laboratory that 'radiation oedema' was in fact 'tumour oedema'. A biological model indicated that small daily increments in dosage from 50 to 100 rads were unsuccessful in relieving obstruction, whereas larger daily doses of 200–1,500 rads at one session were not only well tolerated but uniformly led to rapid relief (*Figure 6*).

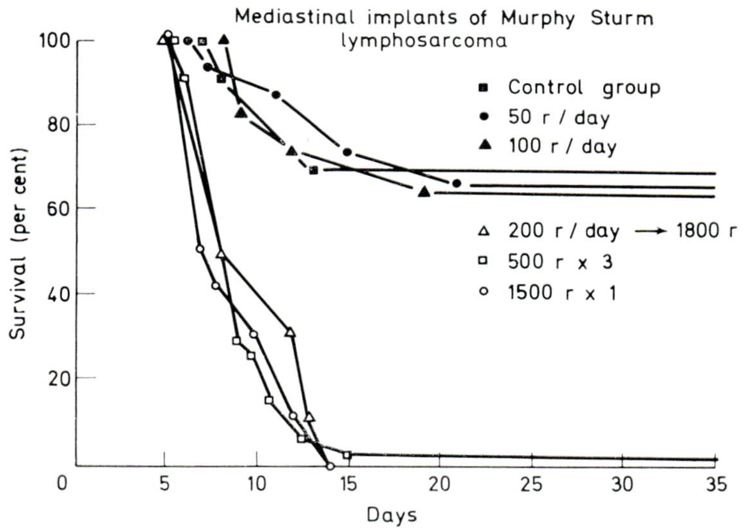

Figure 6. Superior vena caval obstruction—variations in daily dose of x-ray

In the rapid high daily dose treatment, two opposed mediastinal fields are employed, often as large as 15 × 15 cm or 15 × 20 cm, to encompass the mass and the mediastinum. A daily midline tumour dose of 400 rads is given, preferably with supervoltage irradiation. After three such treatments to a total of 1,200 rads, the SVCO symptoms are in most cases relieved and the daily dose is decreased to 150–200 rads. If no alteration in oedema occurs, the rapid dose therapy is terminated at 2,000 rads and the protracted regimen is instituted. The diagnostic work-up for a tissue confirmation proceeds at this time. A split course regimen is utilized if diagnostic procedures such as thoracotomy are indicated. The maximum dose and the shortest schedule used have been 4,000 rads in 10 days. However, this is poorly tolerated due to the large field size, the severe oesophagitis at the completion of treatment and the subsequent risk of radiation pneumonitis. It has therefore been abandoned in favour of a more protracted schedule with final dose levels of 4,000–5,000 rads in 4–5 weeks, depending on the response of the tumour and the associated general condition of the patient.

The rate of response to the two contrasting dose schedules—rapid high versus slow low daily doses—indicates a similar clearance of symptoms by the conclusion of treatment (Table 2—*see also Figures 1* and *2*). However, the rapid high dose regimen offers relief in 79 per cent of cases within the first week, whereas the slow low dose therapy

TABLE 2
Evaluation of Therapy Method Used

	Slow	*Rapid*
Number treated by various methods	19 (40%)	29 (60%)
Relief in first week	2 (11%)	23 (79%)
Number having relief by end of therapy	15 (79%)	23 (79%)
Average day relief started	3–25 range 10 days	2–25 range 5·6 days
Number having worsening of symptoms during therapy	5 (26·5%)	3 (11%)
Average number of days patients lived following start of therapy	156 days	208 days

offers only 10 per cent relief at this time. The average time needed for relief of symptoms was 5·6 days in contrast to 10 days with slower schedules. A similar response rate is seen in both carcinomas and lymphomas.

The most important feature to determine is whether patients worsen with rapid high daily doses more than with slow low doses. The evidence shows that 27 per cent of patients have worsening of their symptoms with the slow dose technique, in contrast to 11 per cent with the rapid dose method. If a patient fails to respond or worsens despite rapid treatment, this suggests that a thrombosis of the superior vena cava has occurred and rapid decompression is not possible. This can be confirmed by serial ^{99m}Tc scintiphlebogram. Usually there is an improved flow associated with clinical improvement in those cases studied following the rapid dose treatment. The argument that true relief of caval compression by tumour regression rather than incidental collateral formation is the mechanism for relief of SVCO has been resolved, on the basis of these studies, in favour of the former.

Although the average number of days patients have survived is greater in the high dose than in the low dose group (Table 2), this depends mainly on problems unrelated as a rule to SVCO. The vital statistics indicate no difference in prognosis between the patient presenting with SVCO and the average patient presenting with bronchogenic cancer. There are associated features which shorten survival for lung cancer patients, but this is not true of caval obstruction *per se*. Long-term survivors with bronchogenic cancer or lymphoma presenting as cases of superior vena caval obstruction are known in our series.

DISCUSSION: RADIATION OEDEMA AND RAPID DOSE SCHEDULES

The spectre of 'radiation oedema' has influenced the rate of delivery of radiation doses in numerous sites and has also been a major argument for the prior use of chemotherapy. The statement of Karnofsky and colleagues (1948) expresses this concern.

> 'Rapidly growing or anaplastic lung tumours do not usually respond satisfactorily to roentgen rays, and irradiation is considered hazardous in patients with obstruction of the superior vena cava. . . . Furthermore, oedema of the diseased area, which may sometimes occur during irradiation, has not attended the use of Mustard . . .'

There is no difference on clinico-pathological grounds between the mechanism of action of alkylating agents and that of radiotherapy. In fact, these chemotherapeutic substances have often been described as radiomimetic. It is not the uniqueness of the action of nitrogen mustard but its rapidity that prevents the oedema from worsening. Rapid dose x-irradiation acts in a similar fashion and has the further advantages of selectivity of action to the tumour site, fewer attendant untoward effects on bone marrow, and a broader range of effectiveness in a larger variety of bronchogenic cancers.

This critical point in management was studied by Levitt and colleagues (1969) in a controlled clinical trial. Twenty-eight consecutive patients with superior vena caval obstruction were randomly assigned either to prior chemotherapy and 200 rads daily irradiation or to rapid high daily doses of 400 rads up to a 2,000 rad level.

In both schemes, total dosages of 4,000–5,000 rads were delivered. The relative times for relief of symptoms were similar. The numbers experiencing complete relief were also similar, with the group given x-irradiation alone having a slight advantage in lower recurrences

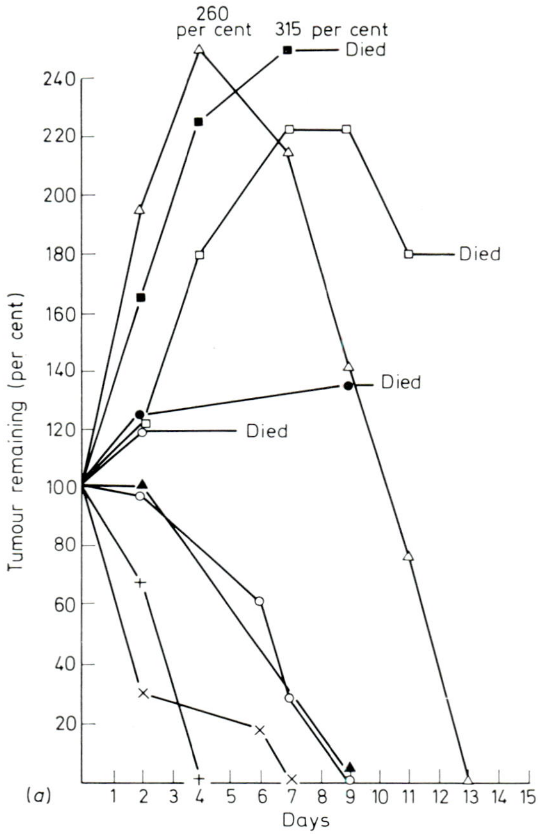

Figure 7. Response of flank tumour to therapy. (a) Rate of regression with 50 r/day

compared with the group receiving NH_2 and x-irradiation. However, the major difference was in the significantly higher mortality and morbidity with nitrogen mustard therapy. Four of fifteen patients died during this combined therapy regimen, and severe drops in leucocyte and platelet counts occurred in 33 per cent of the group.

The laboratory evidence provided by a series of controlled biological studies has exploded the myth of radiation oedema (Green, Rubin and Holzwasser, 1963; Rubin, 1969). When bits of a Murphy Sturm lymphosarcoma were inserted into the mediastinum of

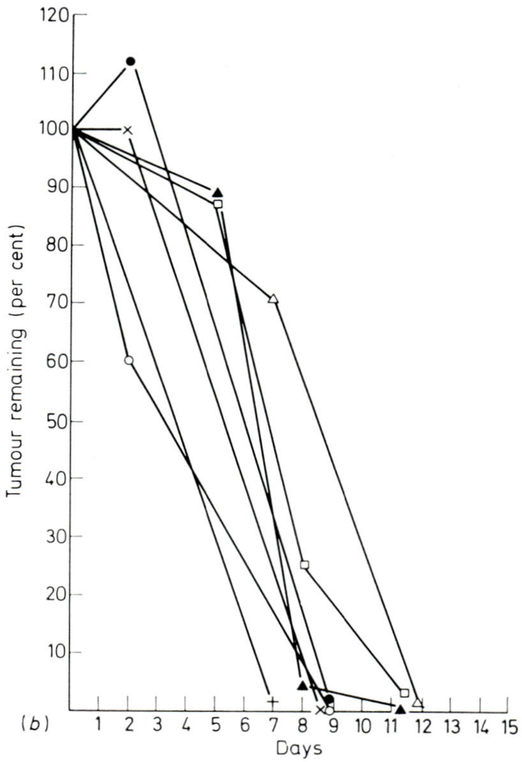

Figure 7b. Flank tumour regression with 100 r/day

Sprague Daley rats, superior vena caval obstruction occurred within 7–10 days and death followed if this was not relieved within two weeks. The study of different dosage schedules indicated that the minimum daily dose required to produce effective tumour regression was 200 rads. If lower doses were used, the tumour increased in size and further contributed to oedema. This has been referred to as 'tumour oedema' (Green, Rubin and Holzwasser, 1963). Measurements of flank tumours treated with exactly the same schedules as the mediastinal tumours indicated that with 50–100 rads, even this exquisitely radiosensitive tumour increased in size (*Figure 7*). Rapid regression and decrease in tumour size were seen with 500 rad and 1,500 rad schedules. Histological control has identified a tissue oedema which appears after 12–24 hours as the tumour is irradiated

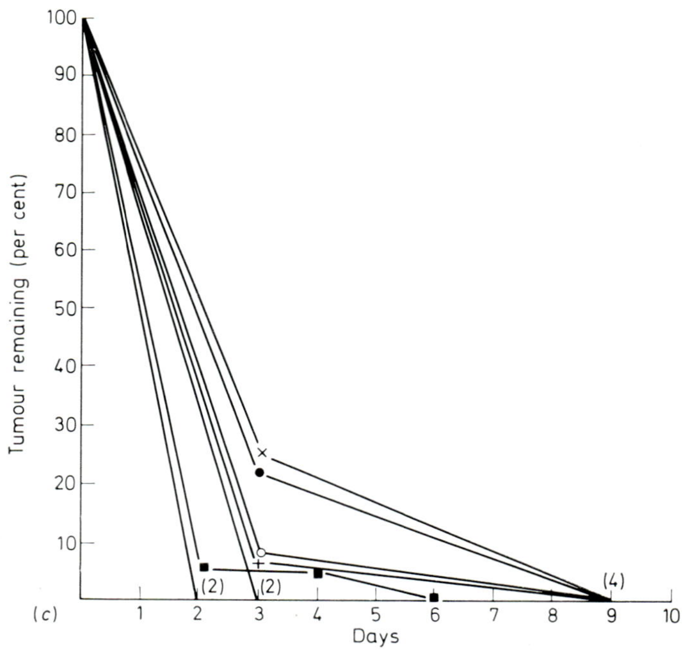

Figure 7c. Flank tumour regression with 500 r/day

(*Figure 8*); however, this intercellular fluid is a replacement of cell loss and does not contribute to an increase in total tumour volume (Green, Rubin and Holzwasser, 1963).

The above studies were repeated with the induction of spinal cord compression (Rubin, 1969) in the same type of rats and with the same tumour. The treatment schedule which proved most effective was again a rapid daily dose rather than a slow dose regimen. No worsening of symptoms or signs occurred with higher doses, and this study again casts doubt on the hypothesis that 'radiation oedema' exists as a true risk or a clinico-pathological entity.

The single massive dose grid technique has been described by Holmes (1963). Utilizing orthovoltage therapy and a grid with 40 per cent transmission and holes of 1 cm diameter, doses of 4,000–5,000 rads were given. The only untoward effect noted was a feeling of tightness in the chest 12 hours afterwards in some cases. Most patients were sent home on the second or third day. There

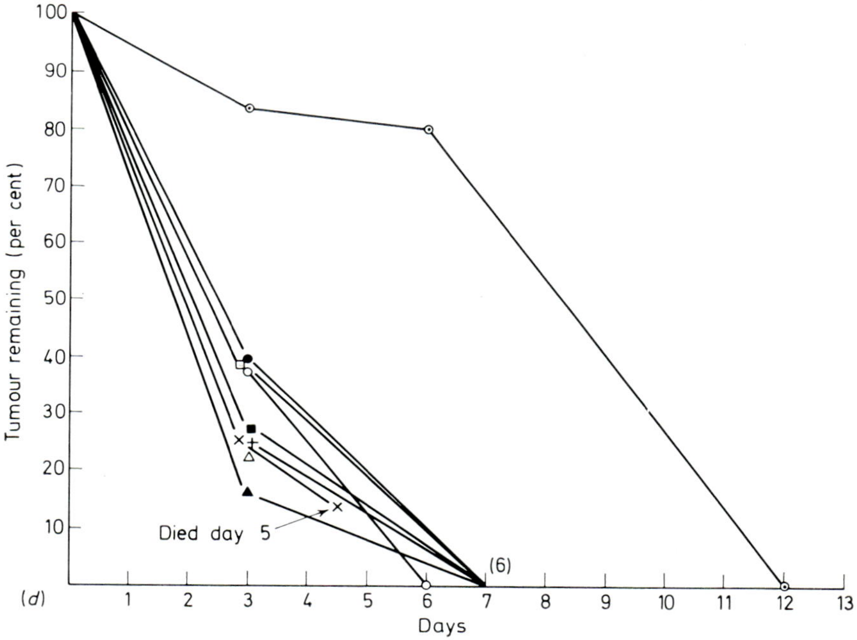

Figure 7d. Flank tumour regression with 1,500 r × 1

was palliation of symptoms in 48 per cent of patients at the 4,500 rad level and in 63 per cent at 5,000 rads. The palliation was ineffective with doses of 4,000 rads or less, again suggesting that higher dose levels are not only tolerated but immediately more beneficial. Although it is difficult to compare standard and grid techniques, it again seems unlikely that with such massive doses, radiation oedema would not have occurred in some instances if it existed as a true radiobiological phenomenon.

The clinical evidence for the effectiveness of rapid high daily dose schedules in SVCO is based on a decade of experience. The method is not only effective but safe. The application of the rapid dose technique to other sites under compression by malignant tumours is

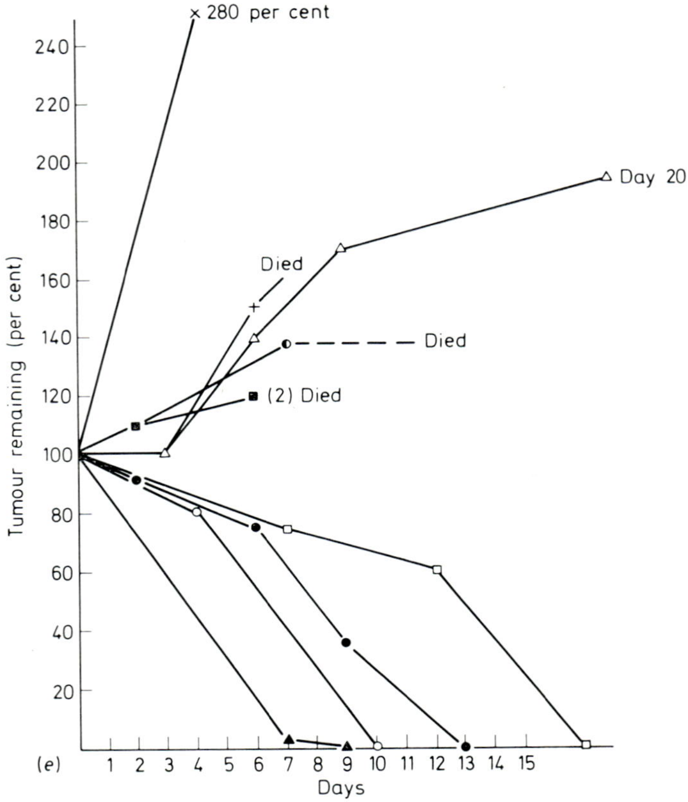

Figure 7e. Flank tumour regression with nitrogen mustard 4 mg/kg intravenously

being more widely accepted. Spinal cord compression by radiosensitive tumours such as lymphoma, Hodgkin's disease, anaplastic carcinoma and sarcoma can be relieved without laminectomy by giving high daily doses of 400–500 rads (Rubin and colleagues, 1969) (*see Figure 5*). In brain metastases, the use of large doses of cortisone

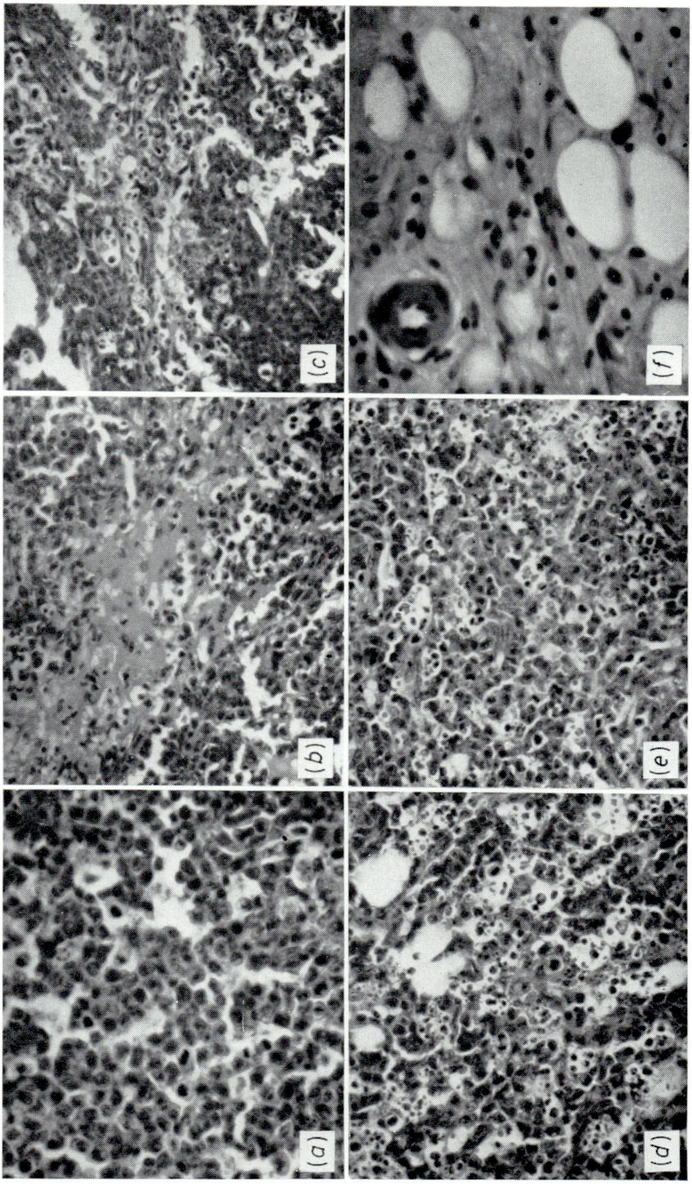

Figure 8. Histological study of flank tumours following 1,500 r × 1. (a) Control tumour (non-irradiated). (b) Four hours after 1,500 r. (c) Five hours after 1,500 r. (d) Fifteen hours after 1,500 r. (e) Twenty-four hours after 1,500 r. (f) Ninety-six hours after 1,500 r

derivatives to reduce intracerebral pressure affords an opportunity to treat the entire brain by midline daily doses of 400 rads to a total of 4,000 rads in two weeks. Tolerance of this approach is excellent, good palliation being achieved in more than 50 cases in our department. A 'field within a field' technique is utilized for lymphomatous nodes compressing ureters or for sudden collapse of a lung by a bronchogenic carcinoma. The small fields permit the delivery of 400 rads daily, while larger fields allow slower treatment to the larger mass. Where decompression of vital viscera or other organs is a major problem, rapid daily doses deserve consideration. The only exception is in treating lymphomatous invasion of the stomach or gut, when high doses may be poorly tolerated and may lead to sudden tumour lysis and perforation.

SUMMARY

(1) The evidence favouring a high daily dose technique for rapid decompression of superior vena caval obstruction has been reviewed.

(2) The radiotherapeutic regimen followed is the delivery of 400 rads $\times$ 3 to the mediastinal midline; when the oedema is relieved, the daily dose is reduced to 150–200 rads.

(3) The success rate of 79 per cent for rapid dosage compared with 10 per cent for slow dosage in relieving obstruction within the first week of treatment, together with the absence of any immediate mortality, substantiates the value of the rapid dose approach.

(4) The value of the isotopic (^{99m}Tc) scintiphlebogram in diagnosing and serially evaluating the relief of obstruction is noted.

(5) The application of high daily dose decompression to other sites, organs or viscera compromised by malignant tumours is briefly discussed.

(6) The myth of so-called 'radiation oedema' is invalidated.

REFERENCES

Farrer, P. A., Ciccio, S. S. and Rubin, P. (1969). '$^{99m}TcO_4$—Rapid sequential thoracic scintiphotography in the diagnosis and management of acute mediastinal obstruction.' *J. nucl. Med.* **10** (6), 332.

Green, J., Rubin, P. and Holzwasser, G. (1963). 'Experimental production of superior vena caval obstruction.' *Radiology* **81,** 406.

Holmes, K. S. (1963). 'The treatment of superior vena caval syndrome by high-dose grid technic.' *Radiology* **81,** 402.

Karnofsky, D. A., Abelmann, W. H., Craver, L. F. and Burchenal, J. H. (1948). 'The use of the nitrogen mustards in the palliative treatment of carcinoma, with particular reference to bronchogenic carcinoma.' *Cancer*, **1,** 634.

Knowles, J. H. and Smith, L. H. Jnr. (1960). 'Extrapulmonary manifestations of bronchogenic carcinoma.' *New Engl. J. Med.* **262,** 505.

Levitt, S. H., Jones, T. K., Kilpatrick, S. J. and Bogardus, C. R. (1969). 'Treatment of malignant superior vena caval obstruction. A randomized study.' *Cancer*, **24,** 447.

Okay, N. H. and Bryk, D. (1969). 'Collateral pathways in occlusion of the superior vena cava and its tributaries.' *Radiology* **92,** 1493.

Rubin, P. (1963). 'Symposium on superior venal caval obstruction: Introduction.' *Radiology* **81,** 377.

— (1971). 'Extradural spinal cord compression by tumor. Part I: Experimental production and treatment trials.' *Radiology* **93,** 1243.

— Paterson E. and Poulter, C. (1971). 'Biassociation of superior vena caval obstruction and spinal cord compression by malignant tumors.' In the press.

— Green, J., Holzwasser, G. and Gerle, R. (1963). 'Superior vena caval syndrome.' *Radiology* **81,** 388.

— Mayer, E., Poulter, C. and Augusta, V. (1969). 'Extradural spinal cord compression by tumor. Part II: High daily dose experience without laminectomy.' *Radiology* **93,** 1248.

Schwartz, W. B., Bennett, W., Curelop, S. and Bartter, F. (1957). 'A syndrome of renal sodium loss and hyponatremia probably resulting from inappropriate secretion of antidiuretic hormone.' *Am. J. Med.* **23,** 529.

15—Palliative Therapy

Daphne Line and Thomas J. Deeley

Many patients seen in the radiotherapy department have lesions too far advanced, because of the presence of distant metastases, for radical radiotherapeutic techniques aimed at a cure. It is disturbing to find that some clinicians think that if the condition in the chest is inoperable, there is nothing that can usefully be done for the patient. Unfortunately, some radiotherapists also tend to adopt this pessimistic view. Some of these inoperable patients, however, have a possibility of survival for some years even when metastases are present; in a large proportion a considerable palliation of symptoms may be achieved and may last the patient for all or most of the time that he still has left. There is little doubt that the palliation from radiation is more certain and lasts longer than that achieved by means of chemotherapeutic agents.

The palliative therapy of carcinoma of the bronchus will be considered from the following aspects: the relief of troublesome chest symptoms, the treatment of symptoms caused by distant metastases, the relief of generalized neurological or endocrinological manifestations, and the treatment of recurrent tumour in the chest.

DISEASE IN THE CHEST

Palliative radiotherapy to the chest may be considered in the patient who has troublesome chest symptoms even in the presence of widespread dissemination of the disease. Haemoptysis is always an upsetting symptom to the patient; he may have had a cough with offensive yellow sputum for many years, he may have increasing dyspnoea of some years' duration or an irritating wheeze, but often he will dismiss these symptoms as negligible or just a nuisance; however, the appearance of blood suggests that something serious is wrong and he is afraid. If this symptom can be relieved, his last few days may be made less distressing to him. Haemoptysis can be relieved completely in the majority of cases. Other distressing symptoms such as cough, dyspnoea and chest pain are relieved to some extent in about 60–70 per cent of patients, and palliative treatment aggravates the symptoms in only a small proportion of cases.

Table 1 shows the palliation achieved in patients treated by a radical course of supervoltage radiation. Similar results have been reported by other workers. Schulz (1966) reported relief of haemoptysis in 75 per cent of cases, and Garland (1960) in 60–70 per cent. Hustu and Nickson (1964) found relief of other symptoms in the

TABLE 1

Palliation Achieved in 513 Patients

Result	*Presenting symptoms (per cent)*					
	Haemoptysis	*Cough*	*Dyspnoea*	*Pain*	*General symptoms*	*Hoarseness*
Improved	95	58	60	72	68	50
No change	5	39	35	24	23	50
Worse	—	3	5	4	9	—

majority of their patients. Rubenfeld and Kaplan (1959) reported relief of cough in 75 per cent of their cases, Garland (1961) in 60–70 per cent, Barton, McGranahan and Jordan in 70 per cent, and Schulz (1966) in 50 per cent. Chest pain was relieved in nearly all patients, but dyspnoea was seldom relieved.

Atelectasis due to obstruction of a main or large bronchus by an intraluminal growth or by extrinsic pressure may be relieved as a result of the treatment, with marked improvement in ventilation and in drainage of retained secretions. Hackenthal (1960) reported re-aeration of the lung collapsed by a blocked bronchus in 25 out of 51 patients.

It is sometimes necessary to decide how much of the improvement in the patient's symptoms can be attributed solely to radiotherapy. The general nursing care, the regular hospital routine and the psychological effect of 'having something done' may all contribute to his general improvement and wellbeing. In addition, patients will often report symptomatic improvement because they think they are doing what is expected of them and pleasing the doctor.

A pleural effusion may distress a patient because of the increased dyspnoea and may require repeated aspiration. Often small effusions are asymptomatic, but if there is dyspnoea or if repeated aspirations are necessary, then further radiotherapy should be considered. Radioactive gold, nitrogen mustard and other cytotoxic agents have been reported to reduce the frequency of the pleural tappings. Dybicki, Balchum and Meneely (1959) found good results in 50 per cent of their patients after injection of radioactive gold. Walter (1960) reported useful palliation in 6 out of 9 patients treated with radioactive yttrium. The instillation of nitrogen mustard into the pleural cavity has given symptomatic relief in from 40 to 65 per cent of reported cases (Weisberger, Levine and Storaasli, 1955; Fullerton and Reed, 1958; Ultmann, 1962; Zelenik, Halpern and Williams, 1964). It is interesting to note that such instillation of nitrogen mustard appears to be effective even in those tumours which do not normally respond to this drug given intravenously. It is possible that a better cancericidal effect may result from the higher concentration of the drug which can be obtained in the pleural cavity. The obvious advantage of using cytotoxic agents is that there are not the problems of protection associated with a radioactive substance.

Often, however, there is a large tumour beneath the fluid. In such cases, measures taken to reduce the amount of fluid do little if anything to the underlying mass which continues to stimulate the pleura, thus producing more fluid, and to encroach on the lung which is capable of aeration. It would appear reasonable to treat the whole hemithorax by two large fields and to angle the posterior field so that an excessive dose of radiation is not administered to the spinal cord. Relatively small daily doses are given initially, and the dosage is slowly increased to give a total tumour dose of about 3,000 rads in four weeks. In our experience, the results are at least as good as those obtained with radioactive or chemotherapeutic agents instilled into the pleura, and some patients have experienced a marked improvement in their breathing capacity.

METASTASES

We have reviewed the necropsy findings in 647 patients who had suffered from carcinoma of the bronchus and had been referred to either the chest clinic or the radiotherapy department. The necropsies had been carried out at various hospitals, and the group is rather heterogenous in that it represents the interpretations of several pathologists. There are, of course, many objections to the analysis of post-mortem results: the cases are selected in that they have died in hospital and have had a necropsy, and also any results obtained may not represent the true incidence of metastases. Even at post-mortem examination it is not possible to gain a true picture of the frequency of metastases. The findings are gross only, and serial sections would be needed to discover small foci invisible to the naked eye. In addition, some structures, especially bones, may not have been routinely examined at necropsy. With these provisos, we must accept that the necropsy findings provide us with the best available evidence of the disease in the body and give us more information than could be obtained clinically.

The histological sections have not been examined by one pathologist, but from the reports available it has been possible to divide the cases into four main groups—squamous, oat cell, anaplastic and adenocarcinoma.

Spread of the carcinoma may occur through the lymphatic system, through the blood stream or by direct infiltration. Although Ackerman and Regato (1947), Onuigbo (1961) and Warner and Gates (1964) considered that lymphatic spread was the common mode of dissemination, in our series spread by the blood stream was found most frequently for each of the different pathological types (Table 2).

TABLE 2

Method of Spread Related to Histological Type of Tumour

	Squamous	*Oat cell*	*Anaplastic*	*Adenocarcinoma*
Number of patients	238	187	171	51
Lymphatic spread	54%	85%	76%	75%
Haematogenous spread	60%	91%	79%	82%

Solitary Metastases

The presence of metastases outside the chest has usually been taken as indicating widespread dissemination of the disease and a hopeless prognosis. It is, however, possible that in some of the patients the metastasis outside the chest may be the only manifestation of dissemination. If this is so and the deposit can be satisfactorily ablated together with the primary growth in the chest, it may be possible to 'salvage' a few patients who would normally be considered hopeless.

Deeley and Line (1969) reviewed 647 necropsies to determine the incidence of solitary metastasis—defined as 'the only deposit found at necropsy outside the chest'. The results are shown in Table 3.

No solitary metastases were found at any other anatomical site examined.

It will be seen that a small proportion of metastases in carcinoma of the bronchus are solitary. It was further found that the proportion of the solitary metastases was higher in squamous cell tumours (Table 4).

TABLE 3

Percentage of Solitary Extrathoracic Metastases

Site of deposit	*Number with secondary at site*	*Number in whom metastasis was solitary*	*Percentage which were solitary*
Brain	109	22	20
Vertebrae	162	6	4
Other bones	94	6	7
Liver	265	24	9
Adrenals	214	14	7
Kidneys	100	8	8
Pancreas	79	2	3
Stomach	18	1	6
Eye	2	1	50
Supraclavicular nodes	87	10	11
Cervical nodes	78	3	4

TABLE 4

Proportion of Solitary Metastases for the Different Histological Types

	Squamous	*Oat cell*	*Anaplastic*	*Adenocarcinoma*	*Total*
Number with metastases outside the chest	144	175	140	43	502
Number of patients with solitary metastases	39	33	19	6	97
Percentage	27	19	14	14	19

It is interesting to speculate on the higher frequency of solitary metastases to the brain. A clump of cells penetrating a small vein in the lungs will be carried to the heart and expelled from the left ventricle into the aorta. The flow of the blood round the arch of the aorta will mean that a greater centrifugal force will operate on a clump of cells than on the individual blood cells, with the result that the cells will be pulled out to the periphery of the aorta and will have a greater chance of entering one of the carotids.

Treatment of Solitary Metastases

A patient who presents with clinical evidence of only one metastasis outside the chest should be considered for a radical course of treatment aimed at a cure because that metastasis may be solitary.

Deeley and Rice-Edwards (1968) reported the results of treatment of cerebral metastases in patients who had no clinical evidence of other metastases. A tumour dose of at least 3,000 rads was given over a period of four weeks to the whole brain, using two opposed lateral fields of 15–17 cm length by 10–12 cm width. Clinically it is impossible to tell whether a lesion is single or multiple throughout the brain, and the authors recommended that in all cases the whole brain should be irradiated. In 29 patients (47 per cent) there was significant palliation. 'Significant' is defined as 'improvement sufficient to enable the patient to return home and live a relatively normal and comfortable life for at least one month after completing the treatment'; in fact, several of these patients were able to return to work. 'Not significant' implies that the patient showed no improvement, that there was some relief of troublesome symptoms but the patient was unable to return to normal life, or that the improvement obtained lasted for less than one month. Significant palliation of three months' duration was found in 30 per cent of cases, of six months' duration in 15 per cent, of 12 months in 7 per cent, 24 months in 5 per cent and 36 months in 3 per cent. The one-year survival rate was 14 per cent, the two-year 6 per cent and the three-year 4 per cent.

Deeley and Line (1969) treated patients with metastases at various sites where there was some evidence to suggest that the metastasis was solitary. In all cases a tumour dose of 3,000 rads was given in 10 treatments in two weeks. The results are shown in Table 5.

TABLE 5

Survival Rates for Metastases at Various Sites

Site	*Number of patients*	*Survival (per cent)* 1 *year*	2 *years*	3 *years*	4 *years*	5 *years*
Supraclavicular nodes	70	22	7	3	1	1
Cervical nodes	16	6	—	—	—	—
Bone	35	6	—	—	—	—

These figures suggest that a more active approach should be made to dealing with cerebral and supraclavicular metastases, but the results of treatment at other sites are not encouraging. The diagnosis of secondary deposits in the kidney, adrenals, pancreas and stomach is seldom made clinically, and small deposits in the liver are difficult to diagnose.

Palliative Therapy of Widespread Metastases

The relief of bone pain is well known, and often single doses of 1,000 rads or 2,500 rads in five treatments will give satisfactory relief. Ulcerating masses or skin deposits, or masses of glands causing distress, are often worth treating if only to give the patient relief for a few weeks. Cerebral metastases in the presence of widespread disease are sometimes worth treating because the terminal care of the patient may thus be made easier for the nurses; a comatose patient may become conscious and co-operative again.

Liver metastases may become very distressing; occasionally a patient is seen with huge liver metastases which cause discomfort by their size and weight, the patient's general condition being fair. We have given cautious doses of radiotherapy, using large fields over the liver, with some relief of symptoms. In some cases the size of the liver has been markedly reduced and the patient has ceased to complain of pain. Treatment is started with very small doses of 20 rads daily, the dosage being gradually increased depending on the patient's response; signs of nausea and vomiting are an indication to reduce the dose rate.

ENDOCRINE AND NEUROLOGICAL DISTURBANCES

It is often worth attempting treatment of patients who present with neurological manifestations or with endocrine or skin changes secondary to a carcinoma of the bronchus. Neuromyopathy may show improvement if the primary lesion in the chest is treated. Endocrine disorders such as hypercalcaemia may improve with treatment to the primary lesion or to a secondary deposit, and the discomfort associated with gynaecomastia may be reduced if the primary tumour is irradiated. We have seen a case of erythema gyratum repens improve with treatment to the chest. The presence of unusual manifestations should not preclude radiotherapy to the primary tumour.

RECURRENT CHEST TUMOUR

The patient with a tumour which recurs after a radical course of radiotherapy presents a problem, it being the generally accepted policy that once radical radiotherapy has been given it is impossible to repeat the treatment. If the patient presents with recurrence producing superior vena caval obstruction, we think that he should receive a further course of treatment and that a sufficient dose should be given to relieve the obstruction. Treatment is stopped when the symptoms are relieved. A patient with haemoptysis should have further treatment, planned on a day-to-day basis, until the bleeding stops. Obstruction of a main bronchus with atelectasis of the distal lobe and increasing dyspnoea due to recurrent tumour can be relieved by further radiotherapy. Such patients have been treated by weekly doses of therapy supplying a dose of 400 rads to the tumour and continuing until there is relief of the symptoms.

These patients with recurrent tumour are dying, and if it is possible to obtain any relief of symptoms, further treatment should be given. The risk of complications from the radiation does not arise, since the patient will not live long enough to develop these.

CHEMOTHERAPY

There is little to suggest that chemotherapeutic agents bring about more than a transitory palliation. In our opinion, palliation can be produced more rapidly by x-ray therapy, and the palliation achieved is of longer duration than that achieved with any of the chemotherapeutic agents.

CONCLUSIONS

Considerable relief from distressing symptoms can often be obtained by means of radiotherapy. Treatment must be short and must be stopped as soon as palliation is achieved; often a single treatment suffices. Protracted courses of therapy to a high dose will only cause further distress to a patient who has no hope of recovery.

REFERENCES

Ackerman, L. V. and Regato, J. W. del (1947). *Cancer: Diagnosis, Treatment and Prognosis.* St. Louis: Mosby.

Barton, H. L., McGranahan, G. M. and Jordan, G. L. (1960). *Dis. Chest* **37,** 170.

Deeley, T. J. and Line, D. H. (1969). *Br. J. Dis. Chest* **63,** 150.

— and Rice-Edwards, J. M. (1968). *Lancet* **1,** 1209.

Dybicki, J., Balchum, O. J. and Meneely, G. R. (1959). *Archs intern. Med.* **104,** 802.

Fullerton, C. W. and Reed, P. (1958). *Can med. Ass. J.* **79,** 190.

Garland, L. H. (1961). *Am. J. Roentg.* **86,** 621.

Hackenthal, P. (1960). *Strahlentherapie* **III,** 190.

Hustu, H. O. and Nickson, J. J. (1964). *Am. J. Roentg.* **91,** 95.
Onuigbo, W. I. B. (1961). *Cancer Res.* **21,** 1077.
Rubenfeld, S. and Kaplan, G. (1959). *Radiology* **73,** 671.
Schulz, M. D. (1966). *J. Am. med. Ass.* **196,** 850.
Ultmann, J. E. (1962). *C.A.* **12,** 42.
Walter, J. (1960). *Br. med. J.* **2,** 1282.
Warner, S. and Gates, O. (1964). *Archs Path.* **78,** 467.
Weisberger, A. S., Levine, B. and Storaasli, J. P. (1955). *J. Am. med. Ass.* **159,** 1704.
Zelenik, J. S., Halpern, A. J. and Williams, D. W. (1964). *Obstet. Gynec., N.Y.* **23,** 703.

16—The Cure of Lung Cancer with Chemotherapeutic Agents

A. M. Jelliffe

EMOTIONAL FACTORS IN CHOICE OF TREATMENT

In 1951 the annual death rate from cancer of the lung for the first time exceeded that from pulmonary tuberculosis, and lung cancer is now by far the commonest type of malignant disease among men in Britain. Its frequency and its highly malignant nature are known to almost everybody through the media of the Press, radio and television. Nearly every family knows of at least one relative or friend who has died of lung cancer. It is inevitable that such an appalling problem should develop emotional overtones which influence not only the man in the street but every member of the medical profession.

This emotional background must influence the treatment of the individual patient with lung cancer, and it is very difficult to assess the true value of any method of management. Exact figures of the survival rates of all patients who develop this disease are almost impossible to obtain because so many patients are too old or too ill for adequate investigation and treatment.

Of those patients who do reach a clinic or hospital for investigation, not more than a quarter are serious candidates for attempted cure by radical surgery. All too often a thoracotomy is all that can be attempted. There is a good deal of evidence that the prognosis after an unsuccessful thoracotomy is worse than the prognosis without surgery. Unnecessary surgical intervention could sometimes be prevented if patients were investigated more fully beforehand. However, the emotional overlay is such that unnecessary operations will continue to be carried out, usually because of the very reasonable and highly creditable desire of the surgeon to do all that he can to help in such a desperate condition. There is, of course, no doubt at all that surgery is the treatment of choice in most operable lung cancers.

Similar emotional illogicality may sometimes be recognizable in the use of radiotherapy in the attempted cure of lung cancer. Some of these tumours are very radiosensitive and respond well to small or moderate doses of radiotherapy. Unfortunately many of these highly sensitive tumours metastasize widely, and local tumour regression is followed all too frequently by the explosive appearance of widespread deposits. Nevertheless, there are a few patients in every large radiotherapy centre whose disease remains controlled ten or more years after irradiation. Not unnaturally, attempts have been made to improve the radiotherapeutic cure rate by treating a larger volume of tissue with a higher dose. This type of approach is usually followed by little improvement in local cure and certainly no increase in the long-term survival rate. What is often seen is a marked increase in the damaging side effects from the irradiation.

Use and Misuse of Chemotherapy

If surgery and radiotherapy in the treatment of lung cancer are so often associated with emotional mismanagement because of the desire to benefit the patient, it is not surprising that this should be seen even more frequently in the case of cytotoxic drugs. Almost every known cytotoxic drug has been tried in the therapy of lung cancer. Sometimes there is considerable temporary improvement, and sometimes the results are disastrous.

Cytotoxic drugs are particularly easy to misuse. There are several reasons for this. First, for years they have been referred to as 'chemotherapeutic agents'—a name which equates them with relatively familiar and harmless agents such as penicillin. Every doctor, the day after passing his final examinations, is qualified to administer 'chemotherapeutic agents' even though he knows little or nothing about the natural history of the cancer growing in the patient under his enthusiastic but inexperienced care. Secondly, all doctors wish to help their patients. This is presumably the main reason why the practice of medicine is adopted as a profession by so many people. And what easier method is there to help the cancer patient than by the administration of 'chemotherapeutic drugs', particularly those which have recently been widely publicized? The patient is delighted that he is not being encouraged to be 'cut about' by a surgeon or 'burnt up' by x-rays, details of which he has learnt from all the exaggerated horror stories circulating in the neighbourhood. If the patient knows the diagnosis, he is bound to be helped psychologically by the use of cytotoxic drugs; the relatives are reassured that everything possible is being done; and a somewhat inexperienced clinician, perhaps not fully aware of the true possibilities of treatment and the chances of cure (however small they may be) by other methods, can continue to look after his patient in the belief that he is doing something that may be of benefit. He is apparently not always aware that what he is doing may also be harmful.

Cytotoxic agents are two-edged swords. They may help dramatically on occasion, but they may also do immeasurable harm. Procrastination may rapidly diminish already slim chances of cure by surgery or radiotherapy. And if the patient is eventually referred for attempted radical treatment while the tumour is still curable by surgery or radiotherapy, this slight possibility of cure may be ruled out completely by a severely damaged bone marrow following the prolonged administration of cytotoxic drugs.

Past and Present Attitudes

When considering the present attitude to these agents, it is interesting to see in papers published in 1948 that the views expressed by eminent authors twenty years ago closely resemble those held today by some clinicians who view with extreme suspicion both surgery and radiotherapy as curative measures. Karnofsky and colleagues (1948) stated: 'The rapidly growing or anaplastic lung tumours do not usually respond satisfactorily to Roentgen-rays, and irradiation is considered hazardous in patients with obstruction of the superior vena cava.' They then indicate that, because of this, nitrogen mustard is the treatment of choice. This statement suggests that at that time the authors had never seen the often dramatic, immediate and very occasionally long-term responses which may follow radiotherapy when used correctly for 'rapidly growing or anaplastic lung tumours', especially those with mediastinal compression of short duration. This strong recommendation in favour of nitrogen mustard is even more difficult to understand because an earlier paragraph in the same paper refers to 'palliative effects in 74 per cent of the patients . . . from two weeks to two months.' 'Improvements' for periods of as little as two weeks are not usually considered to be related to treatment by surgeons and radiotherapists, who would regard an improvement of such short duration as having no significance. In 1948, however, cytotoxic drugs had been in clinical use for only a short time, and such a report was perhaps not only fully justified but also very necessary in order to focus attention on the possible value of this type of agent.

It is essential that this approach should now be abandoned and that the relative value of any cytotoxic drug should be indicated, whenever possible, by comparing its long-term effects with those of surgery and radiotherapy. In order to view the whole problem in perspective, it is perhaps interesting to quote a paragraph from another paper published in 1948. 'Methyl-bis is a useful drug, but so far as we know, it is not curative. One direct benefit from the drug is that the patients are observed more carefully and symptoms are treated as they arise. This in itself helps in raising the morale of those patients who were formerly told to go home and that nothing else could be done for them' (Skinner, Carr and Denman, 1948). This statement still affords an excellent summary of the present emotionally charged situation.

CURABILITY OF CANCER BY CYTOTOXIC DRUGS

That cytotoxic drugs do not eliminate lung cancer has been emphasized frequently over the last twenty years, and it has been recently repeated by Anderson and Hutchison (1969) in a paper comparing the effects of nitrogen mustard with those of a mixture of agents. To date, there is no conclusive evidence that any patient with lung cancer has been permanently cured of his disease by treatment with cytotoxic drugs alone. Far from being of value in this context, they are potentially extremely dangerous. An attempt at total eradication of lung cancer with cytotoxic agents requires extremely high doses with very serious risks of bone marrow depression. This cannot be avoided by intra-arterial perfusion, because the blood supply of primary bronchial carcinoma comes as a rule from the bronchial arteries.

One must therefore conclude that until more effective agents become available, any attempt to eliminate a localized, potentially curable lung cancer with cytotoxic drugs only, in any known combination or separately, cannot succeed. Moreover, efforts of this type must inevitably delay the introduction of other possibly curative methods of treatment, with a reduction of the patient's chance of survival. Under exceptional circumstances, as part of a well-controlled investigation, the radical use of cytotoxic drugs may be permissible in a definite programme which includes surgery or radical radiotherapy when indicated as an additional measure; but the employment of cytotoxic agents alone for this purpose appears to the author to be totally unethical in our present state of knowledge.

It is disturbing to see an increasing number of publications reporting trials of various cytotoxic agents, either carried out on 'all patients referred to the clinic' (Jelliffe, 1966) or else without any indication that the patients in the trial had been examined and considered incurable by a radiotherapist as well as by a surgeon. The overall results of surgery are bad, and the survival rate after radiotherapy is even worse, but these methods of treatment offer the only possibilities of cure of lung cancer.

There is little doubt that a small number of potentially curable patients are being mismanaged at the present time because of excessive pessimism on the part of their medical advisers. Lung cancer is not necessarily incurable, but it certainly cannot be cured if the only treatment is with cytotoxic agents. The use of such methods is a confession of failure by the patient's doctor.

REFERENCES

Anderson, J. M. and Hutchison, J. (1969). *Br. J. Cancer* **23,** 744.

Jelliffe, A. M. (1966). *Proc. R. Soc. Med.* **59,** 1261.

Karnofsky, D. A., Abelmann, W. H., Craver, L. F. and Burchenal, J. H. (1948). *Cancer*, **1,** 634.

Skinner, E. F., Carr, D. and Denman, W. E. (1948). *J. thorac. Surg*. **17,** 428.

17—Forecast of Prognosis after Radiotherapy

I—Perfusion Lung Scanning

William S. Maxfield, Hurst B. Hatch Jnr. and James R. Nelson

Perfusion lung scanning is a safe and accurate method of evaluating pulmonary artery perfusion. It has been used in diseases due to many different types of lung pathology (Taplin and colleagues, 1964; Wagner and colleagues, 1964, 1968; Quinn and Whitley, 1964). The technique usually employed is the intravenous injection of 200–300 μCi of 131-iodinated macro-aggregated human serum albumin (^{131}I MAA). The use of technetium-99m macro-aggregated albumin (Webber, Bennett and Suprenent, 1966) or indium-113m iron hydroxide particles (Stern and colleagues, 1966) has also been reported.

The lung scans in our series were obtained with either a three-inch or a dual opposed five-inch rectilinear scanner. The scans were begun immediately after intravenous injection of the ^{131}I MAA with the patient supine. Routinely, anterior and posterior views were obtained; when the dual five-inch scanner was used, lateral views were also taken. In our series of over 400 lung scans, no complications have resulted. In 20 of these patients, pulmonary function studies before and after the scans showed no alteration in lung function. This test confirmed the safety of lung scanning as reported by Gold and McCormack (1966).

* Based on work performed at The Ochsner Foundation Hospital and Charity Hospital, New Orleans, Louisiana.

Neuhoff, Sussman and Nabatoff (1949), Dotter, Steinberg and Holman (1950) and Nabatoff (1951) reported on angiographic demonstration of pulmonary vessels as an aid in evaluation of patients with bronchogenic carcinoma. Perfusion lung scans, on the other hand, demonstrate arterial blood flow at the capillary level in the normal lung, but they can also demonstrate both pulmonary artery blockage and alveolo-vascular reflex shunting of blood. As the scan is an easier and safer means of evaluating pulmonary artery perfusion, the use of perfusion lung scans for this purpose was substituted for angiographic studies as a screening test. The first report on the use of such scanning in patients with lung cancer was by Haynie and colleagues (1962), with larger series being reported by Wagner and colleagues (1965) and Hatch, Maxfield and Ochsner (1965). Since these initial reports, other investigators have studied the place of perfusion scans in the evaluation of patients with this disease (Oeser and Ernst, 1966; Maxfield, Hatch and Ochsner, 1966; Oyamada and colleagues, 1967; Johnson, Sagerman and Jacox, 1968; Vassallo and colleagues, 1968; Germon and Brady, 1968; Ernst, Krüger and Vessal, 1969; Maynard and colleagues, 1969).

From our experience and that of others, the value of the lung scan in evaluating patients with known or suspected bronchogenic carcinoma can be divided into four categories: (1) detection of disease; (2) staging of extent of disease; (3) evaluation of pulmonary function; and (4) measurement of response to radiation therapy.

DETECTION OF BRONCHOGENIC CARCINOMA

Review of 100 patients with confirmed bronchogenic carcinoma from our series of 400 lung scans demonstrated that the scan showed the lesion in all but 6 cases. In 5 cases where the scan was interpreted as showing no defect, the chest film showed a small to moderate sized peripheral nodule or Pancoast tumour. In one case with a carcinoma involving the carina, both the chest film and the scan were interpreted as showing no abnormality.

The accuracy of the lung scan in detection of hilar lesions has also been noted by Ernst, Krüger and Vessal (1969), who reported 100 per cent accuracy for the scan in central tumours versus 88 per cent for the chest radiograph. In that series the chest film was 100 per cent accurate for peripheral lesions. In our series, however, there were 4 cases in which the chest film was interpreted as normal but the lung scan was positive (*Figure 1*). Johnson, Sagerman and Jacox (1968) and Maynard and colleagues (1969) also noted the greater accuracy of ^{131}I MAA perfusion lung scans in the detection of hilar or central bronchogenic carcinoma in comparison with peripheral lesions.

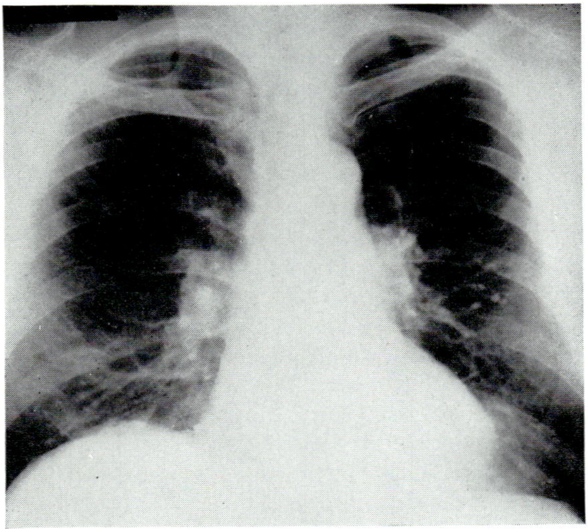

Figure 1a

Figure 1. A 72-year-old white man with intermittent mild haemoptysis for 6 weeks. Bronchoscopy and chest radiograph (a) were interpreted as showing no abnormality. The ^{131}I MAA lung scan demonstrated (b) essentially no perfusion in left upper lobe and (c) moderate decrease in perfusion of left lower lobe. Repeat bronchoscopy showed obstructing lesion to anterior and apical posterior segmental bronchi of left upper lobe. At surgery there were nodes in the left hilum which partially compressed the left lower lobe branch of the pulmonary artery. Patient died of metastatic disease 37 months after left pneumonectomy

STAGING OF BRONCHOGENIC CARCINOMA

In our series of 100 cases, the chest radiographs and lung scan showed similar abnormality in 54 patients. The scan showed a larger defect than the chest film in 36 patients, and was abnormal while the radiograph was interpreted as normal in another 4 cases. Detection of a larger perfusion defect on the lung scan than the mass shown on x-ray in about 50 per cent of cases has been reported by most authors.

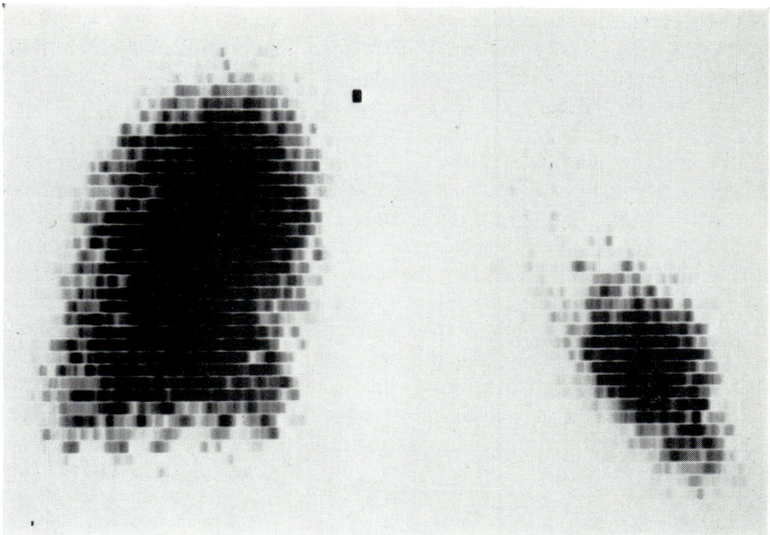

Figure 1b

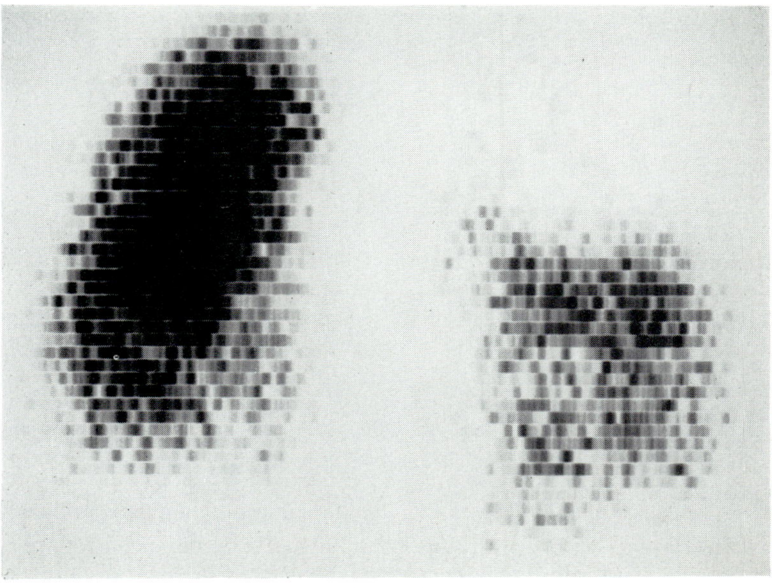

Figure 1c

The greater defect on the lung scan could be produced by obstruction of a bronchus, with reflex shunting of perfusion from the area of poor oxygenation, or by metastasis to hilar nodes which compress the pulmonary artery or its branches. Our experience suggested that if the greater defect on the scan was confined to the same segment of the lung, then obstruction of a bronchus was likely (*Figure 1b*). When a perfusion defect was demonstrated in another segment of the same lung, however, this usually indicated spread to hilar nodes (*Figure 1c*). It must be remembered, though, that emphysema, bronchiectasis and other chronic lung diseases may also cause areas of decreased or absent pulmonary artery perfusion.

Our experience indicated that identification of a perfusion defect which was greater than the mass shown on the radiograph was a sign of a poor prognosis. Only 4 of 36 patients with this finding are alive, as indicated in Table 1, which lists survival statistics for the different patterns. The minimum follow-up period for those

TABLE 1

Comparison of Abnormality Produced by Bronchogenic Carcinoma on ^{131}I MAA Perfusion Lung Scan and Chest Radiograph

Size of lesion	*Number of patients*	*Living*	*Dead*
Scan = x-ray	54	28	26
Scan > x-ray	36	4	32
Scan 0, x-ray 0	1	—	1
Scan +, x-ray −	4	—	4
Scan −, x-ray +	5	3	2
Total	100	35	65

living was six months. Twenty of these patients survived less than one year, 14 less than two years, and only 2 more than two years. The same high mortality is present when the scan is positive and the x-ray negative. Four out of four in this group were dead within the year. Maynard's series (Maynard and colleagues, 1969) suggests a similar outcome when the scan defect is greater than the lesion on the chest film. In 9 out of 18 non-resectable patients this pattern appeared, while only 1 of 6 resectable patients showed a greater defect on the scan.

The treatment in our series was surgical resection for 20 patients and radiation, with or without surgery, in 80 cases. Of the latter group, 55 were inoperable because of associated medical disease or known metastatic spread. Eighteen patients were explored but were found to be non-resectable. In 7 cases, the margin around the resected tumour was deemed inadequate. Thirty-five patients are living 6–36 months after treatment: 12 out of 20 in the surgical group, and 23 out of 80 following radiation therapy. The demonstration of a scan defect greater than the radiographic findings does not make the patient non-resectable, but the survival in our series suggests a grave prognosis regardless of the method of treatment.

EVALUATION OF PULMONARY FUNCTION

The perfusion lung scan can aid in the selection of the method of treatment by providing an accurate means of showing the pattern of pulmonary artery perfusion. The demonstration of this pattern provided a significant aid in determining whether the site of pathology in a patient with borderline pulmonary function studies was in the area of the radiographic findings or in other areas of the lungs.

In 15 of our cases, the lung scan demonstrated a large perfusion defect in the lung opposite to the radiographic lesion. When combined with minimally abnormal pulmonary function, this pattern indicated that the patient would be a poor candidate for surgical resection (*Figure 2*). The defect in the opposite lung was usually due to chronic lung disease, but in four patients it was due to bilateral hilar metastasis. Maynard and colleagues (1969) have reported similar experience with detection of bilateral hilar involvement.

MEASURING RESPONSE TO RADIOTHERAPY

Bronchogenic carcinoma produces an abnormality of pulmonary artery perfusion which is demonstrated by ^{131}I MAA perfusion lung scans in more than 90 per cent of the cases studied by scanning. Re-evaluation of the pattern of lung perfusion after completion of a course of irradiation seemed to offer an objective method of measuring response to radiotherapy. Several authors (Maxfield, Hatch and Ochsner, 1966; Oyamada and colleagues, 1967; Germon and Brady, 1968; Ernst, Krüger and Vessal, 1969) have reported on this approach. The consensus is that about 50 per cent of the hilar lesions will show an improvement in perfusion following therapy (*Figure 3*). Peripheral lesions usually do not show any such improvement and may actually show a larger defect following treatment (*Figure 4*). The timing of the re-evaluation seems important. A scan within two months after treatment is most likely to show the same or a smaller perfusion defect. After this time the effect of the radiation in normal lung tissue, with resultant 'radiation pneumonitis' and 'fibrosis', enlarges the defect. This change, secondary to the radiation, was found most frequently after treatment of peripheral lesions. The enlargement of the perfusion defect following treatment of the peripheral lesions was attributed to these changes in surrounding normal lung tissue. There does not, therefore, seem to be a direct correlation between response of the tumour to radiotherapy and change in the size of the perfusion defect on a follow-up lung scan. This was especially true if the follow-up scan was obtained more than two months after completion of therapy.

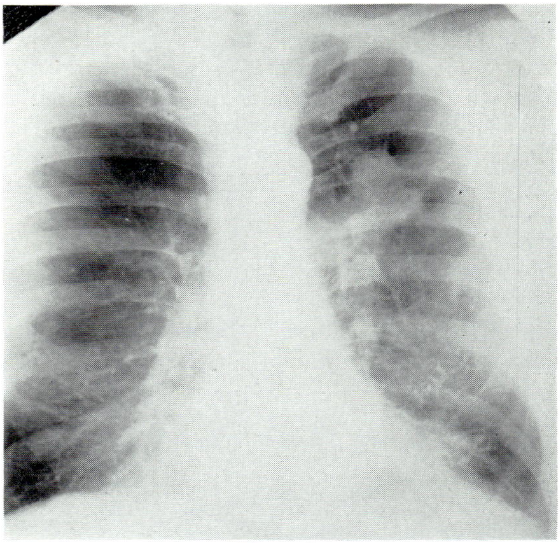

Figure 2a

Figure 2. A 65-year-old white man admitted to hospital because of cough. Chest radiograph (a) showed a mass in the left lung and a prominent left hilum. The right lung was interpreted as showing no abnormality. Pulmonary function studies showed mild hypoxia. However, ^{131}I MAA lung scan demonstrated marked abnormality of perfusion of right as well as left lung (b anterior and c posterior). In addition, liver scan showed a pattern compatible with metastasis to the liver, confirmed by needle biopsy. Liver function tests were normal except for BSP, which was 15. Patient received radiotherapy to mediastinum and to lesion in left lung, but died of metastasis to both lungs and liver 9 months after completion of therapy

The survival of the patient subsequent to radiation therapy showed no definite correlation with improvement in perfusion after treatment. In fact, the reverse seemed to be true. The most frequent

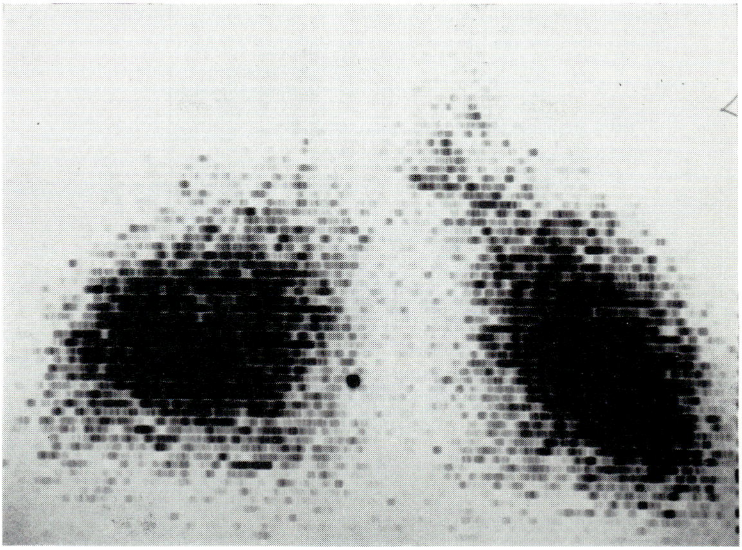

Figure 2b

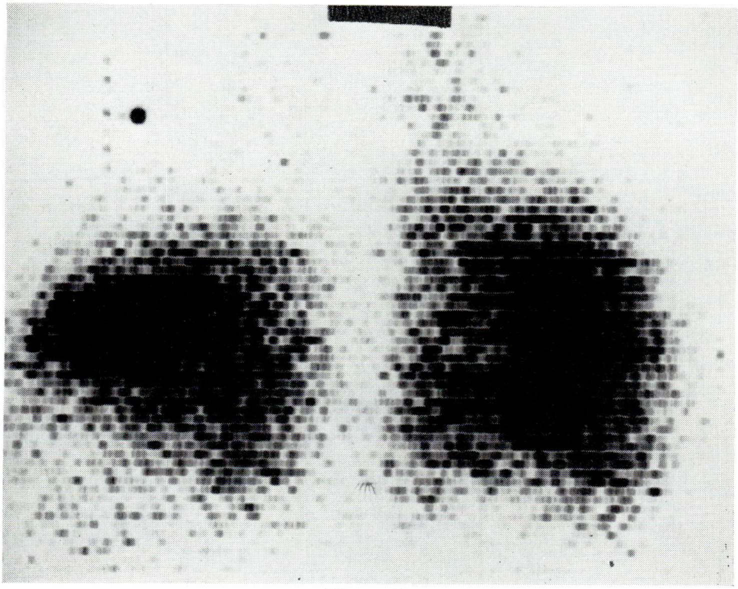

Figure 2c

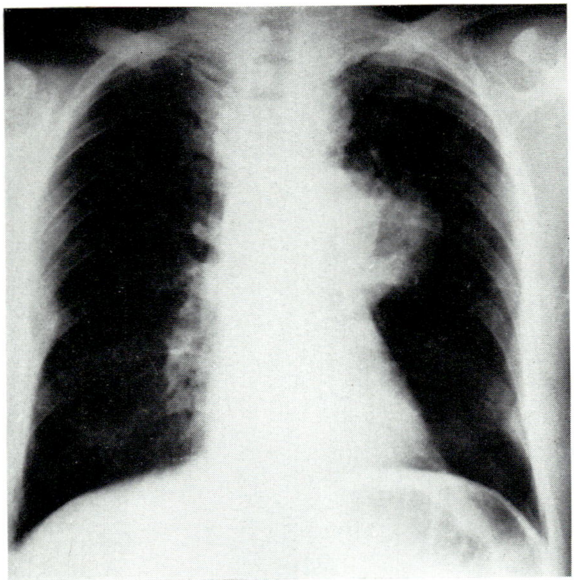

Figure 3a

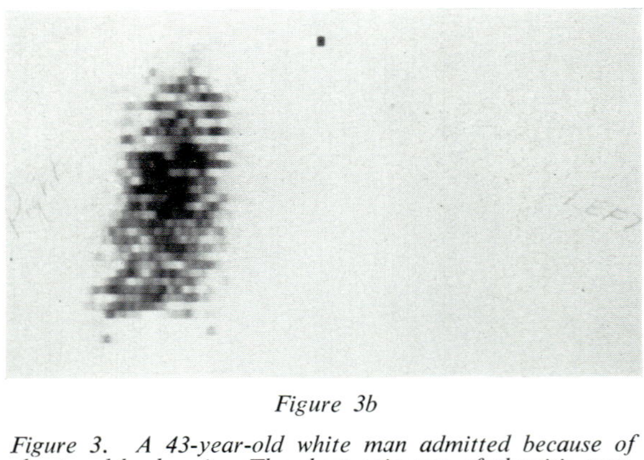

Figure 3b

Figure 3. A 43-year-old white man admitted because of chest and back pain. The chest pain was of pleuritic type. (a) Chest film showed a large left hilar mass and also destruction of right seventh rib. (b) Lung scan demonstrated complete absence of perfusion of left lung. Radiotherapy to left hilum and to right rib lesion produced palliation of pain

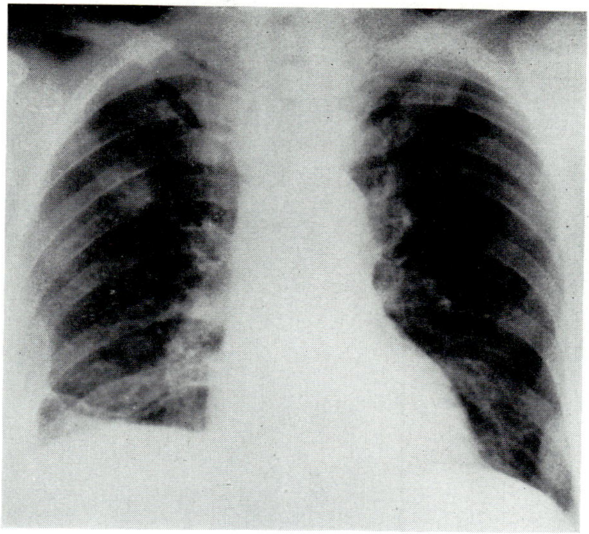

Figure 3c

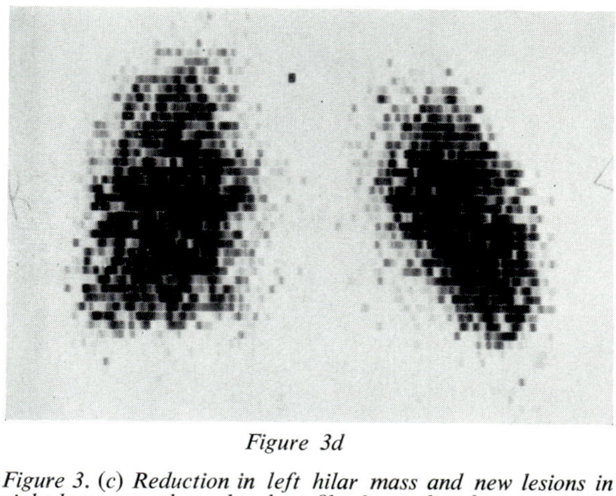

Figure 3d

Figure 3. (c) Reduction in left hilar mass and new lesions in right lung were shown by chest film 2 months after completion of therapy. (d) Follow-up scan at the same time showed return of perfusion to left lung but did not demonstrate the lesion in right lung. Patient died of extensive metastatic disease 4 months after onset of treatment

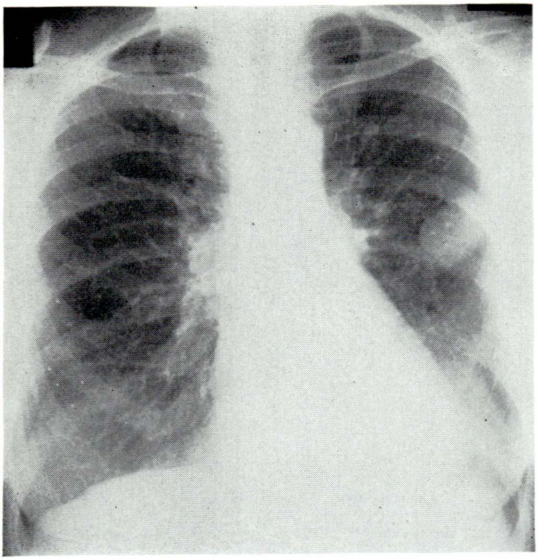

Figure 4a

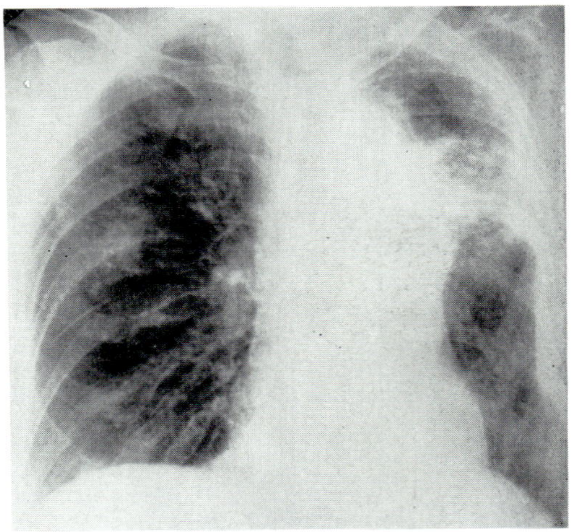

Figure 4b

Figure 4. A 67-year-old white woman who developed enlarging mass in lateral portion of left lung (a). Sputum was positive for malignant cells. Radiotherapy decreased the size of the lesion, but radiation pneumonitis and fibrosis developed as shown on follow-up chest film (b) 18 months after treatment. The ^{131}I MAA lung scan obtained at that time (c and d) shows marked interference of perfusion of left lung, only a small area in the inferior portion of the left lower lobe being perfused. Patient died from distant metastasis 24 months after treatment

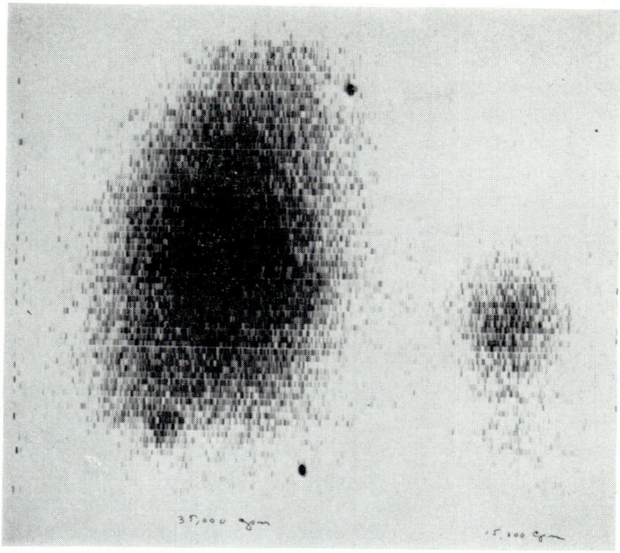

Figure 4c

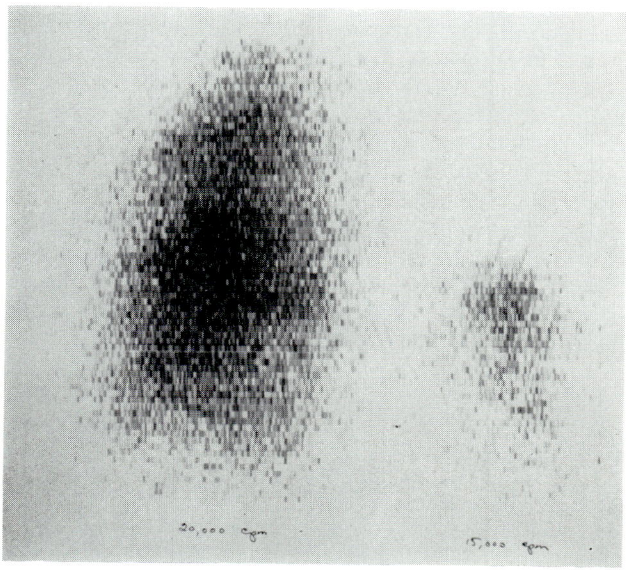

Figure 4d

improvement in the perfusion defect following radiotherapy was in patients with hilar lesions or with a defect greater than the radiological lesions. The survival in this group was markedly shorter than in the cases with small peripheral lesions, whose perfusion defect frequently increased after radiation therapy. The patients showing hilar lesions or perfusion defects out of proportion to the radiographic findings died of metastasis to vital organs, though the area treated frequently remained under control. The ^{131}I MAA perfusion lung scan is therefore an excellent guide to the probable prognosis prior to treatment. It is not effective as an index of response to radiotherapy, because the treatment itself frequently produces its own perfusion defect.

SUMMARY

Iodine-131 MAA perfusion lung scans are an aid in evaluating patients with known or suspected bronchogenic carcinoma. In a small number of cases, the scan has demonstrated the site of pathology when the radiograph was interpreted as showing no significant abnormality. The scan is useful in assessing the risk of surgery by providing information which supplements pulmonary function studies in evaluation of total lung function. It may demonstrate significant perfusion defect in areas of the lungs which radiographically appear normal. If the perfusion defect is in a segment of the lung other than that in which the radiological lesion is located, this pattern is a strong indication of spread to the hilar nodes.

The response to radiation therapy, as measured by improved pulmonary artery perfusion demonstrated on follow-up lung scans, has not been a significant indicator of survival. Central or hilar lesions most often show improvement after radiotherapy but have the shortest survival. The small peripheral bronchogenic carcinoma, with minimal or no initial perfusion defect, has the best survival rate. After radiotherapy, the perfusion defect in this type of case frequently increases due to the effect of the treatment on surrounding normal lung.

REFERENCES

Dotter, C. T., Steinberg, I. and Holman, C. W. (1950). 'Lung cancer operability.' *Am. J. Roentg.* **64,** 222.

Ernst, H., Krüger, J. and Vessal, K. (1969). 'Lung scanning as a screening method for cancer of the lung.' *Cancer, N.Y.* **23,** 508.

Germon, P. A. and Brady, L. W. (1968). 'Physiologic changes before and after radiation treatment for carcinoma of the lung.' *J. Am. med. Ass.* **206,** 809.

Gold, W. M. and McCormack, K. R. (1966). 'Pulmonary function response to radioisotope scanning of the lungs.' *J. Am. med. Ass.* **197,** 146.

Hatch, H. B. Jnr., Maxfield, W. S. and Ochsner, J. L. (1965). 'Radioisotope lung scanning in bronchogenic carcinoma.' *J. thorac. cardiovasc. Surg.* **50,** 634.

Haynie, T. P., Calhoon, J. H., Nasjleti, C. E., Nofal, M. N. and Beierwaltes, W. H. (1962). 'Visualization of pulmonary infarcts and tumors by photoscanning.' *J. Lab. clin. Med.* **60,** 881.

Johnson, P. M., Sagerman, R. H. and Jacox, H. W. (1968). 'Changes in pulmonary arterial perfusion due to intrathoracic neoplasia and irradiation of the lung.' *Am. J. Roentg.* **102,** 637.

Maxfield, W. S., Hatch, H. B. Jnr. and Ochsner, J. L. (1966). 'Perfusion lung scanning in evaluation of patients with bronchogenic carcinoma.' *Surg. Clins N. Am.* **46,** 1389.

Maynard, C. D., Miller, R. P., Heaphy, L. J. Jnr. and Whitley, J. E. (1969). 'Pulmonary scanning in bronchogenic carcinoma.' *Radiology* **92,** 903.

Nabatoff, R. A. (1951). 'Contrast visualization of the pulmonary vessels as an aid in the early diagnosis of pulmonary neoplasms.' *Ann. Surg.* **133,** 270.

Neuhof, H., Sussman, M. L. and Nabatoff, R. A. (1949). 'Angiocardiography in the differential diagnosis of pulmonary neoplasms.' *Surgery, St Louis* **25,** 178.

Oeser, H. and Ernst, H. (1966). 'Die Lungenszinligraphie als Mittel zur Früherkennung des Lungenkrebses.' *Dt. med. Wschr.* **91,** 333.

Oyamada, H., Takeshi, Y., Sakura, M., Tsuboi, E. and Atsumi, K. (1967). 'Estimation of pulmonary blood flow by '^{131}I-MAA pulmogram with special reference to pulmonary carcinoma before and after radiotherapy.' *Tohoku J. exp. Med.* **93,** 79.

Quinn, J. L. III and Whitley, J. E. (1964). 'Lung scintiscanning.' *Radiology* **83,** 937.

Stern, H. S., Goodwin, D. A., Wagner, H. N. Jnr. and Kramer, H. H. (1966). '^{113m}In a short-lived isotope for lung scanning.' *Nucleonics* **24,** 57.

Taplin, G. V., Johnson, D. E., Dore, E. K. and Kaplan, H. S. (1964). 'Lung photoscans with macroaggregates of human serum radioalbumin: experimental basis and initial clinical trials.' *Hlth Phys.* **10,** 1219.

Vassallo, C. L., Gee, J. B. L., Wholey, M. H. and Vester, J. W. (1968). 'Lung scanning in hilar bronchogenic carcinoma.' *Am. Rev. resp. Dis.* **97,** 851.

Wagner, H. N. Jnr., Holmes, R. A., Lopez-Majano, V. and Tow, D. A. (1968). 'The lung.' Chapter X in *Principles of Nuclear Medicine*, p. 472. Ed. by H. N. Wagner Jnr. Philadelphia: Saunders.

Wagner, H. N. Jnr., Lopez-Majano, V., Tow, D. A. and Langen, J. K. (1965). 'Radioisotope scanning of lungs in early diagnosis of bronchogenic carcinoma.' *Lancet* **1,** 344.

— Sabiston, D. C. Jnr., Ilo, N., McAfee, J. C., Meyer, J. K., and Langen, J. K. (1964). 'Regional pulmonary blood flow in man by radioisotope scanning.' *J. Am. med. Ass.* **187,** 601.

Webber, M. M., Bennett, L. R. and Suprenent, E. L. (1966). 'The technique and interpretation of lung scans using technetium-99m labelled macroaggregated albumin.' *J. nucl. Med.* **7,** 353.

II—Blood Cytology

Karl P. Klassen

The long-term survival rate of patients with bronchogenic carcinoma following acceptable resection or irradiation, alone or in combination with chemotherapy or other adjuvant measures, is low (Deeley, 1967; Rubin, 1966). The best results, applying all therapeutic modalities, are obtained in those individuals who present themselves with asymptomatic small lesions, presumably of recent origin, before lymphatic and haematogenous invasion or local extension to adjacent extrapulmonary structures has occurred. In these cases, resection and adequate irradiation should totally remove or destroy the malignancy and prevent local or distant recurrence. In a controlled series of 129 patients in whom the tumour was limited to the lung at the time of resection, a six-year follow-up shows a survival of only 36 per cent (Curreri, 1965). Local recurrence and lymphatic and haematogenous dissemination are responsible for the low survival rate of patients with brochogenic carcinoma.

VALUE OF DIFFERENT FORMS OF THERAPY

Lymphatic spread to peribronchial and mediastinal lymph nodes, direct extension by continuity to the proximal bronchus and trachea, frequently not recognized at the time of surgery, as well as involvement of the pleura may preclude total removal of the malignancy, and local recurrence must be anticipated. It was for this reason that pre-operative irradiation of the primary tumour and adjacent structures in adequate doses to sterilize the tumour was advocated by Bloedorn and Cowley (1960). Subsequent thoracotomy, usually six weeks after irradiation of the area, demonstrated complete sterilization of the involved lymph nodes (Bloedorn and colleagues, 1961). Some early reports indicated a higher survival rate in the patients having irradiation prior to excision of the bronchogenic carcinoma (Bloedorn and colleagues, 1961; Paulson and colleagues, 1962), but others did not confirm this finding (Baker, Cowley and Linberg, 1963). In a large controlled series of 568 cases of primary pulmonary carcinoma, 290 patients received pre-operative irradiation, while 278 had surgery alone (U.S. Public Health Service, 1969). The one-year as well as the life table estimates of three-year survival rates for these two groups were nearly identical. A five-year follow-up report, indicating not only survival time in this group of patients but also the extent of local and distant metastases, should greatly aid our understanding of the mode of dissemination in bronchogenic carcinoma.

Once haematogenous dissemination has taken place, all forms of therapy directed towards the primary tumour and its local extension appear to be of little curative value, although the palliative value of such treatment must not be underestimated. In the majority of cases, dissemination probably occurs before the discovery of the pulmonary tumour and the application of specific therapy. Once the diagnosis of a bronchogenic carcinoma has been established, attempts are made to prevent the entry of malignant cells into the blood stream. The first of these measures is pre-operative irradiation, which may create a local barrier to vascular invasion, destroy the tumour, or alter the nature of the embolic malignant cells and prevent their growth as metastases (Hoye and Smith, 1961). As yet there is no clear-cut evidence of the effectiveness of this therapeutic measure. Ligation of the pulmonary vein of the involved lobe prior to manipulation and biopsy of the tumour and subsequent resection may decrease the number of malignant cells in the blood stream (Klassen and Selbach, 1965).

The third method of preventing metastases is the attenuation of the malignant cells in the blood stream by chemotherapy. A study on these lines was sponsored by the Cancer Chemotherapy National Service Center and conducted by surgeons of 22 university centres from July 1957 to February 1961 (Moore, Ross and Stiver, 1963). Of a total of 1,223 patients undergoing resection, 251 showed no evidence of local or distant spread at the time of surgery and all of the tumour was considered to have been removed. In half of these patients, nitrogen mustard was administered intrapleurally and intravenously at and immediately after surgery, while the remainder received no chemotherapy and served as a control group. Analysis of the results after three years indicated no essential difference in the survival rate of the two groups, which was 44·3 per cent (Curreri, 1962). A subsequent report (Curreri, 1965) on the overall four-year to six-year survival of patients in this trial indicated a rate of 53 per cent in the group treated with nitrogen mustard, compared with 36·6 per cent for the patients in the control group. It appears that the better results in the nitrogen mustard treated cases may be due to the effect of the chemotherapy upon the circulating malignant cells, with possible attenuation of the malignancy.

SIGNIFICANCE OF CANCER CELLS IN BLOOD STREAM

The tendency of malignant tumours to invade the local vascular channels, leading to a haematogenous dissemination and distant secondary tumour as metastases, was recognized by both the clinician and the pathologist prior to the actual demonstration of such circulating cancer cells in the blood stream by Ashworth in 1869. Marcus (1917) found abnormal cells in the blood of a patient with bronchogenic carcinoma. It was not until 1934 that Pool and Dunlop, using a technique of haemolysis and sedimentation, reported on 40 patients with various types of malignant disease, of whom 17 were found to have malignant cells in the blood stream. Cole, Packard and Southwick (1954) reported a high concentration of malignant cells in the mesenteric veins in colonic carcinoma, using an albumin flotation method and the Papanicolaou technique of staining.

Over a period of five years beginning in 1948, Engell (1955) investigated the clinical importance of demonstrating cancer cells, in patients with various malignancies, in the peripheral and venous blood draining the tumour area. Tumour cells were found in 61 per cent of 125 surgical patients. Engell concluded that the degree of differentiation of the tumour was an important factor in dissemination, and that no prognostic information could be derived from the finding of cancer cells in the blood from the draining area. Of those patients surviving resection of the malignancy for five to nine years, 51 per cent had tumour cells in the blood at the time of operation. There were four patients with bronchogenic carcinoma who had curative resection of the tumour. One patient with malignant cells in his blood survived over five years, while three died of recurrence, one with negative blood findings.

The prognostic value of tumour cells in the blood of 98 patients with bronchogenic carcinoma was evaluated by Watne, Sandberg and Moore (1961). Malignant cells were found in the peripheral blood in 7 per cent of these cases, and in the regional vein in 65 per cent of 20 patients undergoing curative resection. The 18 months' survival rate in the latter group was 60 per cent. These investigators concluded that the finding of malignant cells in the peripheral blood was associated with a significant decrease in survival.

In 1962 we reported on the result of an investigation of the significance of finding malignant cells in the blood of 61 consecutive patients with bronchogenic carcinoma in various stages of progression and 40 patients with non-malignant lesions of the lung (Sakurai, Klassen and Selbach, 1962). Blood samples were taken from a peripheral vein and from the draining vein in patients undergoing thoracotomy. The 257 samples were examined by the sedimentation technique of Sandberg and Moore (1957) and by the Millipore filtration method of Malmgren and colleagues (1958), a total of 2,884 slides being prepared. It was found that the Millipore filtration was twice as accurate as the sedimentation method of identifying malignant cells. In the patients with bronchogenic carcinoma, 12 per cent of the samples of peripheral venous blood were found to contain malignant cells compared with 0·2 per cent in the patients with benign lesions. The highest concentration of malignant cells, 42 per cent, was found in the regional vein. Manipulation of the tumour increased this count considerably. On the basis of this study we concluded that the extent of the carcinoma was not reflected in the concentration of malignant cells in the peripheral blood. It was also felt that examination of the peripheral venous blood for malignant cells did not have any practical value as a diagnostic aid.

Twenty-four patients out of the 61 with bronchogenic carcinoma came to resection and were reported upon four years later (Klassen and Selbach, 1965). Of six patients without malignant cells in the peripheral and regional venous blood and with negative regional lymph nodes, five survived and one died of his malignant disease. In five patients with lymph node involvement and negative venous blood, only one survived, suggesting that local extension of carcinoma into lymph nodes was of greater prognostic value than the presence or absence of malignant cells in the blood. Of the patients with malignant cells in the venous blood, peripheral and regional, two out of four without lymph node involvement survived, while of those with lymph node involvement, only one out of seven survived in this group.

Of the nine patients reported by us in 1964, two died four and a half and five years following resection of their malignant neoplasms respectively. The first died of arteriosclerosis at the age of 75 and, at the time of autopsy, tumour was demonstrated in the region of the bronchial stump. There was no evidence of metastases. The second patient died four years later of pulmonary insufficiency due to a gradually increasing tumour of the remaining lung. The exact nature of this growth was not diagnosed and an autopsy was not obtained. The x-ray appearance was that of a second primary tumour of the lung.

Only six patients out of 33 suffering from carcinoma and undergoing a thoracotomy had malignant cells in the peripheral blood. In five of these, malignant cells were also found in the draining pulmonary vein. Two of this latter group have survived for over eight years. There was no regional lymph node involvement in these two cases. One patient with such lymph node extension had malignant cells in the venous blood only and has survived for nine years.

Delarue and colleagues (1964) pointed out the clinical significance of malignant cells in the blood of 46 patients with bronchogenic carcinoma considered curable at the time of resection. Sixty-three per cent of all patients had positive blood samples; of these, 76 per cent died of recurrence within two to five years, while only 47 with negative blood samples died of their disease. In a group of 767 patients with cancer of various organs studied by Roberts and colleagues (1967) over a period of five to ten years, malignant cells were found in 7 per cent. These authors found no difference in the frequency of positive blood samples between the patients considered curable and those with extensive disease. In the entire group the survival rate was 13 per cent in patients with positive and 12 per cent in patients with negative blood samples, while in those with assumed curative resection it was 34 per cent regardless of the presence or absence of malignant cells in the blood stream.

Kuper and Bignall (1966) reported on the significance of tumour cells in the pulmonary veins of 35 patients with bronchogenic carcinoma coming to resection. All five patients in whom malignant cells were demonstrated in the blood, of whom four also had positive lymph nodes, died of cancer within two years. Of the 30 patients without malignant cells in the blood, 21 survived for two years. Nine patients in the latter group had positive lymph nodes, but only four of these died within the two years. It was the impression of the investigators that the presence of malignant cells in the blood of patients with bronchogenic carcinoma was of prognostic significance; however, they felt that the available evidence was insufficient to indicate whether this finding was of greater importance than the presence of regional lymph node extension.

Comparison of Published Results

The available statistics indicating the incidence of malignant cells in the peripheral and regional venous blood in patients with bronchogenic carcinoma, disregarding the extent of the lesion, are shown in Table 1. Although the methods of demonstrating the malignant cells differed and some regional blood samples were obtained following manipulation, it appears that in these 286 cases, malignant cells were found twice as frequently in the regional blood as in the peripheral samples.

TABLE 1

Malignant Cells in Peripheral and Regional Venous Blood in Patients with Bronchogenic Carcinoma

Investigators	*Number of patients*	*Percentage of positive blood samples*	
		Peripheral vein	*Regional vein*
Engell (1955)	4	50	75
Watne, Sandberg and Moore (1961)	98	7	63
Delarue and colleagues (1964)	88	21	39
Klassen and Selbach (1965)	61	12	42
Kuper and Bignall (1966)	35	—	14
Total	286	22	44

An attempt was also made to determine the survival rate after resection of the carcinoma and its possible relation to the incidence of malignant cells in the peripheral and regional blood. The extent of the carcinoma, the method of demonstrating malignant cells and other factors are not comparable and are not valid statistically (Tables 2 and 3). There is a suggestion from this material that no prognosis can be made on the basis of finding malignant cells in the peripheral blood, whereas in the regional samples there appears to be a definite trend, twice as many patients surviving in the group with no malignant cells in the blood of the involved lobe.

Need for Further Studies

The published results of the investigation of the significance of cancer cells in the circulating blood as well as our own experience can be accepted only as a preliminary report, and assessment of the importance of demonstrating malignant cells in the peripheral and regional blood must await more extensive and more uniform studies. Von Haam (1966), following an extensive investigation in his laboratory, has pointed out the wide discrepancy in the published results concerning cancer cells in the peripheral blood. He concludes that malignant cells can be found in the peripheral blood of cancer patients at various times, but that the techniques of identification

TABLE 2

Malignant Cells in Peripheral Venous Blood: Relationship to Survival of Patients with Bronchogenic Carcinoma Following Resection

Investigators	*Number of patients*	*Duration of survival (years)*	*Blood samples of patients*	*Number of patients survived*	*Percentage survival*
Engell (1955)	4	5–9	+2	1	50
			−2	—	—
Watne, Sandberg and Moore (1961)	22	1½	+0	—	—
			−22	11	50
Klassen and Selbach (1965)	33	8	+6	2	33
			−27	5	18
Total	59	1½—9	+8	3	37
			−51	16	31

TABLE 3

Malignant Cells in Regional Venous Blood: Relationship to Survival of Patients with Bronchogenic Carcinoma Following Resection

Investigators	*Number of patients*	*Duration of survival (years)*	*Blood samples of patients*	*Number of patients survived*	*Percentage survival*
Watne, Sandberg and Moore (1961)	35	1½	+22	9	41
			−13	4	30
Klassen and Selbach (1965)	33	8	+16	3	19
			−17	4	23
Kuper and Bignall (1966)	35	2	+5	—	—
			−30	21	70
Total	103	1½–8	+43	12	28
			−60	29	48

must be standardized to permit comparative conclusions. He states that the cells must appear atypical and must resemble the cells of the primary tumour as evidenced by biopsy study, and that such cells must not be present in the blood of patients who do not have cancer. Until a standard technique has been developed and the pathologists are able definitely to identify malignant cells, no conclusions can be drawn as to the prognostic importance of finding such cells in the blood.

We are not aware of any controlled clinical study dealing with the effects of irradiation of bronchogenic carcinoma on circulating malignant cells and their subsequent growth. Experimental work in mice conducted by Hoye and Smith (1961) suggests that irradiation of the primary tumour greatly reduces the growth of the disseminated tumour.

Possible conclusions could be drawn from the study of a large group of patients without regional lymph involvement or adjacent tissue invasion and with examination of the regional and peripheral blood. Only in the series reported by Sakurai, Klassen and Selbach (1962), by Klassen and Selbach (1965) and by Kuper and Bignall (1966) is such analysis suggestive of the importance of finding malignant cells in the blood stream. In our study of six patients with negative lymph nodes and negative blood samples (Klassen and Selbach, 1962), five were alive four years following surgery, while in the series of Kuper and Bignall, 16 out of 21 were alive after two years. In the group with positive blood findings there were four patients of whom two were dead within four years, while in the series of Kuper and Bignall (1966) there was only one patient with positive blood and negative lymph nodes who died within two years. This series is altogether too small for statistical analysis, and these patients were observed only over a period of two to four years, which is not sufficient in carcinoma of the lung. It would appear that a controlled study of a larger series of cases with the disease localized in the lung parenchyma, with concomitant studies of the presence of malignant cells in the peripheral arterial blood observed over a period of at least five years, should aid materially in assessing the prognostic significance of malignant cells in the peripheral blood stream.

SUMMARY

The results of radiation and excisional therapy in bronchogenic carcinoma are poor. This is due to the early lymphatic and haematogenous dissemination of this disease and its extension by direct continuity. Involvement of regional lymph nodes and local extension can usually be determined without difficulty, but haematogenous dissemination still presents problems. Malignant cells which resemble those of the primary tumour can be found in the peripheral venous and regional venous blood of patients with cancer. Such cells are not found in patients with benign pulmonary lesions. A higher incidence of malignant cells is found in the regional veins, and manipulation of the primary tumour can increase this cell count. The finding of malignant cells in the regional venous blood may be of prognostic importance, whereas such findings in the peripheral veins must be questioned.

REFERENCES

Ashworth, T. R. (1869). 'A case of cancer in which cells similar to those in the tumours were seen in the blood after death.' *Aust. med. J.* **14,** 146.

Baker, N. H., Cowley, R. A. and Linberg, E. (1963). 'A follow-up in patients with bronchogenic carcinoma "locally cured" by preoperative irradiation.' *J. thorac. cardiovasc. Surg.* **46,** 298.

Bloedorn, F. G. and Cowley, R. A. (1960). 'Irradiation and surgery in the treatment of bronchogenic carcinoma.' *Surgery Gynec. Obstet.* **111,** 141.

— — Cuccia, C. A. and Mercado, R. (1961). 'Combined therapy—irradiation and surgery in the treatment of bronchogenic carcinoma.' *Am. J. Roentg.* **85,** 875.

Cole, W. H., Packard, D. and Southwick, H. (1954). 'Carcinoma of the colon with special reference to prevention of recurrence.' *J. Am. med. Ass.* **155,** 1549.

Curreri, A. (1962). *Surgical Adjuvant Lung Study—1962 Progress Report.* Chemotherapy Statistical Unit, Roswell Park Memorial Institute, Buffalo, N.Y.

— (1965). *Surgical Adjuvant Lung Study—1965 Progress Report.* Chemotherapy Statistical Unit, Roswell Park Memorial Institute, Buffalo, N. Y.

Deeley, T. J. (1967). 'The treatment of carcinoma of the bronchus.' *Br. J. Radiol.* **40,** 801.

Delarue, N. C., Watters, N., Anderson, W. E., Tompson, D., Brown, T. C., Falk, R. E., Lansky, G. S., Fielden, H. N., Lau, C. and Steele, D. (1964). 'Circulating "cancer cells".' *Archs Surg., Chicago* **89,** 392.

Engell, H. C. (1955). 'Cancer cells in the circulating blood: a clinical study on the occurrence of cancer cells in the peripheral blood and in venous blood draining the tumour area at operation.' *Acta chir. scand.,* Suppl. **201,** 1.

Hoye, R. C. and Smith, R. R. (1961). 'The effectiveness of small amounts of preoperative irradiation in preventing the growth of tumour cells disseminated at surgery.' *C.A.* **14,** 284.

Klassen, K. P. and Selbach, G. J. (1965). 'The prognostic value of cytologic studies of the blood of patients with bronchogenic carcinoma.' *J. thorac. cardiovasc. Surg.* **50,** 127.

Kuper, S. W. A. and Bignall, J. R. (1966). 'Survival after resection of bronchial carcinomas.' *Lancet* **1,** 10.

Malmgren, R. A., Pruitt, J. C., Del Vecchio, P. R. and Potter, J. F. (1958). 'A method for the cytologic detection of tumour cells in whole blood.' *J. natn. Cancer Inst.* **20,** 1203.

Marcus, H. (1917). 'Krebszellen im strömenden Blut?' *Z. Krebsforsch.* **16,** 217.

Moore, G. E., Ross, C. A. and Striver, R. B. (1963). 'Chemotherapy as an adjuvant to surgery.' *Am. J. Surg.* **105,** 591.

Paulson, C. L., Shaw, R. R., Kee, J. L., Mallams, J. T. and Collier, R. E. (1962). 'Combined preoperative irradiation and resection for bronchogenic carcinoma.' *J. thorac. Surg.* **44,** 281.

Pool, E. H. and Dunlop, G. R. (1934). 'Cancer cells in blood stream.' *Am. J. Cancer* **21,** 99.

Roberts, S. S., Hengesh, J. W., McGrath, R. G., Valaitis, J., McGrew, E. A. and Cole, W. H. (1967). 'Prognostic significance of cancer cells in the circulating blood.' *Am. J. Surg.* **113,** 757.

Rubin, P (1966). 'Bronchogenic carcinoma: current concepts in cancer.' *J. Am. med. Ass.* **195,** 653.

Sakurai, A., Klassen, K. P. and Selbach, G. (1962). 'The presence of malignant cells in the blood of patients with carcinoma of the lung.' *Acta cytol.* **6,** 314.

Sandberg, A. A. and Moore, G. E. (1957). 'Examination of blood for tumour cells.' *J. natn. Cancer Inst.* **19,** 1.

U.S. Public Health Service (1969). 'Preoperative irradiation of cancer of the lung.' *C.A.* **23,** 419.

Von Haam, E. (1966). 'Malignant cells in the peripheral blood.' *Am. Acad. gen. Pract.* **34,** 98.

Watne, A. L., Sandberg, A. A. and Moore, G. E. (1961). 'The prognostic value of tumour cells in the blood.' *Archs Surg., Chicago* **83,** 190.

III—Plasma Cortisol Levels

Ivan Lichter

INTRODUCTION

Overt endocrine disorders are known to occur in association with carcinoma of the bronchus (Kovach and Kyle, 1958; Vogel, Keating and Bahn, 1961; Boruchow, 1965). Bronchial carcinoma, especially the oat cell type, may be associated with Cushing's syndrome, and in these cases the tumour produces a substance indistinguishable from pituitary corticotrophin (Meador and colleagues, 1962; Marks, Rosenbaum and Russfield, 1963; Liddle and colleagues, 1965). Cushing's syndrome occurs only rarely, but its occasional presence has stimulated investigations into steroid hormone production in patients with carcinoma of the bronchus in whom there is no clinical evidence of endocrine abnormality.

In patients dying of bronchial carcinoma, an increase in width of the adrenal cortex has been demonstrated at necropsy (Sholiton, Incze and Werk, 1961; Caranasos and Ruebner, 1963). It has been suggested that this is not due to the prolonged stress of the disease, as studies on patients with non-malignant chronic pulmonary lesions have shown no evidence of adrenocortical hyperactivity (Segaloff, Hatch and Rongone, 1962). Werk and Sholiton (1960) reported increased morning plasma 17-hydroxycorticoid levels in 22 patients with carcinoma of the bronchus. Segaloff, Hatch and Rongone (1962) also assessed adrenal function in 26 patients with carcinoma of the bronchus and found plasma corticoid levels generally higher than in 6 control patients who had benign lung lesions. Hatch, Segaloff and Ochsner (1965), investigating 100 patients with bronchial carcinoma, considered 71 to have elevated plasma corticoid levels.

It is now well documented that when compared with a control group, a group with carcinoma of the bronchus shows significantly higher plasma cortisol levels. It has been postulated that these high levels are due to sustained steroid production by the adrenals as a result of stimulation by tumour-produced adrenocorticotrophic hormone (Sholiton, Incze and Werk, 1961). Hatch, Segaloff and Ochsner (1965) considered that abnormally high levels in patients with pulmonary disease provided added evidence that the lesion might be malignant. They reported that after surgical removal of bronchial carcinoma the plasma corticoid levels returned to normal, and that elevation of these levels again occurred with recurrence of the growth before its clinical presence was apparent.

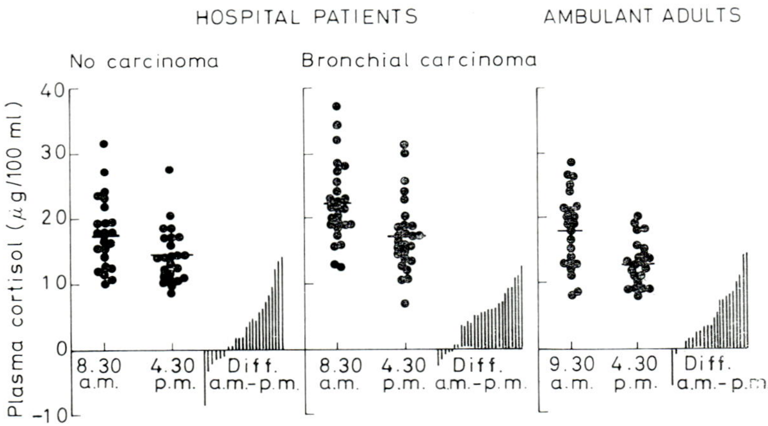

Figure 1. Distribution of morning and afternoon plasma cortisol levels in hospital patients with no bronchial carcinoma (n = 24), those with proven bronchial carcinoma (n = 26), and healthy ambulant adults (n = 23)

The important implications of these findings led to a further study of the diagnostic and prognostic potential of plasma cortisol levels in patients with carcinoma of the bronchus (Lichter and Sirett, 1968). Many factors such as emotional disturbance, pain, stress and drug therapy may influence the cortisol level, and precautions were taken to eliminate the variables as far as possible, to have adequately screened controls and to take account of normal diurnal variations. The study, using a fluorimetric method to measure morning and afternoon levels of plasma cortisol (Purves and Sirett, 1969), confirmed that in patients with carcinoma of the bronchus *taken as a group*, the levels showed a significant elevation as compared with those in a control group. In this series the mean group differences (both in the morning and in the afternoon) between the bronchial carcinoma and no bronchial carcinoma groups were significant. However, as shown in the scatter diagram (*Figure 1*), the variation of the individual levels was so wide that it was impossible to separate patients by their plasma cortisol levels into cancer and non-cancer groups, and few cancer patients showed levels clearly beyond the range found in normal subjects.

The levels found in a group of healthy ambulant adults also showed that single estimations from individuals fell within a very wide range. Observed over the period Monday to Friday, there was a considerable daily variation, the highest individual level being 14 μg/100 ml during the five-day study.

STAGE OF DISEASE

Bronchial carcinoma patients with unequivocally high plasma cortisol levels were often in an advanced stage of the disease. These findings accord with those of Borkowski and colleagues (1966), who reported on 76 patients with carcinoma of the bronchus: 16 patients had evidence of hypercorticism, and 11 of these died within three months of observation, suggesting that high levels were related to the late stage of the disease. In the series of Werk and Sholiton (1960), 18 of the 22 patients had secondary deposits. The bronchial carcinoma patients with high plasma cortisol levels reported on by Sholiton, Incze and Werk (1961) and by Hymes and Doe (1962) were all inoperable, and many survived for only short periods.

Sandberg and colleagues (1956) demonstrated that raised plasma corticoid levels can be expected in patients dying from a variety of illnesses.

DIURNAL VARIATION

McNamara and colleagues (1968) reported a study on patients with bronchial carcinoma. They found normal plasma cortisol levels at 8 a.m., but the 4 p.m. and 10 p.m. levels were elevated, and it was considered that this indicated a loss of normal corticosteroid circadian rhythm.

Lichter and Sirett (1968) reported normal diurnal variation in the group means of patients with bronchial carcinoma, patients without bronchial carcinoma and healthy ambulant adults, but within each group there were individuals who failed to show a reduced level in the afternoon. The incidence of these irregularities appeared to be similar in each group. The mean difference a.m.–p.m. and the standard deviation (in parentheses) were: diagnosed carcinoma of the bronchus, 5·1 (4·4) μg/100 ml; no bronchial carcinoma, 3·5 (5·5) μg/100 ml; ambulant adults, 5·1 (5·1) μg/100 ml. The distribution of plasma 11-hydroxycorticoids in the hospital patients was similar to those reported by others using a fluorimetric method (McGill and colleagues, 1967; McHardy-Young and colleagues, 1967), but was higher than those reported by Liddle (1966), who measured 17-hydroxycorticoids as Porter–Silber chromogens.

Caution is recommended when comparing results of plasma cortisol estimations from different laboratories because of the variability in methods of measurement (James, Townsend and Fraser, 1967).

TUMOUR CELL TYPE

McNamara and colleagues (1968) related plasma cortisol levels to tumour cell type and considered that plasma cortisol elevations were shown most clearly with squamous cell neoplasms. Cushing's syndrome usually occurs in the presence of an oat cell carcinoma (Kovach and Kyle, 1958; Vogel, Keating and Bahn, 1961; Boruchow, 1965). In other series, significantly elevated cortisol levels have been found with all histological types of cancer (Borkowski and colleagues, 1966; Lichter and Sirett, 1969).

SIGNIFICANCE OF RAISED PLASMA CORTISOL LEVELS

Most investigators agree that a definite correlation exists between high plasma cortisol levels and bronchial carcinoma. The series of Lichter and Sirett (1969), when extended to include 44 patients with bronchial carcinoma and 35 with no bronchial carcinoma, showed group means of the same order as the smaller series. The mean plasma cortisol levels, μg/100 ml ± one standard deviation, were: bronchial carcinoma, 8.30 a.m., 23·7 ± 7·7; 4.30 p.m., 18·1 ± 6·5; no bronchial carcinoma, 8.30 a.m., 17·5 ± 5·5; 4.30 p.m. 13·6 ± 4·3. The 8.30 a.m. figures showed that 9 per cent of patients with carcinoma of the bronchus and 29 per cent of those with no bronchial carcinoma had levels less than 15μg/100 ml, while at 4.30 p.m., 30 per cent of those with and 11 per cent of those without bronchial carcinoma had levels above 20 μg/100 ml (Table 1).

Only a small proportion of patients with carcinoma of the bronchus have cortisol levels beyond the normal range. Similar observations were made by Borkowski and colleagues (1966), who reported that 6 of a series of 76 patients with bronchial carcinoma had abnormally high levels. Consequently, plasma cortisol levels are of limited use in the diagnosis of carcinoma of the bronchus in the individual patient. When high levels are found, they appear to indicate an advanced stage of the disease and a short-term prognosis.

TABLE 1
Distribution of Plasma Cortisol Levels in Male Hospital Patients

Time	*Range of plasma cortisol (μg/100 ml)*	*Percentage of patients with no carcinoma (n = 35)*	*Percentage of patients with bronchial carcinoma (n = 44)*
8.30 a.m.	<10	2·9	2·3
	<15	28·6	9·1
	>20	22·8	68·0
	>25	8·6	31·8
4.30 p.m.	<10	17·1	2·3
	<15	65·7	38·6
	>20	11·4	29·6
	>25	—	15·9

RADIOTHERAPY AND PLASMA CORTISOL LEVELS

A study was designed to assess the effect of radiotherapy on patients with carcinoma of the bronchus (Lichter and Sirett, 1969) on the premise that a fall might indicate successful control of the neoplasm and a subsequent rise might presage recurrence.

The series is as yet small. In a control group of patients with cancer in sites other than the bronchus, radiotherapy produced no regular effect on plasma cortisol levels. It appeared to reduce the plasma cortisol levels in patients with bronchial carcinoma. However, to date no reliable predictability of effect based on these estimations has been demonstrated.

REFERENCES

Borkowski, A., Levin, S., Mahler, A. and Verhas, V. (1966). 'A study of adrenal function in seventy-six consecutive cases of bronchial carcinoma.' *Eur. J. Cancer* **2,** 263.

Boruchow, I. B. (1965). 'Endocrine and metabolic aspects of bronchogenic carcinoma.' *Archs Surg., Chicago* **90,** 101.

Caranasos, G. and Ruebner, B. H. (1963). 'Adrenal width and metastasis in bronchogenic carcinoma.' *Archs Path.* **76,** 263.

Hatch, H. B., Segaloff, A. and Ochsner, A. (1965). 'Adrenocortical function in bronchogenic carcinoma: study of 100 patients.' *Ann. Surg.* **161,** 645.

Hymes, A. C. and Doe, R. P. (1962). 'Adrenal function in cancer of the lung, with and without Cushing's syndrome.' *Am. J. Med.* **33,** 398.

James, V. H. T., Townsend, J. and Fraser, R. (1967). 'Comparison of fluorimetric and isotopic procedures for the determination of plasma cortisol.' *J. Endocr.* **37,** XXVIII.

Kovach, R. D. and Kyle, L. H. (1958). 'Cushing's syndrome and bronchogenic carcinoma.' *Am. J. Med.* **24,** 981.

Lichter, I. and Sirett, Nancy E. (1968). 'Plasma cortisol levels in lung cancer.' *Br. med. J.* **2,** 154.

— — (1969). Unpublished data.

Liddle, G. W. (1966). 'Analysis of circadian rhythms in human adrenocortical secretory activity.' *Archs intern. Med.* **117,** 739.

— Givens, J. R., Nicholson, W. E. and Island, D. P. (1965). 'The ectopic ACTH syndrome'. *Cancer Res.* **25,** 1057.

Marks, L. J., Rosenbaum, D. L. and Russfield, A. B. (1963). 'Cushing's syndrome and corticotropin-secreting carcinoma of the lung.' *Ann. intern. Med.* **58,** 143.

McGill, P. E., Greig, W. R., Browning, M. C. K. and Boyle, J. A. (1967). 'Plasma cortisol response to Synacthen (B^{1-24} Ciba) at different times of the day in patients with rheumatic diseases.' *Ann. rheum. Dis.* **26,** 123.

McHardy-Young, S., Harris, P. W. R., Lessof, M. H. and Lyne, C. (1967). 'Single-dose dexamethasone suppression test for Cushing's syndrome.' *Br. med. J.* **2,** 740.

McNamara, J. J., Varon, H. H., Paulson, D. L., Shah, I. and Urschel, H. C. (1968). 'Steroid hormone abnormalities in patients with carcinoma of the lung.' *J. thorac. cardiovasc. Surg.* **56,** 371.

Meador, C. K., Liddle, G. W., Island, D. P., Nicholson, W. E., Nuckton, J. G. and Luetscher, J. A. (1962). 'Cause of Cushing's syndrome in patients with tumours arising from "nonendocrine" tissue.' *J. clin. Endocr. Metab.* **22,** 693.

Purves, H. D. and Sirett, N. E. (1969). 'The fluorimetric estimation of cortisol in human plasma'. *Aust. J. exp. Biol. med. Sci.* **47,** 589.

Sandberg, A. A., Eik-Nes, K., Migeon, C. J. and Samuels, L. T. (1956). 'Metabolism of adrenal steroids in dying patients.' *J. clin. Endocr. Metab.* **16,** 1001.

Segaloff, A., Hatch, H. B. and Rongone, E. L. (1962). 'Elevated plasma corticoids associated with lung cancer.' *Cancer Chemother. Rep.* **16,** 343.

Sholiton, L. J., Incze, J. S. and Werk, E. E. Jnr. (1961). 'Adrenocortical width in carcinoma of the lung.' *Cancer, N.Y.* **14,** 105.

Vogel, M. D., Keating, F. R. Jnr. and Bahn, R. D. (1961). 'Acute Cushing's syndrome associated with bronchogenic carcinoma.' *Proc. Staff Meet. Mayo. Clin.* **36,** 387.

Werk, E. E. Jnr. and Sholiton, L. J. (1960). 'Adrenocortical function in carcinoma of the lung.' *Cancer, N.Y.* **13,** 469.

18—Infection in the Carcinomatous Lung

P. C. Elmes

The development of infection while a patient with carcinoma of the bronchus is under treatment can be very serious. Unfortunately the circumstances which may lead to such infection are many and varied, so that no general rule can be laid down for prevention and treatment. It is necessary to consider the way in which the normal lung is protected from infection, the way in which this protection may become defective, and finally the organisms which are most likely to cause serious lung infections in these patients.

NORMAL DEFENCE SYSTEM

The Larynx

The normal larynx is so efficient that even during sleep, liquid and solid material in the pharynx does not get through into the respiratory tract. Disturbances of laryngeal function are relatively common in carcinoma of the bronchus because of involvement of the recurrent laryngeal nerve on the left side or, less commonly, because of degenerative changes in the central nervous system leading to pseudobulbar palsy. Aspiration of pharyngeal contents during swallowing and sleep invariably leads to basal lung infection and must be avoided. When there is any suspicion of laryngeal incompetence, the patient should be tested carefully for evidence of difficulty in swallowing. Diet and feeding habits should be adjusted so as to minimize the risk. Liquids are most liable to cause aspiration, and the use of drinking straws and 'feeders' can be particularly dangerous in these patients. They should sleep with the foot of the bed raised and with no more than a single pillow (similar to the position for a comatose patient), so that aspiration does not occur during sleep.

A similar but more serious situation arises when a cancer of the lung or main bronchus ulcerates through into the oesophagus and a fistula develops. If the prognosis warrants it, a permanent gastrostomy may be the only method of preventing fatal lung damage.

The Bronchial Filter

Inspired air is brought to body temperature and saturated with water vapour by the time it leaves the trachea to enter the main bronchi. It still contains the dust and droplets from the inspired air which are the chief source of infection of the lung. However, the flow of air along the branching of progressively narrower bronchi ensures that all the particles larger than 0·5 μ in diameter come sufficiently close to the mucous surface for gravitation to cause them to adhere. Particles smaller than this may reach the alveoli but, because of the larger size of these air spaces, the majority go out in the next expirate and few are retained. Once a particle touches the mucous surface, it is caught up and moved towards the larynx by the combination of respiratory movement and the beating of the cilia. All parts of the lung are cleared every 20 minutes in the normal individual.

It is this simple but extremely efficient system which is most likely to be defective in patients with lung cancer. In the commoner types of bronchial lesion (squamous and anaplastic or oat cell), the environmental factors leading to the cancer have already damaged the bronchial filter. Cigarette smoking and atmospheric pollution have usually caused chronic bronchitis. The fundamental defect in this disease is a breakdown of the mucociliary filter system due to proliferation of the goblet cells and the submucous bronchial glands. This thickening of the bronchial wall narrows the airways, which become liable to blockage. Excessive production of mucus leads to overloading of the ciliary clearance mechanism and also increases the tendency for bronchi to become temporarily blocked. Airway obstruction leads to limitation of respiratory movement and increases the mechanical difficulty. Micro-organisms which would normally be removed before they could cause infection are enabled to multiply. They may give rise to episodes of acute infection, cause chronic low grade infection or simply grow as commensals. Recurrent bacterial, virus and mycoplasmal infections in these patients may also be factors leading to the development of chronic bronchitis. It has also been suggested that the failure of the mucociliary clearance system increases the effect of inhaled carcinogens by allowing them more prolonged contact with the mucosa: this would be particularly likely to occur if the mucosal change had progressed as far as squamous metaplasia.

Even in chronic bronchitics, most of the dust-borne organisms do not survive in the bronchial environment. Respiratory pathogens such as the pneumococcus and the haemolytic streptococcus do not survive for long, although they may be responsible for an acute infection. This may be due to the secretion of antibodies in the mucus or simply to the fact that the environment is unsuitable for their growth. The first organisms to become established are those from the nasopharynx, mainly *Streptococcus viridans*. With increasing obstruction and recurrent infection, *Haemophilus influenzae* becomes the prodominant organism, not invading the mucosa to any serious extent at first, but in the later stages of the disease causing a chronic suppurative infection. Also at this later stage, pneumoccocci, coagulase-positive staphylococci and *Klebsiella pneumoniae* (Friedländer's bacillus) may contribute to the active bronchial infection for long periods. Antibiotic therapy at any stage in the illness shifts the population towards those best able to resist its effects: coliforms, proteus, pyocyaneus and yeasts may become residents and may be responsible for maintaining a chronic purulent infection. What is not yet known is whether persistent infection with mycoplasma or viruses is a contributing factor either to the progress of chronic bronchitis or to the development of lung cancer.

Tissue Resistance

The last factor in the system which protects the lung depends for its very existence on the fact that over the years the other two lines of defence are breached. Respiratory virus infections during childhood and adult life cause temporary damage to the mucosa and lung parenchyma and may often be associated with temporary bacterial infection. These infections leave behind them both a local and a systemic immunity which may last for months or for a lifetime. The immunity is usually not complete and may in some cases (for instance, in healed untreated tuberculosis) be associated with persistence of the infecting agent in an inactive form. The very presence of the resident bacteria in the chronic bronchitic may be a defence mechanism in that these organisms may prevent colonization by fresh invaders because they produce antibiotic substances.

DEFENCE SYSTEM IN LUNG CANCER

Effect of the Tumour

The development of a cancer in the lung may disturb the defence system and cause an existing but dormant infection to become active or encourage fresh infection. The position which has been reached by the time the patient comes to the radiotherapist depends on the pre-existing pulmonary condition and the way in which the patient has been treated already.

The indirect effects of the tumour on the larynx have already been discussed (*see* page 343). The more direct effects are due to ulceration of the bronchi, impairment of the blood supply and restriction of ventilatory movement. To some extent these overlap in that ulceration of the mucosa not only lays bare tissue which can become infected directly, but also obstructs the movement of mucus up the airway. Restriction of ventilatory movement, caused by tumour infiltrating the pleura or the pulmonary lymphatics or by painful lesions of the thoracic cage, will also result in failure of the mucociliary clearance mechanism. Tumour damage to the blood supply to the bronchi or lung leads to a breakdown of tissue resistance to infection. If the occlusion occurs gradually at a time when there is no frank infection or airway obstruction, then fibrosis with shrinkage occurs, which may even help by destroying large areas of tumour. However, if pathogenic organisms are present, a pneumonitis will develop. Sudden vascular occlusion leads to tissue necrosis and abscess formation.

In vascular insufficiency and occlusion, antibiotics cannot be expected to reach the area in sufficient concentration to be effective. As radiotherapy might make the condition worse, this is a situation where palliative excision of the tumour and the ischaemic lung should be considered if the patient's condition permits.

Effect of Radiation

Although there is a great deal of experimental data on the effects of radiation on the lung, there is very little useful information regarding its effect on infection in human lungs. One must suppose that the therapeutic doses may impair ciliary action, slow the mucociliary clearance mechanism and damage tissue resistance to infection. However, the human situation is always complicated by other factors such as temporary swelling and then shrinkage of the tumour, which may first increase and then relieve the bronchial obstruction which may have been the chief cause of a pulmonary infection. There is no doubt that if shrinkage of the tumour improves the blood supply and relieves pain, this will help to control any infection.

Except when there is well-established bronchial obstruction or ischaemia with abscess formation, it is probably advisable to proceed with radiation and attempt to deal with concomitant or subsequent infection as it arises. As in the ischaemic lesion, palliative surgery is probably indicated when an abscess has developed behind a well-established obstruction.

MANAGEMENT

Prophylaxis

The prevention of serious infection is a very important aspect of the care of patients undergoing radiotherapy, because treatment of established infection with antibiotics may be relatively ineffective and radiotherapy may have to be abandoned. It is the practice in many units to use prophylactic antibiotic therapy, just as antibiotics have also been used as a cover for many surgical procedures. Under current hospital conditions, however, it is doubtful whether prophylactic antibiotics are useful, and they may lead to secondary invasion of the damaged area by resistant organisms from the hospital environment. These may be more dangerous than the patient's own flora. The conjunction of tumour irradiation and antibiotic therapy can lead to fatal systemic infection by yeasts and similar organisms of low pathogenicity. As far as possible, the patients should be kept out of the hospital environment; if in-patient treatment is necessary for other reasons, they should be nursed in protective isolation and the staff should be screened for carriers of dangerous strains of bacteria.

Patients with a long history of bronchitic symptoms and a cough productive of mucoid sputum should be taught to do deep breathing and postural drainage, especially for the area of lung under treatment, and should preferably sleep in a position which drains this area. An adequate fluid intake and stopping smoking are also helpful.

Patients with purulent sputum but with no other overt signs of infection do not necessarily require antibiotic treatment provided there is free drainage. A specimen should be sent for culture so that appropriate antibiotic therapy can be instituted if fever or signs of pneumonia develop.

Antibiotics should be used when there is fever and radiological evidence of pneumonia or abscess formation.

Choice of Antibiotic

Obstruction Absent or Incomplete

If the patient has not received previous antibiotic therapy or been exposed for a long time to the hospital environment, then crystalline penicillin is usually effective. If the sputum is purulent and contains only 'upper respiratory flora' or 'no pathogens', 600 mg (1 mega-unit) crystalline benzyl penicillin 12-hourly is sufficient. If the sputum grows *Haemophilus influenzae*, the dose of penicillin should be doubled and streptomycin should be given twice daily. Alternatively, ampicillin can be used in a dose of 4 g daily by mouth. The safe dose of streptomycin depends on age and renal function, varying from 0·5 g twice daily for a fit middle-aged man to 0·25 g twice daily for patients over 65 years of age. If the blood urea is twice the normal, the dosage should be halved. Streptomycin should also be used for Klebsiella (Friedländer) infection.

If the sputum grows a staphylococcus sensitive to penicillin, then crystalline penicillin alone is sufficient; but if, as is usually the case in patients who have been in hospital for long, the organism is resistant to penicillin, cloxacillin or methicillin should be used. If there are severe systemic symptoms and presumptive evidence of a septicaemia, the cloxacillin or methicillin should be given parenterally combined with benzyl penicillin 600 mg six-hourly.

When the sputum cultures a mixed respiratory flora or a flora containing coliforms or Proteus, a combination of sulphonamide and an antifolic agent should be considered. The preparation marketed (Septrim or Bactrim) is very effective and can be used for up to ten days in normal people. The combined effect of the antifolic agent and radiation is not known, and without careful haematological supervision the combination should not be used for more prolonged treatment until more information is available. This combination, or tetracycline in a dose of 2 g daily by mouth, can be used instead of penicillin in patients allergic to that group of drugs.

Obstruction Present

When there is infection behind an obstructed bronchus, the causative organism can be only guessed at. If the patient was already a bronchitic with purulent sputum, there may well be previous cultures indicating the flora in the bronchus at the time of obstruction. However, particularly if the patient has already had antibiotic treatment, such cultures may be misleading. Especially when there is ischaemic as well as bronchial obstruction, anaerobic organisms similar to those found in putrid lung abscess may be responsible for the infection. Large doses of benzyl penicillin (2·4 to 3·6 g—4 to 6 mega-units per day in divided doses) should be tried. If the clinical response is not apparent within the first two days, the treatment should be changed to ampicillin or tetracycline.

Duration of Treatment

Five to seven days of high dosage antibiotic therapy produce the greatest benefit, and more prolonged treatment, even when abscesses are present, seldom results in further improvement. Prolonged high dosage carries an increasing risk of superinfection with antibiotic-resistant bacteria and yeasts and creates an increasingly dangerous ward environment. Although combinations of two antibiotics can be used to prevent the emergence of resistant strains of staphylococci, as a policy this can cause more serious damage by increasing the incidence of toxic side effects of drugs and of superinfection by organisms such as pyocyaneus, Proteus and yeasts which have a great capacity for becoming resistant to antibiotics.

Persistent fever in a patient who initially responded well to antibiotic drugs is an indication for stopping treatment so as to establish whether the fever is due to drug allergy and to see what organisms grow in the absence of antibiotic. If pus reappears in the sputum and an organism such as *Haemophilus influenzae* reappears, treatment can be resumed either with the same drug as before or with alternatives such as tetracycline or the sulphonamide–antifolic acid combination. If relapses of clinical significance continue to occur, then maintenance suppressive therapy with either ampicillin or tetracyclines should be considered. The smallest dose which keeps the sputum mucoid should be used, and this is usually 1–2 g daily of either drug.

SUMMARY

The management of patients receiving radiotherapy for lung cancer should be directed towards prevention of infection without prophylactic antibiotic therapy. The treatment arrangements should be such that patients are not brought into contact with infected cases, and every effort should be made to maintain free drainage of the bronchial tree. Should infection occur, a 5–7-day course of the appropriate antibiotic should be given. Surgery should be considered for suppurating lesions beyond an obstructed bronchus and in cases where there is evidence of vascular occlusion. Under these circumstances, radiotherapy may have to be abandoned. Prolonged, especially broad-spectrum, antibiotic therapy carries an increasing risk of superinfection with resistant bacteria and yeasts which prove more harmful than the original infection.

Index

Page numbers in italics denote illustrations